AGGRESSION

RESEARCH PUBLICATIONS
ASSOCIATION FOR RESEARCH IN
NERVOUS AND MENTAL DISEASE

World List Abbreviation: Res. Publ. Ass. nerv. ment. Dis.

VOLUME 52

Editor:

SHERVERT H. FRAZIER, M.D.

A list of previous issues in the Series of Research Publications will be found on verso of title page

AGGRESSION

PROCEEDINGS OF THE ASSOCIATION

December 1 and 2, 1972

NEW YORK, N. Y.

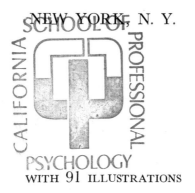

WITH 91 ILLUSTRATIONS

AND 18 TABLES

BALTIMORE

THE WILLIAMS & WILKINS COMPANY

1974

Research Publications

* Out of print in original edition. Some out-of-print volumes available in reprint editions from Hafner Publishing Co., 866 Third Ave., New York, N.Y. 10022. Current in-print volumes available from The Williams & Wilkins Company, 428 E. Preston St., Baltimore, Md. 21202.

Library of Congress Cataloging in Publication Data Association for Research in Nervous and Mental Disease. Aggression; proceedings of the association, Dec. 1 and 2, 1972, New iYork. (Its Research Publications, no. 52) Bibliography: p. 1. Aggressiveness (Psychology)—Congresses. 2. Violence—Congresses. I. Title. [DNLM: 1. Aggression—Congresses. 2. Violence—Congresses. W1AS481 v. 52 1974/BF575.A3 A849a 1972] BF575.A3A85 1974 152.4'32 74-1317 ISBN 0-683-00245-7

Printed at the Waverly Press, Inc., Baltimore, Md., United States of America 21202

PROGRAM COMMITTEE

SHERVERT H. FRAZIER, M.D., *Chairman*

MURRAY GLUSMAN, M.D. LAWRENCE C. KOLB, M.D.

DAVID HAMBURG, M.D. FRANK OCHBERG, M.D.

COMMITTEE ON ARRANGEMENTS

FLETCHER H. McDOWELL, M.D., *Chairman*

HOWARD P. KRIEGER, M.D. ARCHIE R. FOLEY, M.D.

COMMITTEE ON NOMINATIONS

FRANCIS J. BRACELAND, M.D., *Chairman*

LAWRENCE C. KOLB, M.D. JOSEPH RANSOHOFF, M.D.

COMMITTEE ON ADMISSIONS

SIDNEY MALITZ, M.D., *Chairman*

WILLIAM AMOLS, M.D. WILLIAM K. HASS, M.D.

COMMITTEE ON PUBLIC RELATIONS

FRANCIS J. HAMILTON, M.D., *Chairman*

ROBERT E. BARRETT, M.D.

CONTRIBUTORS AND DISCUSSANTS, VOLUME 52

BARD, PHILIP, PH.D., Department of Physiology, Emeritus, Johns Hopkins University School of Medicine, Baltimore, Maryland

BENDER, LAURETTE, M.D., Department of Psychiatry, College of Physicians and Surgeons, Columbia University, New York, New York

CLARK, RAMSEY, L.L.B., Former Attorney General of the United States, Private Law Practice, New York, New York

DINITZ, SIMON, PH.D., Department of Sociology, Ohio State University, Columbus, Ohio

EIBL-EIBESFELDT, IRENÄEUS, PROF. DR., Arbeitsgruppe Für Humanethologie, Am Max-Planck-Institut für Verhaltensphysiologie, Deutschland

FALCO, MATHEA, L.L.B., Chief Council and Staff Director, Senate Subcommittee on Juvenile Delinquency, Washington, D. C.

FERRACUTI, FRANCO, M.D., Department of Criminology, Instituto Di Diritto Penale, Universita Degli Studi de Roma, Roma, Italia

FLOODY, OWEN R., B.A., The Rockfeller University, New York, New York

FRANK, JEROME D., M.D., Department of Psychiatry, Johns Hopkins University School of Medicine, Baltimore, Maryland

FRAZIER, SHERVERT H., M.D., Department of Psychiatry, Harvard Medical School, McLean Hospital, Boston, Massachusetts

GEEN, RUSSELL G., PH.D., Department of Psychology, University of Missouri, Columbia, Missouri

GLUSMAN, MURRAY, M.D., Department of Psychiatry, College of Physicians and Surgeons, Columbia University, New York State Psychiatric Institute, New York, New York

GREENE, HENRY F., L.L.B., Executive Assistant, United States Attorney for the District of Columbia, Washington, D. C.

HAMBURG, DAVID A., M.D., Department of Psychiatry, Stanford University School of Medicine, Stanford, California

KELLY, DENNIS D., PH.D., Department of Psychiatry, College of Physicians and Surgeons, Columbia University, New York State Psychiatric Institute, New York, New York

KETY, SEYMOUR S., M.D., Department of Psychiatry, Harvard Medical School, Massachusetts General Hospital, Boston, Massachusetts

KOLB, LAWRENCE C., M.D., Department of Psychiatry, College of Physicians and Surgeons, Columbia University, New York State Psychiatric Institute, New York, New York

MACLEAN, PAUL D., M.D., Laboratory of Brain Evolution and Behavior, National Institute of Mental Health, Rockville, Maryland

MARK, VERNON H., M.D., Department of Surgery, Harvard Medical School, Boston City Hospital, Boston, Massachusetts

MELLO, NANCY K., PH.D., Laboratory of Alcohol Research, National Institute on Alcohol Abuse and Alcoholism, National Institute of Mental Health, Bethesda, Maryland

MENDELSON, JACK H., M.D., Department of Psychiatry, Harvard Medical School, McLean Hospital, Boston, Massachusetts

OCHBERG, FRANK, M.D., Associate Regional Health Director for Mental Health, San Francisco, California

PFAFF, DONALD W., PH.D., Department of Psychology, Rockefeller University, New York, New York

PURPURA, DOMINICK P., M.D., Department of Anatomy, Albert Einstein College of Medicine, Rose Fitzgerald Kennedy Center for Research in Mental Retardation and Human Development, Bronx, New York

RAISMAN, GEOFFREY, M.A., D.PHIL., B.M., B.CH., Department of Human Anatomy, Oxford University, Oxford, England

REIS, DONALD J., M.D., Department of Neurology, Cornell University Medical College, New York Hospital, New York, New York

ROSE, JAMES, PH.D., Department of Psychology, Dartmouth College, Hanover, New Hampshire

SHAH, SALEEM, PH.D., Center for Studies of Crime and Delinquency, National Institute of Mental Health, Rockville, Maryland

SIEGEL, ALBERTA E., PH.D., Department of Psychiatry, Stanford University School of Medicine, Stanford, California

SILBERT, EARL J., L.L.B., Principle Assistant United States Attorney for the District of Columbia, Washington, D.C.

SPIEGEL, JOHN P., M.D., Lemburg Center for the Study of Violence, Florence Heller School for Social Welfare, Brandeis University, Boston, Massachusetts

SUTIN, JEROME, PH.D., Department of Anatomy, Emory University, Atlanta, Georgia

SWEET, WILLIAM H., M.D., D.Sc., Neurosurgical Service, Massachusetts General Hospital, Boston, Massachusetts

THALMANN, ROBERT, PH.D., Department of Anatomy, Baylor College of Medicine, Texas Medical Center, Houston, Texas

TINKLENBERG, JARED R., M.D., Department of Psychiatry, Stanford University School of Medicine, Palo Alto Veterans Administration Hospital, Stanford, California

VANATTA, LOCHE, PH.D., Department of Psychology, Oberlin College, Oberlin, Ohio

WOODROW, KENNETH M., M.D., National Institute of Mental Health, Division of Special Mental Health Research, St. Elizabeth's Hospital, Washington, D.C.

FOREWORD

With the increase in evidences of human aggression, the Trustees of the Association felt it wise to try to correlate ethology, the scientific study of animal behavior, in the natural state as well as in the laboratory, with the clinical studies of human aggression. With the aid of Dr. Murray Glusman and Dr. Frank Ochberg, each of whom has a long and distinguished history in the study of aggression in both laboratory and clinical situations, it was possible to bring outstanding ethologists, laboratory and animal experimentors, researchers on the human brain, as well as fine researchers with expertise in applied clinical trials of various drugs, and to evolve a two-day program which extended from the anthropological through the biological, psychological and psychosocial indices of human aggression. Finally, we were honored by the presence of The Honorable Ramsey Clark, former Attorney General of the United States, who has an extraordinary insight into the problems of crime and criminal justice in our society.

The timeliness of the topic discussed at the 52nd annual meeting of the Association for Research in Nervous and Mental Disease was emphasized several months later by the awarding of the Nobel Prize in Medicine/Physiology for the first time in the area of behavior to two comparative ethologists. Both men have examined extensively the question of instinctive aggression in man and in other species.

It is the purpose of the presentations at the annual meeting and the contents of this book to review the current status of our knowledge about various aspects of aggression and to assess the impact and implications of violence in our culture.

To the Program Committee and to the Commission, as well as to the Trustees and Officers of the Association, I express my sincere gratitude for the many excellent suggestions, much time consuming and helpful understanding, but most of all to each of the presentors. To the publishers, and to Mrs. Harriette Bailie, Miss Rosalie Frazier, Mrs. Alice Nelson, Mrs. Rose Schwartz Oberstein, Miss Laurie Reich and Mrs. Alan Woodward, I express my greatest gratitude. Dr. Alan Bateman assisted in the finalization of the copy and Mrs. Paul Meyerson acted as editor of this important volume. To all my gratitude.

S.H.F.

CONTENTS

Chapter 1

AGGRESSION IN THE !KO-BUSHMEN

IRENAEUS EIBL-EIBESFELDT

The question whether the aggressive behavior of man is solely a result of learning processes, or whether phylogenetic adaptations preprogram it to any significant extent is a matter of controversy. Proponents of the learning theory of aggression repeatedly point to the existence of allegedly nonaggressive peoples (1–4). In a recent publication Schmidbauer, although admitting that territorial defense occurs, says that what is lacking, however, is a "territorial imperative" pressing the hunters and gatherers toward conquest of new already occupied areas. Again this seems a gross oversimplification. But since ethologists did not coin the term "territorial imperative" and since Schmidbauer has never seen a hunter and gatherer alive so far, I do not feel obliged to try to understand what he actually means. If he implies that hunters and gatherers would never fight for the possession of territories under population pressure, he certainly jumps to conclusions. So far, there are no facts backing such a statement. These statements, however, do not stand critical examination. The allegedly peaceful Eskimos actually perform a rich variety of aggressive acts, although most tribes settle their disputes in a fashion that does not result in bloodshed. The tribes of Siberia, Alaska, Baffinland and Northwest Greenland settle their disputes by wrestling, and only occasionally does one get killed. The Eskimos in Central Greenland slap each other's faces. In West and East Greenland, song duels are favorite means to settle conflicts.

The myth of the aggressionless society is old, actually dating back to Rousseau, but it pops up again and again. Nansen, by creating the myth of the aggression-free Eskimos, wanted to create a favorable picture of his beloved people. Koenig (5) pointed to this fact already in 1925: "Um zunaechst einmal das letztere (the alleged peacefulness) zu beleuchten, so ist seine Quelle, auf die er dieses Urteil ueber das Volk stuetzt, einzig und allein Nansen. Dieser hat aber die Eskimos im Naturzustande nur sehr wenig kennengelernt, und sein moralisches Urteil ueber sie—das er besonders in seinem 'Eskimoleben' kundgibt—ist durchaus tendenzioes gefaerbt, da er Mitleid erwecken wollte." ("In order to throw some light on the latter point, his source on which he has based his conclusions concerning

1

this tribe is only and solely Nansen. Nansen, however, has gotten to know the Eskimos in their natural state only very little, and his moral judgment about them—as described in part in his "The Life of the Eskimo"—is colored because he wants to rouse compassion.")

Although this correction was published in 1925, the myth is not at all dead. On the contrary, it serves to blame our industrial achievement society for all aggression, by depicting the members of hunting and gathering societies as noble, noncompetitive and therefore nonaggressive savages. The argument runs like this: If human aggressiveness is a phylogenetically determined disposition, rooted in the human's inherited genetic disposition, then it must be especially evident in those cultures which characterized the stage occupying 99 percent of the human evolutionary timetable. The stage here in question is designated as the Stone Age, characterized by the patterns of roaming hunters and gatherers. If such groups of hunters and gatherers existed for approximately 1 million years, one can assume that the psychological and physical properties of (present) man became deeply ingrained at this time. The mere 10,000 years in which man became a farmer could have hardly changed the genetic biological basis of the human. If, therefore, there exists any reason to assume that the life patterns of hunters and gatherers were stamped into our heredity, then the theory of an inborn, aggressive drive would have some support. If it could be proved to the contrary that hunters and gatherers in general are more peaceful than the latter and have more highly developed culture forms, then the hypotheses of an aggressive drive would be totally unbelievable. (6)

After this introduction, Schmidbauer concludes on the basis of the data of cultural anthropology, that the majority of hunters and gatherers are very unaggressive and, most notably, that they would not defend territories. His statement, however, is not supported by a thorough count of the known hunters and gatherers and an examination of their aggressiveness. It is based on a selection of some allegedly nonaggressive hunters and gatherers. In addition to the Eskimos which we already mentioned, the Hadza and the Bushmen of South Africa are quoted as examples. In doing so, Schmidbauer relied primarily on the articles by Lee and DeVore (7). In one of the papers Woodburn (8) claims that the Hadza defend no territories, show no aggression and also live in open groups. Woodburn, however, studied this group in 1958 and thereafter, when the group, which had formerly occupied approximately 5000 km.² of land, was pressed into an area of 2000 km.². The group had certainly been uprooted and, consequently, changes in their original behavior and social structure are to be expected. Indeed, Kohl-Larsen (9), who visited the Hadza between 1934 and 1936, and later between 1937 and 1939, in respect to this recorded a noteworthy story told him by a Hadza friend. The protocol of August 7, 1938, reads as follows:

"In the old times the Hadzapi fought amongst one another. One tribe which was located in Mangola went to another tribe over in Lubiro. When they arrived there, a man was picked out. He went to the Lubiro band and said. 'We have come to you today to fight you!' Now someone from the Lubiro tribe said, 'Yes, if you have come here to wage a war with us, we are satisfied'. The people in Lubiro come together and discuss among each other. They pick a man who is to fight with the man from Mangola. He is chosen, each of the men get two sticks. With them they beat each other. If no one is victor over the other, both tribes begin to battle each other with arrows and spears. As they are battling each other, an old lady steps out of the crowd and out of the other crowd an old man. Both of them place themselves in the middle of the two fighting tribes and say, 'Sit down and rest a bit!'. Having rested a bit, they begin hitting each other again. They fight each other for a long time. One tribe is beaten and runs away. The others, the victors, follow them a stretch, then go back again into their camp and sleep. The next day the tribe that won goes to the losers. They stay overnight with them. In the morning all the strong men and youths go hunting. When they kill a few animals, they take its meat, which is fatty, and sit down and eat it. Only the men may be around then. If a woman goes to the men, she can be killed. However, if the woman has a child which she carries on her back, she pinches him so he cries. When the men hear a crying child they cannot hit the woman. When they (all) eat the meat the friendship between them is reestablished. Having lived many days like this and seeing that they are living for no good purpose (no work and nothing to do), they look for another tribe to fight with. They hit each other so badly that a few people often are killed. Whoever loses goes then into the big crowd of the victor."

The protocol is noteworthy not only because of its numerous interesting details, but also because it demonstrates that it is a grossly false generalization to conclude, on the basis of the current behavior of the Hadzas, that they, or hunters and gatherers in general, were originally peaceful peoples.

THE CONTROVERSY ON BUSHMEN TERRITORIALITY

In recent publications (3, 10, 11) the Bushmen have been referred to as living in open nonexclusive bands and as not expressing territoriality in the sense it is usually defined, namely, as intolerance confined to space. For example, this is explicitly stated by Lee (11) concerning the !Kung: "The camp is an open aggregate of persons which changes in size and composition from day to day. Therefore, I have avoided the term band in describing the !Kung-Bushmen living groups. Each waterhole has a hinterland lying within a six mile radius which is regularly exploited for vegetables and animal food. These areas are not territories in a zoological sense, since they are not defended against outsiders."

Such statements are puzzling in view of the overwhelming evidence on territoriality of the same Bushmen published by older authors. Thus, Passarge (12) describes the !Kung-Bushmen as belligerent, and he emphasizes that not only the bands but every family owns their particular collecting grounds, and he writes in this context: "Die Einteilung der Buschmaenner in Familien ist bereits seit langem bekannt ... Dagegen habe ich noch nirgends eine Notiz darueber gefunden, das auch der Grund und Boden gesetzmaesig verteiltes Eigentum der Familien ist. Das ist aber ein Punkt von ungeheurer Wichtigkeit. Denn erst bei Beruecksichtigung dieser Tatsache kann man einen klaren Einblick in die soziale Organisation der Buschmaenner gewinner." ("The subdivision of the Bushmen into families has been known for a long time. However, I have nowhere noticed that the soil too is legally distributed property of the families. This, however, is a point of tremendous importance, and only by taking this fact into consideration, is it possible to give a clear insight into the social organization of the Bushmen.")

Zastrow and Vedder (13) report that the Bushmen are not allowed to hunt or collect food in the land of another band: "Wo das Buschmanngelaende noch nicht in Farmen aufgeteilt ist, sondern Sippengebiet sich an Sippengebiet schliesst, weiss jeder Buschmann, dass er in fremdem Gebiet nicht jagen oder Feldkost sammeln darf. Wird ein Wiudjaeger angetroffen, so hat er sein Leben verwirkt. Es ist nicht damit gesagt, das man ihn auf jeden Fall umbringt. Die Blutrache ... haelt vielleicht davon ab..." ("Where the Bushmen territory has not been subdivided into farms but is included in the territory of the clan, each Bushman knows that he is not allowed to hunt in strange territory to collect fruit. When a poacher is caught, his life is in danger. This does not mean that he is killed in every case. There is a blood feud perhaps keeping them from it.")

Lebzelter (14) reports of the great distrust the !Kung show when meeting members of foreign bands: "Jeder Bewaffnete, dem sie begegnen gilt von vornherein als Feind. Fremde Stammesgebiete darf der Buschmann nur unbewaffnet betreten. Selbst am Rande der Farmzone ist das gegenseitige Misstrauen so gross, dasein Buschmann, der als Bote auf eine Farm geschickt wird, in deren Bereich eine andere Sippe sitzt, den Fahrweg, der als eine Art neutrale Zone gilt, nicht zu verlassen wagt. Naehern sich zwei fremde bewaffnete Buschleute einander, so legen sie zunaechst auf Sichtweite die Waffen ab." ("Each armed man whom they encounter is considered at first as an enemy. The territory of a strange tribe may be entered by a Bushman only if he is unarmed. Even at the perimeter of the farm there is great mutual mistrust. A Bushman who is sent as a messenger to another farm, in the area of another clan, does not dare to deviate from the established route which is considered to be a sort of neutral zone. When two strange armed Bushmen approach each other, they put down their arms.") Similar reports can be found in Brownlee (15), Vedder (16) and Wilhelm (17). Also, Marshall (18) reports on territoriality: "The !Kung say that one cannot eat the ground itself, so it does not matter to whom it belongs. It is these patches of veldkos (wildfruit) that are clearly and jealously owned and the territories are shaped in a general way around these patches ... The strange concept of ownership of veldkos by the band operates almost like a taboo. No external force is established to prevent one band from encroaching on anothers veldkos or to prevent individuals from raiding veldkos patches to which they have no right. This is just not done." Tobias (19) emphasizes that the Bushmen move strictly within their territory: "Territoriality applies among bands of the same tribe and between different tribes. Intribal bounds are sometimes reinforced by social attitudes, such as the traditional enmity between the Auen and Naron. Under special conditions such as an abundance of food these bounds and the accompanying enmity are forgotten."

In view of all these reports, we have to assume that the group studies by Lee no longer show the typical pattern, probably because of the fact of acculturation. In addition, they may not have been aware of the possible existence of the nexus system, which bonds several bands to a larger unit in the !Ko-Bushmen.

TERRITORIALITY AND AGGRESSION IN THE !KO-BUSHMEN

The !Ko-Bushmen belong to the central Kalahari. Bushmen live in the area south of Ghanzi. Many of the bands are still living as hunters and gatherers. Heinz (20) gave a detailed report on this group, and I had the opportunity to visit repeatedly one of his groups in 1970, 1971 and 1972 and live with these people, documenting unstaged social interactions by film. These studies not only shed light on Bushmen aggression and aggression control, but also contribute to the more general problem of phylogenetic adaptations in human aggressive behavior.

1. Territoriality

This subject has been dealt with extensively by Heinz (20, 21). I will therefore review his findings. My observations are in complete agreement. Heinz distinguishes three levels of social organization: a) the family and extended family, b) the band and c) the band nexus. All of these units have a definite pattern of bonding *and* spacing. The sitting position of family members around the fire is less formalized than in the !Kung (18). The wife can sit anywhere at the house side of the fire, but the proper place, according to Heinz, is on the right side of her husband. Parents settle at least 12 m. away from their married children, and the entrance is always arranged so that they are not able to watch their married children sleeping. "Though all band territory is accessible to everyone in the band, nevertheless the family's area of activity is recognized. When hunting alone, a man is expected to hunt on the side of the village on which his house is built, a rule applying to women collecting veldkos or firewood as well. Only collective activity, which is most prevalent, breaks this rule" (20). Heinz reports furthermore, that the bands periodically split in family groups, each family then moving to a family place which is respected by the others.

Although families have no direct territorial claims, the band definitely has. A band considers a piece of land as its territory. The control over it is exercised by the "headman" (21, 22) on behalf of the band with a group of older men and women acting as consultants. The band hunts and collects wood and veldkos within its territory. In case of emergency they may ask for permission to hunt and collect in another band's territory. To members of the same nexus, permission in normally readily granted.

I consider the nexus system as the most important discovery of Heinz, since it may explain, at least to a certain extent, how some of the controversial statements on Bushmen arose. The nexus constitutes a group of bands. Members refer to themselves as "our people." The people are bonded by friendship and kinship ties, by ritual bonds (for example, by coming together for trance dances) and they share slight peculiarities in their dialect. There is extensive intermarriage within the nexus. The band nexus is a territorial group which is more exclusive than the band territories. The nexus territory is demarcated from the land of another nexus by a strip of "no man's land," which is generally avoided by the members of both sides. It would not occur to a !Ko-Bushman to seek permission to hunt in the land of another nexus.

Access to territory is acquired by birth, admission to a band or by marriage. If the parents come from different bands, dual band membership is the result. When marrying, the groom resides for a certain period of time with the bride's band and has access to this territory. Thereafter the couple moves to the man's band, where the bride receives access to the band's territory. "It is this phenomenon which gives parents rights in each other's land, and which is transmitted to the children and which might in certain cases blur band territoriality" (2).

2. Patterns of Aggressive Behavior

Being interested in the universals in human behavior, I spent many hours studying and filming unstaged social interactions. In total, approximately 12,000 m. of 16-mm. film were taken on the !Ko-Bushmen and about 2000 m. on the !Kung. On the basis of this documentation it can be proved that a) aggressive behavior patterns are fairly frequently observed and b) many of the patterns are identical in form with those observed by people of other cultures in the same context. Aggressive acts in this context are defined as all of those that lead to spacing or to the establishment of a dominance-subordination relationship. Whether or not the person involved hurt another person physically does not enter the definition. If one were to speak of aggression only when damage results, one would have to omit all the patterns of aggressive threat and other ritualized patterns of aggression. I see no reason to do this.

a. Sibling Rivalry

Intersibling rivalry can be observed at a very early age. I documented a most dramatic example during my stay with the !Kung. The parties involved were two brothers. The younger was approximately 1 year old, the elder perhaps 5 years old. The elder son tried fairly frequently to harm his younger brother. He attempted to scratch and beat him on several occasions and tried to poke him with sticks (Fig. 1.1). The mother had to be on the alert to keep both brothers from fighting. The older brother also tried to interfere with his younger brother's play, teasing him by taking his toys and throwing them away. But the younger brother, too, was aggressive. For example, while drinking, he was observed giving his brother a well aimed kick with one foot. The older brother certainly was suffering quite a lot, and in his frustrated efforts of contact seeking with the

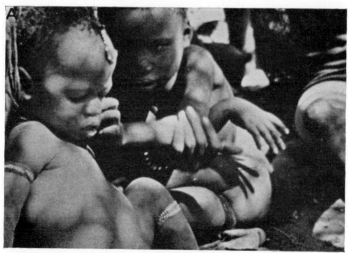

Fig. 1.1, A to C. Sibling rivalry can be observed at a very early age.

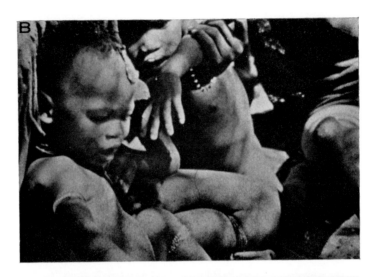

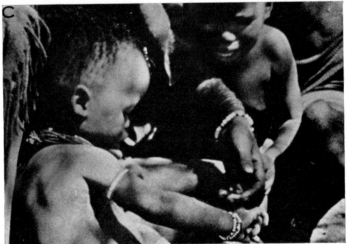

Fig. 1.1 B anb C.

mother, he often cried. His mother did not respond to him very eagerly. When her small son was away on a playing excursion, she allowed contact but she did not invite it. Rather, she seemed fed up with him.

Less dramatic cases of sibling rivalry were observed in the !Ko-Bushmen. In view of the fact that hunters and gatherers are so often reported as growing up without any frustration, these observations are of importance in correcting such ideas. In general, babies show aggressive behavior at a very early age. In one instance, a 10-month-old boy attacked other babies by pushing them over and by scratching them (Fig. 1.2).

b. Aggression in Playing Groups of Children

1. PLAYFUL AGGRESSION. Patterns which normally lead to spacing sub-ordination and the cutoff of contact are often performed during play. Although the motor patterns in such a case are often difficult to distinguish from real aggressive acts, additional signals like laughing and smiling allow us to recognize that the aggressive interaction is actually play. And so does the fact that the roles of attacker and defender or pursuer and pursued change freely. We do not want to deal here with play aggression, inasmuch as this will be dealt with by one of my students (H. Sbrzesny, in preparation).

2. SERIOUS AGGRESSIVE INTERACTIONS. Serious aggressive interactions are fairly common within playing groups of children. The acts of aggression are: slapping with the palm, beating with a stick or another object, throwing objects toward a child, throwing sand, punching with the fist, kicking with the foot, pushing the other with one or both hands, ramming a child with the shoulder, pushing with the hip, pinching, biting, pulling the hair, scratching, wrestling, spitting and stealing objects (Fig. 1.3). All of these patterns have been described in detail in my monograph (23). There are some remarkable patterns of threat and submission which I want to describe. When threatening, the person frowns, clenches the teeth while often exposing them at the same time and stares at the opponent. Sometimes a hand with or without an object is raised. Both opponents may get engaged in such a threat-stare duel. When such a display leads to the submission of one, the loser lowers his head, tilts it slightly and

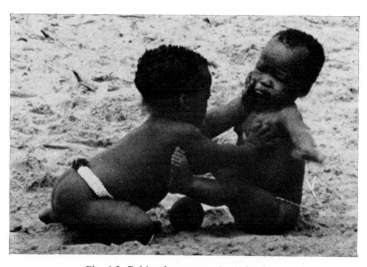

Fig. 1.2. Babies show aggressive behavior.

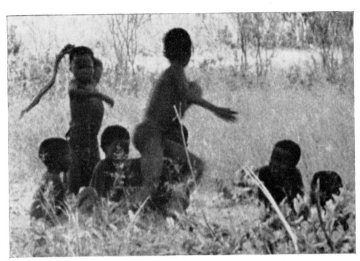

Fig. 1.3. Serious aggressive interactions are fairly common within playing groups of children.

turns sideways. At the same time the child pouts. This behavior strongly inhibits further aggression; but not only that. One can observe the the aggressor quite often tries to comfort his victim, seeking friendly contact. The victim normally responds to the effort by clear, cutoff behavior, for example, by turning away. Another aggression-inhibiting behavior is crying. Both submissive behaviors are to be found in all cultures I have visited so far (Figs. 1.4 and 1.5).

Aggressive interactions are fairly common in groups of playing children. Within 191 minutes, I counted in a group of 7 girls and 2 boys 166 aggressive and defensive acts: slapping, punching with the fist or beating with an object 96 times; kicking with the foot 23 times; throwing sand 8 times and a number of other acts. Ten times a child cried loudly during this observation period, which indicates clearly that many of the aggressive acts lead to serious conflicts. Only about one-third of the interactions were clearly playful aggression by the criteria mentioned above. Not all play sessions are disturbed by so many aggressive acts. Another time 12 children played for 88 minutes together and seven aggressive acts were counted.

There were a number of typical situations in which aggression did occur.

1. Quarrelling about the Possession of Objects. Children like to play ball with melons, and the ball is often the object of a quarrel. In particular, boys try to rob others of the ball. Pursuits and fights for and in defense of the object develop. The loser often shows all of the signs of

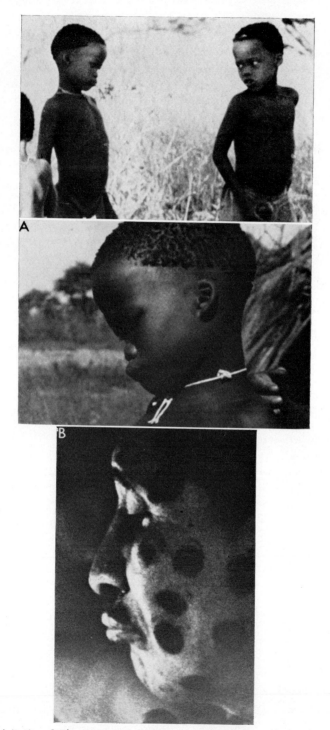

Fig. 1.4 (top) and *Fig. 1.5,* A and B *(bottom)*. Threatening and submissive patterns of behavior strongly inhibit further aggression.

11

serious anger and sometimes even cries. Children rob each other also of other objects, sometimes even of food, which is considered a more serious offense. Refusing to share food is an offense which invites punishing attack. Once a girl gave a morsel to an 8-month-old baby, expecting that the infant would return part of it. The baby crawled away with all of it and immediately was beaten by the girl. Robbing another child of an object is often a means of teasing a playmate and enticing him into a fight.

2. *Punishment of Offenses.* Older children often interfere with the quarrels of their younger playmates, for example, by punishing the attacker. In one play group, the oldest prepubertal girl regularly acted in such a way that she practically controlled the play activity. She initiated many of the play activities and demanded obedience. If a child was breaking a rule of the game, or sometimes even if he or she behaved in an unskilled way, she attacked. We called her the "Spielleiterin" for this reason.

3. *Demonstrative Aggression.* The "Spielleiterin" sometimes attacked another child without evident reason. In the morning, when she came to the already assembled group of the other children, she kicked the melon out of the hand of a child, or boxed another. Indeed, all of the children showed signs of respect to her by approaching and showing their melon, even at the danger of being robbed of this prized object. It seems to me that the function of this aggression is to achieve and keep rank and respect, which are prerequisites for functioning as a mediator and soothing quarrels between the other playmates.

4. *Unprovoked Spontaneous Attacks.* Children often attacked others without apparent reason. The patterns were of particular interest, since it was evident that a child is inhibited from starting a full attack against an innocent bystander. If a child seeks a fight, he or she incites it by a pattern of provocation. Teasing, by offering something and then withdrawing it when the other child tries to grasp it, is a common way. A slight slap, a kick, showing the tongue or stealing an object and throwing it away are all typical small insults that provoke the other child. And once the other child attacks, heavy retaliation follows. It looks as if the provoking child seeks an excuse to attack by provoking aggression which allows him to retaliate.

5. *Escalation of Play.* Rough and tumble play occasionally developed into a fight. If one child accidentally or by intent hits the other slightly more strongly than expected, he invites retaliation and a fight may start.

c. Quarrels between Children and Adults

Children sometimes responded violently when parents admonished them. Once a girl was scolded by her father for carelessly kicking against a pot, causing part of its contents to spill. Upon this reprimand, the girl grasped the pot and threw it against the floor, spilling it completely. The father did not say anything further. On another occasion a girl kicked her mother after she had been scolded for begging too greedily for food. Once a girl robbed a small boy of a piece of meat. When the boy cried out, his father came, took the meat back to the boy and slapped the girl slightly on the head. The girl retaliated by throwing sand at the man, who in turn slapped her a second time. This did not subdue her at all, for she answered by throwing sand at the man, who in turn slapped her a third time. A final example: A man hid a little object to prevent a baby from swallowing it. The baby and another boy, approximately 6 years of age, were searching for the object. They were body searching the man with much laughter, and finally the man and the little boy started in a playful fashion to exchange slappings. This escalated, however, and when the man slapped stronger, the boy started to cry out, ran away and returned with large bones and antelope horns, threatening to throw them at the male. At this moment the boy's father intervened, soothing the excitement of his son.

d. Aggression in the Adult

Within a band, aggressive behavior of the adult is under good control. The cultural ideal of the Bushmen is indeed to live a peaceful life. Should tension arise between two families of one band, the problem is solved by splitting. One family moves for a while to another place, and this relieves the tension (21, 22). I myself had no opportunity to observe serious aggression between adults but saw many playful aggressive acts. Young men wrestle; married couples engage in teasing and mock fighting. An element of aggression is certainly to be observed in the numerous games. Heinz described that males tease and maltreat "underdogs," that is, low ranking members of the group. Verbal threats of murder are often uttered ("I will kill you with my medicine"). Males, after insulting each other, occasionally use their weapons, and Heinz reports a case of manslaughter. He also describes the temper fits which occasionally overcome the Bushmen: "An angry Bushman finally settles down with a face that shows an unbelieveable degree of anger. It takes very little for this anger to cause a wrestling and punching encounter with sticks and knobkerries. If the reasons are serious, the fight will deteriorate into one in which knives and spears are used ... " (20). Married couples fight for reasons of jealousy, and so do women. Adultery may lead to bloodshed among the males.

e. Teasing and Mocking

By testing and mocking, group homogeneity is enforced and an outlet for aggression provided. Heinz describes the existing joking relationships in detail and I will not describe the subject in depth here. However, I want to discuss some patterns of mocking. These patterns are released by behaviors of individuals that deviate from the group's norm. The mocking puts outsiders under pressure to conform, and certainly has an educational function. Mocking is done by imitating the patterns which provoked the hostility of the group and thus ridiculing it. I furthermore found that female genital display, showing the tongue and showing the rear, are used during mocking. Several ways of female genital display can be observed. Kids repeatedly mocked me while I was filming with my mirror lens. They imitated my behavior, and if I did not pay attention, they approached, dancing and singing, and, at close distance, lifted their genital apron (Fig. 1.6). Often the girls posed with their hands on their hips, posturing in a characteristic way with their legs (Fig. 1.7). In addition to this frontal genital display, there was also a genital display from the rear. When the mocking girl turned her rear and bent deeply (Fig. 1.8), the pubic region was exposed in a very conspicuous way, particularly since this race as a characteristic feature shows a strong lordosis. Also, the enlarged labia minora contribute to the marked visibility of the vulva. I assume that this posturing is indeed homologous to primate sexual presenting. In fact, the Bushmen copulate from the rear lying on their side.

The widespread use of patterns of sexual presenting (24) in mocking displays may be explained by the fact that sexual inciting is taboo except in certain circumstances. To use it outside its original context is therefore a demonstration of disregard. Not to be confused with the pattern of genital presenting are patterns of showing the rear. This pattern is more often used as an aggressive threat. I observed that this was the way that girls mocked boys who were teasing them. They shoved sand between their buttocks and then approached the boys, turned in front of them, and bending, let the sand go as if defecating. Sometimes wind is passed. Both are clear indications that this pattern is a ritualized form of defecation.

Tongue showing is another pattern used in mocking. It is difficult to interpret, since it occurs in various forms. In derogatory tongue showing, the tongue is stuck out and turned down, as if the person were about to vomit. Even spitting can occur in this context, and, interestingly enough, the German word "spotten" (mocking) is related to the word "spucken" (spitting). There exists, furthermore, a sexual tongue flicking, and to complicate matters further, there exists a friendly tongue showing derived

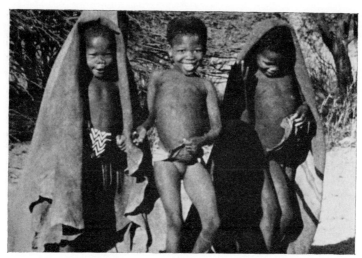

Fig. 1.6. Teasing and mocking are patterns of behavior which provide an outlet for aggression.

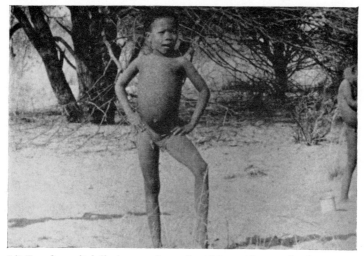

Fig. 1.7. Female genital display as a form of mocking: girl posturing in a characteristic way with the legs.

from licking which I will not discuss here. I want to mention, however, that the tongue flicking is often used in a teasing fashion.

SUMMARY

The much quoted cross-cultural "evidence" for man's primarily peaceful and nonaggressive nature on examination proves to be a weak point

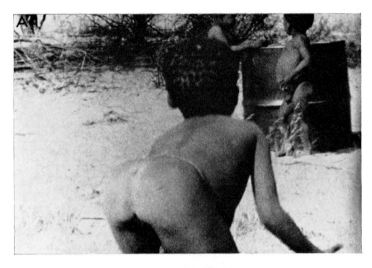

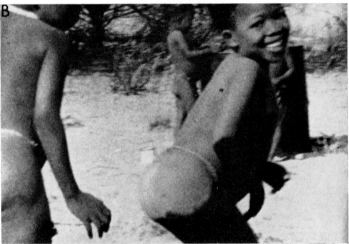

Fig. 1.8, A and B. Patterns of showing the rear are more often used as an aggressive threat.

in the environmentalist's argument. Among others, the often quoted Bushmen certainly do not lack territoriality nor do they fail to be aggressive. Even within the band, numerous aggressive acts can be observed. The situations and most of the movement patterns are identical with the aggressive patterns in other cultures. They are universals concerning the releasing situations and the motor patterns of aggression, and although the similarity of many of the movements can be explained on a functional basis (hitting, kicking and so forth), and thus be acquired independently in a similar way, this certainly does not hold for the more elaborate aggressive displays, such as the facial expressions of threat, the threat stare, the patterns of submission (pouting, head lowering, gaze avoidance, crying) or some of the patterns of mocking (genital presenting, tongue showing). We can assume that many of these patterns are phylogenetic adaptations ritualized in the service of spacing and aggression control.

It is true, however, that Bushmen are not belligerent. Their cultural ideal is peaceful coexistence, and they achieve this by avoiding conflict, for example by splitting and by emphasizing and encouraging the numerous patterns of bonding. This way they achieve a peaceful life. Most of the socialization of aggression takes place within the playing groups of children. In interaction with others, children learn to control their aggression. It should be mentioned that many of the patterns of bonding and the urge to bond are inborn to man. Man is, so to speak, by nature a bonding as well as a spacing creature. Culture puts emphasis on one or the other and may unbalance man for better or worse. The Bushmen certainly belong to those people whose culture shapes man according to a peaceful idea. What is striking when observing the Bushmen is not their lack of aggression, but their efficient way of coping with it. Friendly bonding behavior predominates in the interaction of adults, and these people spend many hours a day grooming each other, chatting, sharing the pipe and playing with their children, to mention but a few of their social interactions. Since wood and food gathering consumes only 2 to 3 hours a day for the women, and since men hunt only occasionally, the Bushmen have plenty of time for intimate social interactions. One could say that these people have more time at their disposal to be "human" in a friendly way, while we are losing this capacity to a greater and greater extent.

REFERENCES

1. HELMUTH, H: Zum Verhalten des Menschen: die Aggression. Ethnol 92: 265, 1967.
2. SCHMIDBAUER, W: Methodenprobleme der Human-Ethologie. Stud Gen 24: 462, 1971.
3. SCHMIDBAUER, W: Die Sogenannte Aggression. Hamburg, Hoffmann & Campe, 1972.
4. MONTAGU, A: Man and Aggression. New York, Oxford University Press, 1968.
5. KOENIG, H: Der Rechtsbruch und sein Ausgleich bei den Eskimo. Anthropos 20: 276, 1925.
6. SCHMIDBAUER, W: Zur Anthropologie der Aggression. Dynam Psychiat 4: 36, 1971.
7. LEE, RB, DeVORE, I, eds: Man the Hunter. Chicago, Aldine Publishing Co., 1968.
8. WOODBURN, J: Stability and flexibility in Hadza residential groupings, in Man the Hunter, edited by Lee, RB, DeVore, I. Chicago, Aldine Publishing Co., 1968, p. 103.
9. KOHL-LARSEN, L: Wildbeuter in Ostafrika. Die Tindiga, ein Jaeger-und Sammlervolk. Berlin, Reimer, 1958.
10. SAHLINS, MD: The origin of society. Sci Am 204: 76, 1960.
11. LEE, RB: What hunters do for a living, in Man the Hunter, edited by Lee, RB, DeVore, I. Chicago, Aldine Publishing Co., 1968, p. 30.

12. Passarge, S: Die buschmaenner der Kalahari. Berlin, Reimer, 1907.
13. Zastrow, BV, Vedder, H: Die buschmaenner, in Das Eingeborenenrecht: Togo, Kamerun, Suedseekolonien, edited by Schultz-wert, E, Adam, E. Stuttgart, Strecker u. Schroder, 1930.
14. Lebzelter, V: Eingeborenenkulturen von Sued- un Suedwestafrika. Leipzig, Hiersemann, 1934.
15. Brownlee, F: The social organization of the Kung (!Un) Bushmen of the North-Western Kalahari. Africa 14: 124, 1943.
16. Vedder, H: Uber die Vorgeschichte der Voelkerschaften von Suedwestafrika. J SW Afr Sci Soc 9: 45, 1952/53.
17. Wilhelm, JH: Die !Kung Buschleute. Jahrb Museums Voelkerkunde Leipzig 12: 91, 1953.
18. Marshall, L: Sharing, talking and giving. Relief of social tensions among !Kung Bushmen. Africa 31: 231, 1961.
19. Tobias, P von: Bushmen-hunter-gatherers. A study in human ecology, in Ecological Studies in Southern Africa, edited by Davis, DHS, reprinted in Man in Adaptation, edited by Y. A. Cohen, Chicago, Aldine Publishing Co. 1968, p. 196.
20. Heinz, HJ: Conflicts, tensions and release of tensions in a Bushmen society. The Institute for the Study of Man in Africa, Isma Papers, No. 23, 1967.
21. Heinz, HJ: The social organization of the !Ko bushmen. Master's Thesis, Dept of Anthropology, Univ of South Africa, Johannesburg, 1966.
22. Heinz, HJ: Territoriality among the Bushmen in general and the !Ko in particular. Anthropos. 67: 405, 1972.
23. Eibl-Eibesfeldt, I: Ethology: The Biology of Behavior. New York, Holt, Rinehart and Winston, 1970.
24. Eibl-Eibesfeldt, I: Die !Ko-Buschmanngesellschaft: Aggressionskontrolle und Gruppenbindung. Monographien zur Humanethologie 1. Muenchen, Piper, 1972.

DISCUSSION

Dr. David Hamburg (Stanford, California): We're indebted to Dr. Eibl-Eibesfeldt for calling our attention to a new way of studying hunter-gatherers. Anthropologists working in Australia, New Guinea and Africa over the past decade have, on the whole, done more careful and systematic studies of hunter-gatherers than we've ever had before. These would include Lee, DeVore, Draper and Harperding on the Kung Bushmen, Hyder and Freeman working in New Guinea, Mettick in Australia and Woodburn and Turnbull in Africa.

The reason this work is so important has to do with the time scale of evolution. Perhaps 99 percent of distinctively human existence has been in hunter-gatherer societies over a period of several million years, until the advent of agriculture, perhaps only 10,000 years ago. So it is quite possible, indeed likely, that some of what we are today, some of the biological characteristics of *Homo sapiens*, were shaped by the selection pressures that operated during the faraway time. The issues, therefore, of the universality of aggressiveness, the instigators of aggressiveness and the means of conflict resolution, all have some bearing on possible biological and social heritages brought with us into the contemporary world.

Eibl touched on one of the very difficult methodological problems, the problem of sympathetic identification. Most observers, both early and more recent, wish to identify in a compassionate way with their subjects. The studies, then, tend to give the impression that the people have many admirable characteristics, that, for example, they may be very good natural botanists and zoologists, or that they are tender and kind to visiting anthropologists. There is a distinct effort, one might say, in all these studies, to detoxify the stereotype of the wild savage by playing down the episodes of aggressiveness. This has contributed to what Eibl very well called the myth of the aggressionless society.

Typically, as these studies go along, the later estimates of violent conflict are a good deal higher than the earlier estimates. For example, Eibl says that DeVore and Lee present the Kung in a very nonaggressive light. While that is true of their earlier reports, Lee, in fact, went back and, looking more closely at that same peaceful group, found that their homicide rate was considerably higher than the rate in Houston, Texas, let alone New York. Such reevaluation is, I think, fairly general. While these groups do not justify the myth of the wild savage, there are circumstances and occasions in which even violent conflict does occur and, certainly, verbal conflict occurs very commonly.

The more frequent instigators of verbal conflict have to do with status. Others arise from questions on sexual prerogatives and generosity or the lack of generosity, the latter, of course, a fundamental value in societies living close to subsistence. The more serious conflict tends to occur between adult males, who usually have a near monopoly on the lethal weapons, and very commonly, although not always, seems to center around women.

There are also interesting problems about conflict resolution. These people typically do not have powerful political leadership, like a headman who can settle disputes. Yet they manage, for the most part, to regulate the disputes, partly by the technique of group fission, with the hostile subgroups dividing temporarily for some weeks or months, only to reunite later after passions have cooled. In many of these societies, intervention of immediate family members also seems important in conflict resolution.

The argument about whether our ancestors were wild beasts or pleasant, compassionate creatures is virtually fruitless. Almost certainly they were both, as are we. It will prove much more profitable to work at sorting out the conditions under which serious conflict occurs and the conditions under which it can be resolved than to portray us and our ancestors either as saints or as sinners.

DR. PAUL D. MACLEAN (Bethesda, Maryland): I wonder if Dr. Eibl-Eibesfeldt would comment on the aggressive genital display behavior which is very similar to what Carleton Gynechek observed in the Melanesian tribes, and to that which Pluge and I described in the squirrel.

DR. IRENÄEUS EIBL-EIBESFELDT (Percha bei Starnberg, West Germany): This mocking behavior with sexual display is a reaction toward an outsider. If someone's behavior does not conform to the group's, he gets mocked. It serves the function, by ridiculing him, of bringing him into the group. It's an educational mechanism.

Even though I had been introduced into the group by Heinz, who worked there for 13 years and was accepted to a certain extent, I still was a stranger. My filming activities bothered them. You're there, and they don't know what you're doing. At first the girls ridicule what you're doing by imitating it, and then they dance toward you, but only if you don't look at them. Then they present their rear and bend deeply, making the vaginal opening very visible. It is clearly a sexual presentation.

To Hamburg I would say that lack of time didn't allow me to get into that subject, which is a hobby of mine. What normally causes aggressive behavior to occur in a group and what normally shuts it off is a question of conflict resolution. Biological conflict resolution and culture conflict resolution, both very interesting, would need another hour of discussion.

DR. RENICK (Detroit, Michigan): Did you observe any actually destructive attacks?

DR. EIBL-EIBESFELDT: Not between children's groups. Heinz observed it between adults, even a case of manslaughter, and there are some earlier reports also, as Hamburg pointed out.

Chapter 2

THE EXPERIMENTAL IMPERATIVE: LABORATORY ANALYSES OF AGGRESSIVE BEHAVIORS

DENNIS D. KELLY

Many studies into the biological bases of aggressive behaviors take place in a laboratory, if for no other reason than that only in such controlled surroundings can the more refined biological techniques be applied to the problem. The proposition of this paper is that there now exists an experimental imperative to accelerate the development of behavioral procedures for measuring aggression in the laboratory whose quality will match that of the biological procedures. It seems virtually axiomatic that the sophistication with which one evokes and then measures aggressive behaviors must equal in precision the other techniques applied to the study of aggression, or otherwise the quality of this interdisciplinary research will simply reflect the variability inherent in the weaker of the two technologies.

This is not to say that the only call for laboratory analyses of aggressive behaviors is to be able to match, decimal for decimal, the improving quality of data in nonbehavioral disciplines. The experimental analysis of aggression is valuable in its own right. Just as the study of aggression in natural settings suggests the role of aggressive behavior in the evolution of a species and its adaptation to a particular environment, controlled (if sometimes contrived) laboratory analyses help us understand the factors that affect aggression within the lifetime of a single organism (1–3). Despite differing traditions of method and vocabulary, ethology and experimental psychology offer complementary, not conflicting, approaches to behavior.

The current crop of experimental procedures for inducing aggressive fighting in the laboratory seems to represent a rather severe set of methods. These normally involve either an extreme physical provocation, such as an electric shock (4), or entail a serious compromise of the health of the subject whose physiology is under investigation, such as the practice of destroying certain brain regions so as to obtain an abnormally hostile subject that in turn becomes a "model" of aggression (5). Admittedly, there are some techniques available that may be less intrusive, like prolonged isolation (6, 7), but to the outsider it must seem that it is often the experimenter who has been the most aggressive participant in these studies.

This paper reviews a promising line of studies which have demonstrated that measurable aggressive behaviors can result from types of stimuli other than physically painful ones. The phenomenon behind these studies is called extinction-induced aggression, and the approach is similar to, if more empirical and less theoretically inclusive than, the frustration-aggression work of Dollard and others (8). Unlike the frustration-aggression hypothesis, extinction-induced and schedule-induced aggressive behaviors do not represent a global model for all aggressive behavior. The simple fact is that not all aggressive behavior results in this way. However, that some reliable aggression can be caused by extinction-like manipulations in the laboratory is an empirical fact that is both methodologically heartening and theoretically important. Hopefully some of these implications will become evident as the basic phenomenon of extinction-aggression is explained and its generality explored.

THE ACQUISITION-EXTINCTION CYCLE

As is perhaps widely appreciated, certain behavioral responses can be conditioned, that is, can be made more likely to recur, simply by rewarding their performance. Thus in the laboratory the rate of lever pressing of a hungry rat can be lifted above its spontaneous level if a pellet of food is delivered into the chamber every time the rat presses the lever. Similarly this behavior can be extinguished, or returned to its original level of unimportance, simply by severing the relation between the animal's act and its effect, in other words, by breaking the link between behavior and its rewarding consequence. However, what is not widely appreciated, perhaps because it is not widely measured, is that aggressive behavior is a very reliable byproduct of this simple sequence of conditioning and extinction. Before examining the emotional side effects of extinction, however, it may be useful to consider some of the basic properties of the unlearning process as expressed in terms of the response that was originally conditioned.

Figure 2.1 illustrates four typical extinction curves of a rat's lever pressing which have been reproduced from an experiment performed in 1933 by B. F. Skinner (9). Prior to these extinction periods, each of the four rats was accustomed to receiving a pellet of food for each lever press, in fact, each rat had received 100 such rewards (reinforcements). Undeniably the primary effect of the extinction procedure is the gradual decline in strength of the response that is no longer rewarded (reinforced), so that the net final result is a very low rate of lever pressing which results in a cumulative record that runs almost parallel to the abcissa. (In a cumulative curve each response produces a small increment along the ordinate, and the rate of responding can be read from the slope of the curve.) A

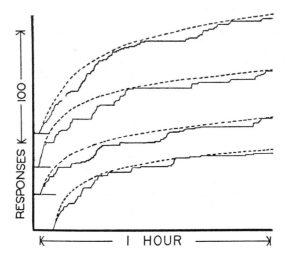

Fig. 2.1. Four typical extinction curves of rats pressing levers. (Reprinted by permission from Skinner, The Behavior of Organisms. © 1938, Appleton-Century-Crofts.)

close look at these records reveals that the initial effect of extinction is actually an unprecedented acceleration in responding followed by extensive fluctuations in response rate. Intermediate extinction behavior is a composite of alternating bursts of activity about the lever interspersed with progressively longer periods of suppression (10). Later in extinction the rat responds less often, and the record becomes smoother and flatter.

It is interesting that Skinner should have superimposed upon these irregular raw data the idealized, smooth functions (shown in dashed lines) to represent an underlying and presumably orderly extinction process. He was otherwise unusually wary of the potential danger of clouding the analysis of individual behavior through recourse to inferred processes. Yet Skinner's early writings (9, 11) also reveal a very special concern for the apparent law*less*ness of the fine grain of extinction behavior, and this curve fitting reflects his attempt to deal with that variability in what might be described as a two-factor theory of extinction. In brief, Skinner considered the smooth theoretical curve as representing the actual decline in strength of the extinguished response. But he acknowledged the act of withholding reinforcement as an "emotional operation" (11, p. 409) and thus saw the erratic deviations from the smooth curve as emotional disturbances. It is particularly interesting that in fitting the curves of Figure 2.1 Skinner chose to project the ideal function along the peaks of the actual extinction record, rather than the troughs. For in so doing, he identified the emotional deviations of extinction as *depressions* in the curve, which in turn were followed by what he called "compensatory increases in rate," these corrective response bursts on the lever serving to return the rat to its normal course of extinction (11, p. 74). It may be valuable to later discussion, however, to point out here that, with little effect upon the shape of this function, a theoretical curve could just as well have been projected along the low points in each experimental record, effectively connecting with a smooth line the closing moments of all of the long pauses in responding recorded during extinction. Such a curve would run under, instead of above, the experimental records in Figure 2.1. Then by analogous reasoning, one might identify as the emotional component of extinction those *bursts* of lever pressing that wrench the subject up away from the ideal curve, with these active deviations continually tempered by compensatory depressions in rate, rather than *vice versa*. With 35 years of hindsight, this version of the two-factor formulation also would seem to be the better of the two for incorporating the recent extinction-induced aggression data which we will consider in a moment. However, the point here is not to evaluate the adequacy of fit of either curve but to suggest that, theoretically at least, any "emotional deviations" from an ideal course of unlearning, or extinction, can as likely be expected to occur in the direction of exaggerated responding as in the form of exaggerated suppression.

EMOTIONAL BY-PRODUCTS OF EXTINCTION

Extinction effects are not confined to frequency changes in the selected response. For example, Joseph Notterman (12) has shown that whereas the force with which the rat presses the lever decreases steadily during training and continued rewarded performance (in a sense the task becomes more stereotyped and less effortful as it is learned), response force increases dramatically again at the onset of extinction with the discontinuation of reinforcement. In other words, a rat hits the lever harder during extinction, occasionally much harder in fact, than at any other time in its experimental history (12). Finally, if one peers into the chamber at the rat generating these cumulative curves, one obtains the rapid intuitive understanding that the extinction process entails far more than the weakening of a single response class, like pressing a lever. The average rat shows a flurry of general activity including a good amount of gnawing and biting of the uncooperative lever. Also those extinction responses of great force more resemble attacks upon the lever, as Mowrer and Jones (13) observed, than they do some weakened version of the previously rewarded behavior.

Lest this phenomenon be thought peculiar to the white rat, the next figure (Fig. 2.2) suggests that the experimental situation as described above is not unlike a gambler dueling with a slot machine which has not paid

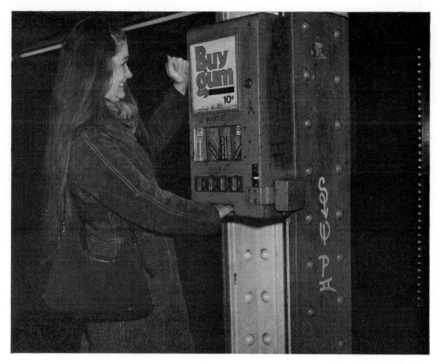

Fig. 2.2. Extinction-induced aggression programmed on a subway platform.

off in some time, or as here, a New York City commuter attempting to extract gum from a subway vending machine.

Other animals besides the white rat and man respond similarly in similar situations. Nearly thirty years ago, Donald Hebb (14) provided a very colorful account of the violent behavior of chimpanzees when a routine chain of their behavior that normally culminated in reinforcement was broken abruptly. Attacks upon the apparatus and Hebb himself ensued; the chimps screamed violently and even pounded their heads upon the floor inflicting self-injuries. Hebb described these behaviors with the terms "sulking," "rage" and "temper tantrums," and it is most interesting that he characterized the initiating circumstances of these emotional behaviors as "the removal of a desired object," the "failure to get something" and "the frustration of an expectation."

As Keller and Schoenfeld (15) have noted, these observations have their counterpart in the aggressive behaviors of angry humans. Georgina Gates (16) interviewed over 50 women students at Barnard College asking them to list for 1 week the circumstances that typically led them to become angry. The women cited as the most common precipitators: refusals of requests; tardiness of friends keeping dates; getting a wrong number on the telephone; failure in operation of watches, pens and typewriters; delays in buses, subways or elevators; and the loss of money. The common thread running through these admissions, of course, is that each cited cause implies a sudden extinction of previously reinforced behavior, an abrupt breaking of a behavioral chain. Each of these situations, the women reported, produced strong tendencies to make verbal retorts, do physical injury to someone else, damage objects, vigorously withdraw from the situation, scream and swear.

Another early and very touching example of the extinction-induced aggression phenomenon can be found in the 19th century journal of Jean Marc Gaspard Itard (17), *The Wild Boy of Aveyron*. This account carries with it as well a very interesting, if dated and typically 18th century, interpretation of the significance of extinction-aggression for the human condition. The journal recounts Itard's attempts to socialize, to educate and to teach language to a feral child who had evidently been discarded for dead with a slashed throat. The boy had miraculously managed to survive living like and with animals for many years until discovered in 1803 in a forest near Aveyron in the south of France. François Truffaut has made a beautiful film, *The Wild Child,* which recreates the journal of Itard and from which the four panels of Figure 2.3 are taken. The scene is that of an extinction test deliberately staged by Itard "as a test of the boy's humanity," about which fact Itard despaired at times because of the boy's failure to learn to talk despite otherwise obvious intelligence. In this learning situation the feral boy's task was to select from among an array of common household items (Fig. 2.3B) the object matching the word pointed to by Itard in a long list of nouns (Fig. 2.3A). Normally Victor was deliberately rewarded with a glass of water and a kind gesture for correct retrievals (Fig. 2.3C). However, during the extinction test, "an act as odious as it was unjust" in Itard's words, Victor was instead lead to a closet to begin an enforced, unmerited "time-out" period. The child replied to this attempt by struggling furiously with Itard, finally biting his arm (Fig. 2.3D).

As Humphrey admitted in the introduction to his English translation of Itard's journal (17, p. xvii), it is difficult to read with dry eyes the passage relating Itard's own reaction to the extinction-induced display:

"It would have been sweet to me at that moment could I have spoken to my pupil to make him understand how the pain of his bite filled my heart with satisfaction and made amends for all my labor. How could I be other than delighted? It was a very legitimate act of vengeance; it was an incontestible proof that the feeling of justice and injustice, that eternal basis of the social order, was no longer foreign to the heart of my pupil. In giving him this feeling, or rather in provoking its de-

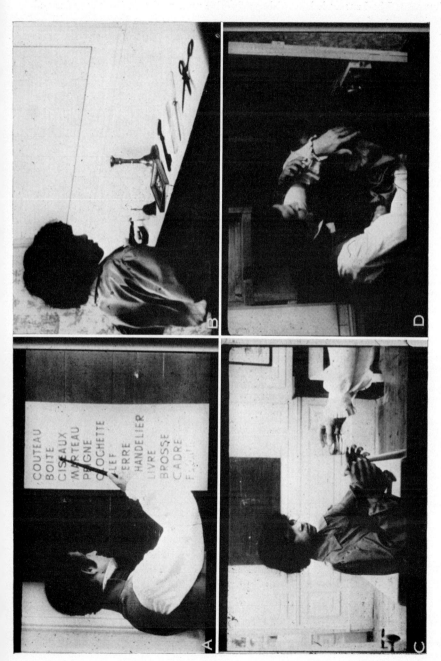

Fig. 2.3. Extinction-induced aggression in a feral child. (A) Itard, played by François Truffaut, points to the French word for "scissors." (B) The boy's task is to select the matching object. (C) Correct responses are reinforced. (D) The child furiously resists being put in a closet after a correct retrieval. (Scenes from the movie "The Wild Child", reprinted by permission from United Artists Inc., © 1970.)

velopment, I had succeeded in raising primitive man to the full stature of moral man by means of the most pronounced of his characteristics and the most noble of his attributes" (17, pp. 95–96).

MEASURING EXTINCTION-INDUCED AGGRESSION

To return to the laboratory example of the rat attacking a newly uncooperative lever, we might ask whether the rat would prefer to launch attacks during extinction periods against some target other than the response lever. Azrin and co-workers (18), in asking the same question, devised a clever technique for quantifying the duration and frequency of aggressive behaviors that result from breaking up a chain of previously reinforced behavior. In their technique, as illustrated in Figure 2.4, a hungry bird was first trained to peck a disk for food. Then, when the experimental pigeon had acquired the key-pecking response, a second "target" bird was introduced. The box holding the target bird was mounted on an assembly with a switch underneath that closed whenever the box jiggled. The whole assembly was balanced so that normal spontaneous movements of the target bird were insufficient to close the microswitch, whereas any forceful attacks by the experimental bird coupled with the evasive reactions of the target bird would be recorded.

In this situation vicious attacks occurred predictably under certain antecedent conditions. Whenever the reinforcement contingency upon the

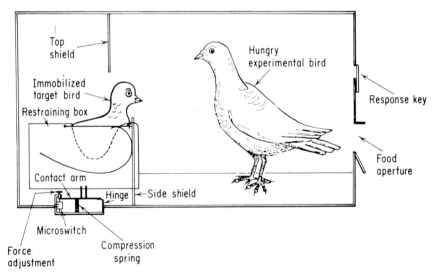

Fig. 2.4. Apparatus for quantifying extinction-induced aggression in the pigeon. (Reprinted by permission from Azrin, Hutchinson & Hake. Extinction-induced Aggression, © 1966, The Society for the Experimental Analysis of Behavior, Inc.)

disk was changed from continuous reinforcement (every peck rewarded) to extinction, the experimental bird invariably turned and mounted an attack upon the target bird as indicated in Figure 2.5. These records are from 19 consecutive sessions of one bird which have been rearranged for considerations of space. Each record shows the 5 minutes preceding and the 5 minutes after a period of continuous reinforcement for key pecking, during which time the experimental bird was allowed 60 food deliveries. The daily extinction curves on the far right in Figure 2.5 bear a remarkable resemblance to the extinction curves shown in Figure 2.1 that were generated by a rat's lever pressing. The important point of Figure 2.5,

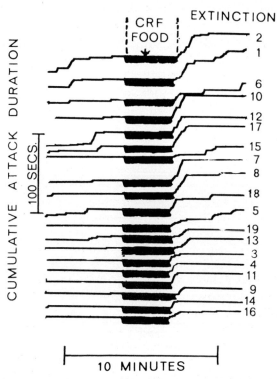

Fig. 2.5. Cumulative records of attacks by experimental bird upon the target bird. The pen steps up during attacks and is deflected downward with each food reward. The apparently solid bar in the middle of each record reflects 60 closely spaced food rewards obtained by the experimental bird through pecks on the response key during a restricted period of food availability. The numbers to the right indicate the actual chronological sequence of the records, which have been rearranged to save space. CRF, continuous reinforcement (Reprinted by permission from Azrin, Hutchinson & Hake. Extinction-induced Aggression, © 1966, The Society for the Experimental Analysis of Behavior, Inc.)

however, is that these are not cumulative curves of the extinguished key-pecking response learned by the pigeon, but of attack behavior upon the target pigeon. Just like lever pressing during extinction, the total number of these attacks was found to be a direct function of the number of preceding reinforced responses. As seen here, extinction-induced attacks were long lived, lasting up to 10 minutes, and were observed to be particularly vicious, aimed most often at the throat, head and eyes of the target. Fortunately an extinguished pigeon will also attack stuffed target birds prepared by a taxidermist. This inanimate target method for measuring extinction-aggression has proven equally successful when adapted to squirrel monkeys (19) and teenage humans (20).

There is even some evidence that the very opportunity for aggression directed elsewhere than at the response key is a highly reinforcing event in itself (21, 22). For example, if a guillotine door is dropped in front of the target bird, the experimental bird can be taught to perform a second response, which it will exercise during extinction periods only, just to gain access to the target bird to carry out these attacks. This stands as operational evidence that a target for aggression becomes reinforcing during periods of transition from conditions of continuous reinforcement to extinction.

In many ways this demonstration in normal subjects of the reinforcing properties of the opportunity for aggression is reminiscent of the findings of Roberts and Kiess (23) in cats that were implanted with perifornical hypothalamic electrodes. When stimulated, these placements would produce directed attack behavior if an appropriate target were present. Under the motivational influence of such stimulation, cats even learned to turn into the correct arm of a two-choice maze, with access to a target rat being the sole reinforcing consequence of the choice. Substitute sudden extinction of learned behavior for hypothalamic stimulation and the paradigms of the two experiments look quite similar. Both sets of results seem to establish the rewarding value for a "provoked" animal of the opportunity to exercise directed aggression against a target. The corollary inference, of course, is that aggression induced by extinction procedures and that elicited by electrical stimulation of attack sites in the diencephalon possess some overlapping functional properties, despite qualitative differences in the methods by which they are produced and in the level of experimenter intervention.

STIMULUS CONTROL OF EXTINCTION-INDUCED AGGRESSION

Another property of extinction-related aggressive behaviors is that it may be feasible to bring such responses under discrete, explicit, time-locked stimulus control, and perhaps also under certain types of unsignaled, but predictably periodic, schedule control. The first of these, stimulus control of emotional behavior, is illustrated by the photographs of Terrace (24) which are reproduced in Figure 2.6. These show the gross behavioral reactions of four pigeons to the onset of a stimulus, the horizontal bar projected upon the response disk, correlated with an extinction contingency. These photos were all taken within 5 seconds of the stimulus change on the disk. Although all four birds had been exposed to the extinction stimulus by this juncture in the experiment, the behavior of one of these pigeons is quite different from the rest. Normally following discrimination training, the extinction signal evokes various emotional responses such as wing flapping (birds A and B) or turning away from the key (bird C). Bird D, on the other hand, is seen here calmly settling down under the response key which bears for him the same bad

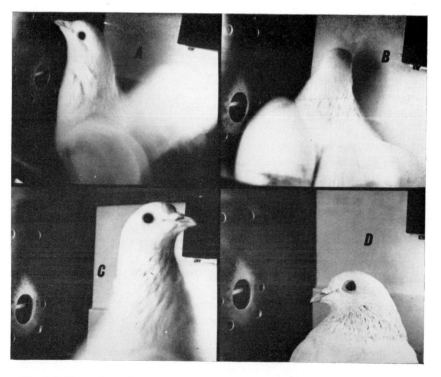

Fig. 2.6. Pigeons' reactions to onset of a stimulus (horizontal line on key) signaling a period of reinforcement unavailability. Birds A, B and C learned the horizontal-vertical discrimination with errors. Bird D learned the same problem without errors. (Reprinted by permission from Terrace. Stimulus control, in Operant Behavior: Areas of Research and Application, edited by Honig, © 1966, Appleton-Century-Crofts)

tidings as for the others. What is different about this bird is its history, and in it lies a possible lesson. Bird D is one of Terrace's flawless learners which has acquired the visual discrimination without errors, that is, without ever having made any, or at least not many, unreinforced pecks at the extinction stimulus (24). Thus, it may be that a history of unproductive extinction behavior, however brief, must precede a subject's aggressive responding. The procedures used by Terrace to train errorless discriminations are not basic to this discussion, and so will not be detailed here. Briefly, they involve a gradual "fading-in" of the extinction stimulus both in terms of its duration and intensity from the very beginning of key-peck training. In fact, technically speaking, it is probably simpler to bring the emotional behaviors of pigeons A, B and C under stimulus control than it is to engineer a stoic bird like D.

Much of importance remains to be learned about the stimulus control of aggressive behaviors. For instance, little can be said currently about the durability of such control, or whether unreinforced responses still have to precede aggression when extinction-correlated cues are presented repeatedly. Although it has yet to be firmly established, it seems likely that if a target were present during traditional discrimination training, an erring subject would probably attack it when the cue for reinforcement unavailability was turned on (18, 25) in much the same manner as it would if shocked (26). The relation of extinction- and pain-induced aggressive reactions is not fully understood either, but at least one report suggests that the combined effectiveness of these operations in eliciting aggression may be additive (27). In this limited, perhaps superficial, sense both the signaled withdrawal of a positive reinforcer, termed time-out, and the presentation of a severe negative reinforcer, like shock, may act as functional equivalents. The two operations have already proven similarly aversive in their ability to suppress behavior that is instrumental in producing either (28, 29). Operationally both are forms of punishment; both prompt aggressive reactions.

SCHEDULE-INDUCED AGGRESSION

Aggression is not only a by-product of transition periods between the rewarding of every response and the subsequent extinction of all responses, as described thus far. This type of aggression may also come under the more subtle cyclic control of certain schedules of reinforcement, where extinction as such is not programmed, but where the rules for obtaining reinforcements are expressed so as to allow the subject to predict certain periods of reinforcement unavailability (30, 31). With simple schedules of reinforcement, there are no explicit cues for periods of reduced reinforcement density except those provided by the reinforcements themselves and the feedback the animal might receive from its own behavior. Consider a differential reinforcement of low rate (DRL) or "timing" schedule, where an animal's task is to delay its next response by some minimum time from its last in order to obtain reinforcement. Here each response the subject makes, as well as each reinforcement it receives, serves as a reliable cue, or predictor, of a minimum period (the DRL interval) during which further reinforcement will be unavailable. As another example, reinforcements delivered according to a fixed-ratio schedule also possess signal properties for the performing subject. On a fixed-ratio schedule a subject is required to respond a preset number of times for each reinforcement. From past experience we know that the number of responses required can be stretched quite high, into the thousands, in fact, if conditions are otherwise favorable (11, 32).

As Figure 2.7 indicates, responding on a fixed-ratio schedule typically

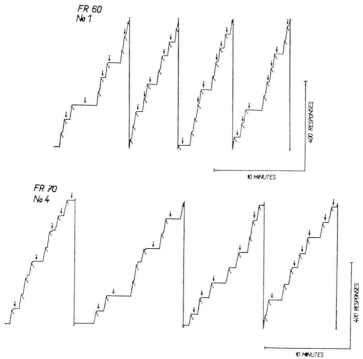

Fig. 2.7. Cumulative records of two rats' lever pressing for reinforcing brain stimulations on fixed-ratio schedules. The pen is deflected diagonally at each reinforcement. Each arrow represents an attack upon a live frog cornered in the chamber. (Reprinted by permission from Huston & DeSisto. Interspecies aggression during fixed-ratio hypothalamic self-stimulation in rats, Physiology and Behavior, © 1971, Brain Research Publ., Inc.)

follows a very stereotyped pattern. The subject almost always satisfies the ratio requirement in one burst of activity, obtains the reinforcer and then pauses. In this particular pair of records, two rats are responding on fixed ratios of 60 and 70 responses, respectively, for trains of reinforcing lateral hypothalamic brain stimulation. The rewarding stimulations are indicated by the downward deflections of the response pen. The pauses that typically intervene between the completion of one burst of responding and the beginning of the next well exceed the time required by a subject to savor the last traces of rewarding brain stimulation, or to consume a tiny food pellet, if that were the reinforcer. It is a matter of current dispute whether this stereotypical pause is linked to the preceding reinforcement or to the succeeding work required to obtain the next reinforcer. Although usually called a postreinforcement pause, this break in lever pressing might also represent a prework or pre-ratio-run delay (33). However, whether forward or backward looking, it is certain that the fixed-ratio pause represents something more to the rat than simply a rest period. For, if an appropriate target is available in the chamber, the subject will attack the target during these self-imposed work delays (34–36) just as it would during an explicitly signaled extinction period (18). In fact, in Figure 2.7 the arrows indicate attacks launched by the experimental rats upon target frogs freshly exchanged after every attack. Most often these were lethal attacks with 4 of the 6 subject rats in this study by Huston and DeSisto (36) averaging more than 1 frog killed per every two fixed-ratio reinforcements earned. The regularity of these attacks upon an alien species is not extraordinary *per se,* for frog killing is a strong response in rats (37). Of interest here is when the killings occurred during the trained schedule performance. All attacks occurred during pauses following reinforcements, and never did the rats interrupt their bursts of lever pressing to aggress against the frog. It is probably useful to recall that in terms of the fixed-ratio schedule, postreinforcement pauses occur at times when the animal has just been signaled (by the reinforcer) that the next reinforcement is as far away in time and effort as is possible.

The psychopharmacology of the varied behaviors involved in this complex performance is also quite intriguing. Low doses of common tranquilizing and antianxiety agents, such as meprobamate (Miltown) and the benzodiazepines, such as chlordiazepoxide (Librium), are known to shorten postreinforcement pauses on fixed-ratio, fixed-interval and differential-reinforcement-of-low-rate schedules (38). Interestingly, these same drugs, tested under different circumstances, have also proven effective in decreasing many aggressive behaviors, including both spontaneous and isolation-induced fighting. They also exert taming effects upon hypothalamically elicited attack behavior and upon the septal hyperirritability syndrome (39). As yet their effects upon schedule-induced aggression have not been reported.

AGGRESSION AS AN ADJUNCTIVE BEHAVIOR

One of the more interesting facts about schedule-induced aggression is that such attacks are not the only behavioral by-product of the recurring weak periods in schedule performance. In fact, it seems that aggression may be only one of a virtually interchangeable set of behaviors that have been called by John Falk (40) "adjunctive" or "displacement" behaviors. Among others this list appears to include drinking (41, 42), air licking (43), wheeling running (44) and pica feeding (45). At first glance these behaviors would seem to have little in common with aggressive acts, yet any one of these responses, given the supporting circumstances and opportunity to occur, can emerge to a similarly exaggerated degree during similar moments in the cyclic control of instrumentally conditioned responding. Stated simply, the antecedents of this type of aggressive behavior are not specific to aggressive responses.

For example, if instead of a target a water tube were made available to an animal responding on a fixed-ratio schedule for food, there is reliable evidence (40) that collateral drinking would occur at the same junctures in responding as indicated by the arrows in Figure 2.7 for collateral aggression. In fact the animals would doubtlessly *over*drink or become polydipsic. Just such an example is presented in Figure 2.8. This chaired rhesus monkey was required to press a rather heavy lever 40 times to obtain each pellet of food delivered at the pen deflections (a fixed-ratio 40 schedule). The format of this record is the same as Figure 2.7 except that the monkey's drinking is recorded by the event pen in the lower record, while its lever pressing is followed by the upper cumulative pen. Drinking occurs in this situation during the same postreinforcement pauses in ratio responding that prompted attacks upon the frog in Huston and DeSisto's experiment. In fact, the only two instances in this record when the monkey's drinking was not fully confined to the postreinforcement period seemed to be associated with an unusually gradual resumption of lever pressing, as shown by the arrows. Normally the transition from pausing to responding is abrupt, and the cutoff in collateral drinking complete.

To one unfamiliar with the schedule-induced polydipsic phenomenon it might seem perfectly normal for a monkey to have something to drink with its meal. Indeed some investigators have considered this exaggerated water intake as a natural form of prandial drinking (46, 47). However, in light of the detailed empirical similarities between this phenomenon and schedule-induced aggression (48) and the relation of both to "emotion-producing" operations, there is likely more to the polydipsic phenomenon

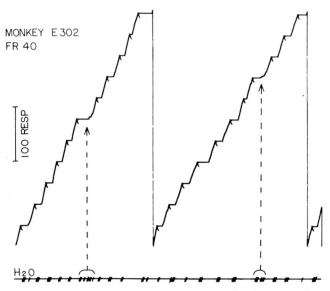

MONKEY E302
FR 40

Fig. 2.8. Schedule-induced polydipsia in a rhesus monkey lever pressing on a fixed-ratio schedule for food pellets, delivered at the pen deflections in the upper record. Nose key presses to obtain squirts of water are shown by the lower pen. Record covers the middle 30 minutes of a 1-hour long session.

than simply a dry mouth. This, too, seems to be the feeling of Falk (41), for he called the drinking "psychogenic polydipsia." Take the monkey in Figure 2.8, for instance, which was maintained on a fixed-ratio schedule for just 1 hour each day, but which drank during that hour roughly 10 times again its previous normal 24-hour *ad libitum* intake. Perhaps even more telling is that this particular rhesus monkey was a "pouch feeder" and rarely ate its food pellets as it earned them, but rather stored them in its cheek pouches for latter consumption, in between experimental sessions (49). Although it ate at a later hour (and drank moderately with its meal), the monkey *over*drank only during the session while it was earning its food. In fact, it would seem that whenever food-seeking behavior is thwarted, however momentarily (as in the case of the preratio work pause), drinking occurs to a greater degree than it otherwise would. Rats drink excessively when starved (50) as well as when a learned, food-motivated response of theirs is extinguished (51). In both the latter situations, there is no food present to dry the subject's mouth.

Under similar fixed-ratio and differential-reinforcement-of-low-rate schedule conditions, not only aggression and polydipsia may occur but, if the experimental environment so provides, one may also observe repetitive licking at a hissing stream of air (43), pecking at self-reflections in a mirror (52), increased alcohol consumption (53, 54) and even, in monkeys, the ingestion of unappetizing sawdust or wood shavings, called pica feeding (45). The latter behavior would seem particularly unrecommended for relieving a dry mouth. In all these instances of exaggerated adjunctive behaviors, it seems to be the predictable, spaced presentations of a positive reinforcer that serves as the explicit "releasing stimulus," to borrow an ethological term. However, it is probably safe to conclude, as does Segal (55), that the presentation of a reinforcer on these schedules functions as a releasing stimulus for aggression and other adjunctive behaviors not in its capacities as a reinforcer, but as a signal for the onset of periods during which reinforcement will not be available.

Admittedly the set of adjunctive behaviors mentioned here is not thoroughly interchangeable merely by the manipulation of the subject's opportunities to engage in the various activities, like aggression, drinking, air licking and so on (56). There is evidence that although fixed-ratio lever pressing for brain stimulation will result in predictable bouts of aggression in the presence of an appropriate target as in Figure 2.7, this method of rewarding fixed-ratio performance apparently will not result in polydipsia, even if a water spout is present and a target is not (57). It is therefore not the intent of this brief discussion to argue the boundary conditions of that class of behaviors called adjunctive, but merely to point out the striking communality that exists among the conditions that can give rise to other unusual behaviors as well as to aggression.

To anticipate the inevitable question of how this form of aggression all started, some closing remarks on the currently uncertain conceptual status of extinction-related aggression might seem in order. At this early stage in data gathering, it is simply not clear whether this form of aggression can be learned or whether it reflects a thoroughly innate mechanism that arises in each individual independently of past experience. Clouding the issue in part is the common observation that at times this sort of aggressive behavior serves a clearly useful function, and hence is open to reinforcement. Occasionally the irritated subway rider back in Figure 2.2 will actually jar loose some Chiclets from the vending machine. We are familiar, too, with the example of the computer in an Apollo space capsule which, before millions on global television, was repaired by a firm whack. On the other hand, teleological explanations for extinction-aggression can also be generated with ease, but are probably no less premature. For instance, if occupation of well staked out personal territory is considered reinforcing, then defense against a trespasser could be considered as less a biological imperative than a simple example of extinction-induced aggression. An intruder programs extinction in a natural setting by breaking a previously reinforcing bond of privacy. Similar interpretive possibilities are virtually limitless, as the tenacity of the frustration-aggression hypothesis aptly illustrates. Such theories are obviously more easy to come by than are the facts which will resolve them.

ACKNOWLEDGMENTS

I would like to thank Drs. John Gibbon, J. R. Millenson and Michael Potegal for their helpful readings of an earlier version of this manuscript.

REFERENCES

1. SCHOENFELD, WN, BARON, S: Ethology and experimental psychology. Science 147: 634, 1965.
2. SKINNER, BF: The phylogeny and ontogeny of behavior. Science 153: 1205, 1966.
3. NEVIN, JA: Problems and methods, Ch 1, in The Study of Behavior, edited by Nevin, JA, Reynolds, G. Glenview, Ill., Scott, Foresman, 1973, p. 3.
4. ULRICH, R, SYMANNEK, B: Pain as a stimulus for aggression, in Biology of Aggressive Behavior, edited by Garattini, S, Sigg, EB. New York, Wiley, 1969, p. 59.
5. MALICK, JB: A behavioral comparison of three lesion-induced models of aggression in the rat. Physiol Behav 5: 679, 1970.
6. ALLEE, WC: Group organization among vertebrates. Science 95: 289, 1942.
7. VALZELLI, L: Drugs and aggressiveness. Adv Pharmacol 5: 79, 1967.
8. DOLLARD, J, DOOB, L, MILLER, N, MOWRER, O, SEARS, R: Frustration and Aggression. New Haven, Yale University Press, 1939.
9. SKINNER, BF: "Resistance to extinction" in the process of conditioning. J Gen Psychol 9: 420, 1933.
10. HURWITZ, HMB: Periodicity of response in operant extinction. Q J Exp Psychol 9: 177, 1957.
11. SKINNER, BF: Behavior of Organisms: An Experimental Analysis. New York, Appleton-Century-Crofts, 1938.
12. NOTTERMAN, J: Force emission during bar pressing. J Exp Psychol 58: 341, 1959.
13. MOWRER, OH, JONES, HM: Extinction and behavior variability as functions of effortfulness of task. J Exp Psychol 33: 369, 1943.
14. HEBB, DO: The forms and conditions of chimpanzee anger. Bull Can Psychol Assoc 5: 32, 1945.
15. KELLER, FS, SCHOENFELD, WN: Principles of Psychology. A Systematic Text in the Science of Behavior. New York, Appleton-Century-Crofts, 1950, p. 343.
16. GATES, GS: An observational study of anger. J Exp Psychol 9: 325, 1926.
17. ITARD, JMG: The Wild Boy of Aveyron (Rapports et mémoires sur le sauvage de l'Aveyron), translated by Humphrey G, Humphrey, M. New York, Appleton-Century-Crofts, 1932.
18. AZRIN, NH, HUTCHINSON, RR, HAKE, DF: Extinction-induced aggression. J Exp Anal Behav 9: 191, 1966.
19. HUTCHINSON, RR, AZRIN, NH, HUNT, GM: Attack produced by intermittent reinforcement of a concurrent operant response. J Exp Anal Behav 11: 489, 1968.
20. KELLY, JF, HAKE, DF: An extinction-induced increase in aggressive response with humans. J Exp Anal Behav 14: 153, 1970.
21. AZRIN, NH, HUTCHINSON, RR, MCLAUGHLIN, R: The opportunity for aggression as an operant reinforcer during aversive stimulation. J Exp Anal Behav 8: 171, 1965.

22. CHEREK, DR, THOMPSON, T, HEISTAD, GT: Effects of Δ'-tetrahydrocannabinol and food deprivation level on responding maintained by the opportunity to attack. Physiol Behav 9: 795, 1972.

23. ROBERTS, WW, KIESS, HO: Motivational properties of hypothalamic aggression in cats. J Comp Physiol Psychol 58: 187, 1964.

24. TERRACE, HS: Stimulus control, in Operant Behavior: Areas of Research and Application, edited by Honig, WK. New York, Appleton-Century-Crofts, 1966, p. 271.

25. COLE, JM, LITCHFIELD, PM: Stimulus control of schedule-induced aggression in the pigeon. Psychonomic Sci 17: 152, 1969.

26. ULRICH, RE, AZRIN, NH: Reflexive fighting in response to aversive stimulation. J Exp Anal Behav 5: 511, 1962.

27. TONDAT, LM, DALY, HB: The combined effects of frustrative nonreward and shock on aggression between rats. Psychonomic Sci 28: 25, 1972.

28. FERSTER, CB: Control of behavior in chimpanzees and pigeons by timeout from positive reinforcement. Psychol Monogr 72: 1, 1958.

29. HOLZ, WC, AZRIN, NH, AYLLON, T: Elimination of behavior of mental patients by response-produced extinction. J Exp Anal Behav 6: 407, 1963.

30. FERSTER, CB, SKINNER, BF: Schedules of Reinforcement. New York, Appleton-Century-Crofts, 1957.

31. MORSE, WH: Intermittent reinforcement, in Operant Behavior: Areas of Research and Application, edited by Honig, WK. New York, Appleton-Century-Crofts, 1966, p. 52.

32. FINDLEY, JD, BRADY, JV: Facilitation of large ratio performance by use of conditioned reinforcement. J Exp Anal Behav 8: 125, 1965.

33. GRIFFITHS, RR, THOMPSON, T: The post-reinforcement pause: A misnomer. Psychol Rec 23: 229, 1973.

34. GENTRY, WD: Fixed-ratio schedule-induced aggression. J Exp Anal Behav 11: 813, 1968.

35. FLORY, RK: Attack behavior in a multiple fixed-ratio schedule of reinforcement. Psychonomic Sci 16: 156, 1969.

36. HUSTON, JP, DeSISTO, MJ: Interspecies aggression during fixed-ratio hypothalamic self-stimulation in rats. Physiol Behav 7: 353, 1971.

37. DeSISTO, MJ, HUSTON, JP: Effects of territory on frog-killing by rats. J Genet Psychol 83: 179, 1970.

38. SCHECKEL, CL: Preclinical psychopharmacology, in Principles of Psychopharmacology, edited by Clark, WG, delGuidice, J. New York, Academic Press, 1970, p. 235.

39. MARGOLIN, S, KLETZKIN, M: Pharmacological properties of anti-anxiety drugs, in Principles of Psychopharmacology, edited by Clark, WG, delGuidice, J. New York, Academic Press, 1970, p. 303.

40. FALK, JL: The nature and determinants of adjunctive behavior. Physiol Behav 6: 577, 1971.

41. FALK, J: Production of polydipsia in normal rats by an intermittent food schedule. Science 133: 195, 1961.

42. FALK, JL: The behavioral regulation of water-electrolyte balance, in Nebraska Symposium on Motivation, Vol. 9 edited by Jones, MR. Lincoln, Neb., University of Nebraska Press, 1961, p. 1.

43. MENDELSON, J, CHILLAG, D: Schedule-induced air licking in rats. Physiol Behav 5: 535, 1970.

44. LEVITSKY, D, COLLIER, G: Schedule-induced wheel running. Physiol Behav 3: 571, 1968.

45. VILLARREAL, J: Schedule-induced pica. Paper read at Annual Meeting of Eastern Psychological Assoc., Boston, April 1967.
46. STEIN, L: Excessive drinking in the rat: Superstition or thirst? J Comp Physiol Psychol 58: 237, 1964.
47. LOTTER, EC, WOODS, SC, VASSELLI, JR: Schedule-induced polydipsia: An artifact. J Comp Physiol Psychol 83: 478, 1973.
48. FLORY, R: Attack behavior as a function of minimum interfood interval. J Exp Anal Behav 12: 825, 1969.
49. KELLY, D: Long-term prereward suppression in monkeys unaccompanied by cardiovascular conditioning. J Exp Anal Behav 20: 93, 1973.
50. OATLEY, K, TONGE, DA: The effect of hunger on water intake in rats. Q J Exp Psychol 21: 162, 1969.
51. PANKSEPP, J, TOATES, FM, OATLEY, K: Extinction-induced drinking in hungry rats. Anim Behav 20: 493, 1972.
52. COHEN, PS, LOONEY, TA: Schedule-induced mirror responding in the pigeon. J Exp Anal Behav 19: 395, 1973.
53. LESTER, D: Self-maintenance of intoxication in the rat. Q J Stud Alcohol 22: 223, 1961.
54. MEISCH, RA, THOMPSON, T: Ethanol intake during schedule-induced polydipsia. Physiol Behav 8: 471, 1972.
55. SEGAL, E: Induction and the provenance of operants. in Reinforcement: Behavioral Analyses, edited by Gilbert, RM, Millenson, JR. New York, Academic Press, 1972, p. 1.
56. HYMOWITZ, N: Schedule-induced polydipsia and aggression in rats. Psychonomic Sci 23: 226, 1971.
57. COHEN, I, MENELSON, J: Schedule-induced drinking with food but not ICS reinforcement. Behav Biol, 1973, in press.

DISCUSSION

QUESTION: I wonder if Dr. Kelly would care to speculate on the possible biological utility of that act of one pigeon attacking another pigeon. Does this mean that in real life the chief frustrator from getting food is a member of the same species competing for the food? Will a pigeon attack other creatures besides another pigeon?

DR. DENNIS KELLY (New York, New York): I must admit that I have no special basis for speculating upon the teleology of this aggressive reaction. This research approach focuses upon the proximate antecedent conditions of aggressive behavior, not upon its long term survival value. However, personally I would doubt that behind a pigeon's every extinction experience in nature that there stands another pigeon.

Regarding the phrasing of the question, it seems to me that, at least for experimental analyses of aggression, the frustration-aggression language has probably added very little to our knowledge. I think it's important to point out that the scientist's job is exactly the same whether he believes the hypothesis or not. Even if the experimentalist accepts that aggression is mediated by a state of frustration, be it defined as cognitive, physiological or whatever, he still must set about identifying those antecedent conditions that induce the frustration. He does this in the same manner as he would to study the aggression itself.

DR. SEYMOUR S. KETY (Boston, Massachusetts): Is it possible that what occurs during extinction-aggression is not necessarily an activation of aggressive patterns but an arousal of optional behaviors of many types, aggression being the one which happens to have been elicited in the experimental situation? If, for example, instead of having the animal exposed only to levers or to another animal against which aggression might be appropriate, what would happen if there were an estrous female in the box during an extinction period?

DR. KELLY: I frankly don't know but, like you, would guess that a male animal would attempt to mount the female. It seems to me that the adjunctive behaviors, as Falk calls them, as a class do occur under "arousal" conditions or stressful points in the environmental control of learned behavior. I would also agree that such activities as overdrinking, aggression, air licking and even sexual behavior (though this has not yet been proven a member of this group) may often constitute an interchangeable set of behaviors, and that the one elicited on a given occasion might depend principally upon environmental options. Relevant to your example, in fact, is the interesting observation on the cormorant made by Tinbergen and quoted by Falk: If approached or threatened by another member of its species, the bird may become aroused and take certain defensive postures; but should the intruder flee, its aggressive behavior may shift abruptly into sexual activity with a mate.

DR. BRUCE BERNARD (Storrs, Connecticut): A frog killing occurs in only a small percentage of rats. Will frustration induce killing in rats who normally do not kill or just an increased percentage of killing in animals that do kill?

DR. KELLY: I don't know. I'd like to point out, though, that a frog target is not necessary for the phenomenon of schedule-related aggression to occur. Inanimate targets appear to work well: bite tubes, levers, gum machines, and so forth. If a frog is there, the rat will attack the frog. I doubt that the success of Huston and DeSisto's experiment depended upon presenting a frog.

Chapter 3

EVIDENCE FOR A SEX DIFFERENCE IN THE NEUROPIL OF THE RAT PREOPTIC AREA AND ITS IMPORTANCE FOR THE STUDY OF SEXUALLY DIMORPHIC FUNCTIONS[1]

GEOFFREY RAISMAN

Tell me where is Fancy bred,
Or in the heart or in the head?
How begot, how nourished?
Reply, Reply.
It is engender'd in the eyes,
With gazing fed; and Fancy dies
In the cradle where it lies.
Let us all ring Fancy's knell:
I'll begin it, — Ding, dong, bell! (1)

The purpose of this Conference is to talk not about the location of Fancy and its morphogenesis, but about its opposite—aggression. In this communication I am going to ask the following questions: 1) What part of the brain is involved in this function? 2) What is the structure of that part of the brain? 3) How is this structure engendered—or as we would say, How does it develop?

Neuroanatomical research is undertaken because we feel that a knowledge of the structure of the brain is important for understanding its function. However, in practical terms a direct relationship between structure and function is not easy to establish. We can say that the lateral geniculate body has a visual function and that it has a similar structure from one individual to another. We can say that it has a different structure from the medial geniculate, which is auditory. However, the ultimate proof that structure reflects function would require the demonstration that if the *same* part of the brain functioned *differently* in different individuals, then it should have appropriate differences in structure. It is not easy to devise experimental situations in which this hypothesis can be tested, but in one case Nature herself has provided a ready made experiment. In what follows I will be referring principally to work on small laboratory rodents such as the rat. The brain of the female is

[1] This work was supported by Grants G969/546/B and G970/668/B from the Medical Research Council and 70-472 from the Foundations Fund for Research in Psychiatry.

42

capable of initiating the cyclic surge of gonadotrophin secretion which results in ovulation. At the same time the animal becomes sexually receptive. The male does not usually exhibit these functions (at least to the same degree) and in most species displays a greater amount of aggressive behavior.

There is considerable evidence that the hypothalamus is the part of the brain ultimately responsible for the control of the secretion of the pituitary gland (and hence the gonad), but that a small region just in front of the hypothalamus—the preoptic area—is essential for triggering the prolonged burst of neural activity which leads to the preovulatory surge of gonadotrophin secretion (2–4). Furthermore, the integrity of the preoptic area is essential for the performance of the normal pattern of mating behavior (5). There is also experimental evidence that the amygdala—a region of the brain which sends fibers through the stria terminalis to both the preoptic area and the hypothalamus (Fig. 3.1)—is in some way involved in the control of ovulation, mating behavior and aggressive behavior (5–7). This was the background for our experimental investigations. We asked the following question: Is there any structural difference between the preoptic area in the female and its functionally different counterpart (8), the preoptic area of the male? The purpose of the investigation was to study that part of the preoptic area which contains synapses established by axons of amygdaloid origin traveling through the stria terminalis. We have called this the strial part of the preoptic area.

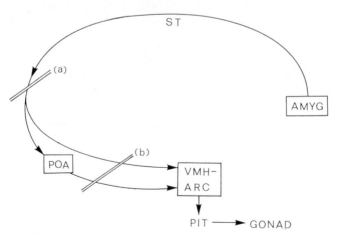

Fig. 3.1. A schematic diagram showing the fibers of the stria terminalis (ST) originating in the amygdala (AMYG) and projecting to the preoptic area (POA) and to the ventromedial (VMH) and arcuate (ARC) nuclear region of the hypothalamus, which in turn is responsible for the control of the secretion of gonadotrophins from the pituitary (PIT). In the rat, spontaneous cyclic ovulation is prevented by cuts at (b) but not at (a).

In order to assess the nature of the neural circuitry in the preoptic area, we studied sections in the electron microscope and counted and classified all of the synapses present in a measured area of section. The results are derived from total counts of more than 100,000 synapses in 82 rats of both sexes. Ninety-eight per cent of the synapses in the strial part of the preoptic area are axodendritic; the remaining 2 per cent are axosomatic. About 90 per cent of the axodendritic synapses are on dendritic shafts (Fig.

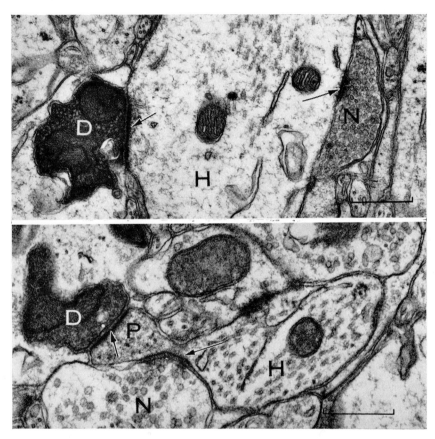

Fig. 3.2 (top). A dendritic shaft (H), identified by its content of microtubules, is contacted (at arrows) by two axon terminals, one of which (N) is normal, and the other (D) shows the electron dense reaction of orthograde degeneration 2 days after cutting its parent axon by transecting the stria terminalis. Scale bar = 0.5 μ.

Fig. 3.3 (bottom). A dendritic shaft (H) containing microtubules bears a small spine (P) characterized by its dense cytoplasm. The spine is contacted (at arrow) by an axon terminal (D) showing the electron dense reaction of orthograde degeneration 2 days after cutting the stria terminalis. A second axon terminal (N) forms a synaptic contact (at arrow) with the neck of the dendritic spine. Scale bar = 0.5 μm.

3.2) and 10 per cent on dendritic spines (Fig. 3.3). The synapses of amygdaloid origin were identified by cutting the stria terminalis 2 days before killing the animal. This results in orthograde terminal degeneration, which is seen as a marked increase in electron density and shrinkage of the amygdaloid fiber terminals. This enables them to be identified in the electron microscope (Figs. 3.2 and 3.3). About half of the spine synapses are of amygdaloid origin, but only a small proportion of the shaft synapses. We have, therefore, four categories of synapse. The two major categories of synapse, synapses on dendritic shafts and synapses on dendritic spines, can each be subdivided into a further two categories: synapses of amygdaloid origin and synapses of unknown, but not amygdaloid, origin.

When we compare the numbers of these four different types of synapses in different animals we find that there is a striking degree of consistency from one animal to the next. This applies to rats of either sex. There is one exception: the number of nonamygdaloid synapses on dendritic spines (Fig. 3.4) is twice as high in the female as in the male (9). No such

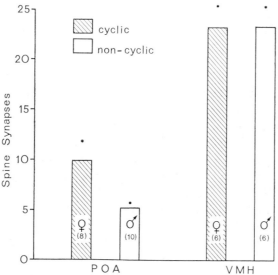

Fig. 3.4. The number of nondegenerating spine synapses per unit area (one grid square of approximately 1800 μ^2) in the preoptic areas (POA) in 8 female and 10 male rats, and in the ventromedial hypothalamic nuclei (VMH) of 6 female and 6 male rats. There are roughly twice as many nonamygdaloid spine synapses per unit area in the female as in the male. No such difference occurs in the ventromedial nuclei. The number of rats in each group is shown in parentheses. Scatter is indicated by the standard error of the mean (dots above bars), although because of the distribution of the data, nonparametric (ranking) tests were used to assess the significance of differences. Crosshatched bars are used to designate animals with a cyclic (female) pattern of gonadotrophin release.

difference occurs in any of the other three categories of synapse. No such difference was found in the surrounding parts of the preoptic area (which do not receive amygdaloid connections). Furthermore, no such difference was found in the part of the ventromedial hypothalamus which does receive amygdaloid connections through the stria terminalis (Fig. 3.4). In other words: whereas the amygdaloid fibers themselves are not sexually dimorphic, they do have access to a sexually dimorphic area of tissue which is located specifically in the preoptic area.

Therefore, it is perhaps of interest to mention here that although destruction of the amygdaloid fibers in the stria terminalis (a, Fig. 3.1) does not prevent cyclic ovulation in the rat, destruction of the preoptic area or cuts between the preoptic area and the hypothalamus (b, Fig. 3.1), cause an anovulatory state with polyfollicular ovaries and persistent vaginal cornification (7, 10, 11).

It is tempting to correlate this sexually dimorphic part of the preoptic area with sexually dimorphic functions such as the control of ovulation and with sexually dimorphic behavior patterns. In attempting to provide experimental confirmation of this hypothesis we were able to take advantage of another fact about sexual differentiation. The female pattern of gonadotrophin secretion does not depend directly on the genetic sex of the animal, but depends on the absence of androgen during a critical perinatal period of development which, in the rat, consists principally of the 1st week after birth (12). Under normal circumstances, the female pattern of gonadotrophin secretion develops in the female but is prevented from developing in the male by the secretion of androgen by its own testes during the 1st week of postnatal life (Fig. 3.5). Treatment of the normal genetic female with a single dose of exogenous androgen on the 4th day of postnatal life permanently abolishes the ability to ovulate in the adult. This is called androgen sterilization. Conversely, castration of the male within 1 day of birth results in an adult which, if transplanted with ovaries, can exhibit cyclic ovulation and behavioral estrus. The same manipulations carried out after the critical period are ineffective. Thus, androgen treatment of the female on the 16th day of life (after the critical period) or castration of the male on the 7th day of life (after the testes have had time to secrete androgen during the critical 1st week) do not affect the normal development and expression of the adult functions proper to the genetic sex of the animal.

If the anatomical differences in the preoptic area do reflect functional differences then they too should be appropriately affected by endocrine manipulations during the early postnatal period. We prepared six groups of 64 adult rats which had been subjected to the endocrine manipulations

GENETIC SEX	AGE (days)					ADULT FUNCTION
	0	5	10	15	20	
	Critical —————▷					
FEMALE	—		—			CYCLIC
	1·25 mg TP Day 4					NON-CYCLIC
	—		1·25mg TP Day 16			CYCLIC
MALE	—	—				NON-CYCLIC
	CASTR. Day 1	—				CYCLIC
	—	CASTR. Day 7				NON-CYCLIC

Fig. 3.5. A summary of the adult pattern of gonadotrophin secretion (cyclic or non-cyclic; right hand column) in the six groups of animals subjected to the neonatal endo-crine manipulations mentioned in the text. Genetic females were either untreated (cyclic gonadotrophin release pattern as adults) or treated with a single subcutaneous dose of 1.25 mg of testosterone propionate (TP) either on the 4th day of life (during the critical period for neonatal differentiation) or on the 16th day of life (after the critical period). Males were either intact (top row) or else castrated on either the 1st or the 7th day of life.

described. As adults these animals were tested for the occurrence of ovulation and for the ability to show a progesterone-facilitated increase in sexual receptive behavior after estrogen priming. Electron microscope sections were taken from each animal 2 days after cutting the stria termin-alis. The sections were coded and the identity of the animals not revealed until all of the counts were completed. When decoded, the morphological data (Fig. 3.6) turned out to be an exact parallel of the functional observa-tions (13). Regardless of the genetic sex, there were high incidences of nonamygdaloid spine synapses in the strial part of the preoptic area in: 1) normal females, 2) females treated with androgen after the end of the critical period (on day 16) and 3) males castrated within 12 hours of birth. All of these three groups show a cyclic pattern of gonadotrophin release in the presence of ovaries. They all show a progesterone-facilitated in-crease in sexual receptivity (14). The remaining three groups consisted of: 1) the normal males, 2) the females treated with androgen on the 4th day

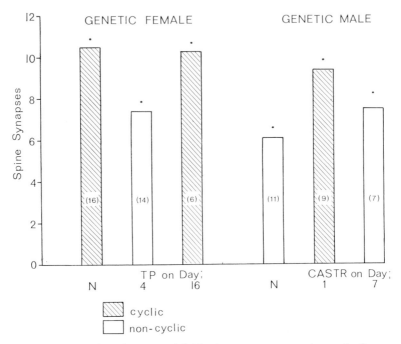

Fig. 3.6. The number of nonamygdaloid spine synapses per unit area in the preoptic area of the six groups of animals (see Fig. 3.5). The genetic females were either normal (N) or treated with testosterone propionate (TP) on either the 4th or the 16th day of life. Genetic males were either normal (N) or castrated (CASTR) on either the 1st or the 7th day of life. Numbers of animals in each group are shown in parentheses. Cross-hatching indicates groups of animals with a cyclic (female) pattern of gonadotrophin release as adults. Dots indicate one standard error of the mean (see note in legend to Fig. 3.4). A high incidence of nonamygdaloid spine synapses is associated with a cyclic adult pattern of gonadotrophin release, regardless of the genetic sex of the animal. Conversely, a low incidence is associated with a noncyclic release pattern, regardless of genetic sex.

of life and 3) the males castrated on the 7th day of life. These all had low incidences of spine synapses and did not show the gonadotrophin release patterns nor the receptivity characteristic of the first three groups.

Our results show that the neuropil of the strial part of the preoptic area is sexually dimorphic and suggest that it is concerned with sexually dimorphic functions such as the control of ovulation and mating behavior. This is supported by two independent lines of evidence. Firstly, the sexually dimorphic neuropil is located specifically in that part of the brain which is essential for these functions. Secondly, the sexually dimorphic neuropil undergoes neonatal differentiation under the influence of androgen in exactly the same way as the sexually dimorphic functions.

REFERENCES

1. SHAKESPEARE, W: The Merchant of Venice, Act III, Scene 2, 1596.
2. EVERETT, JW: Neuroendocrine aspects of mammalian reproduction. Ann Rev Physiol 31: 383, 1969.
3. HALASZ, B: The endocrine effects of isolation of the hypothalamus from the rest of the brain, in Frontiers in Neuroendocrinology, edited by Ganong, WF, Martini, L. New York, Oxford University Press, 1969, p. 307.
4. HILLARP, NA: Studies on the localization of hypothalamic centres controlling the gonadotrophic functions of the hypophysis. Acta Endocrinol 2: 11, 1949.
5. LISK, RD: Sexual behavior: hormonal control, in Neuroendocrinology, Vol. 2, edited by Martini, L, Ganong, WF. New York, Academic Press, 1967, p. 197.
6. KLING, A: Effects of amygdalectomy on social-affective behaviour in nonhuman primates, in The Neurobiology of the Amygdala, edited by Eleftheriou, BE. New York, Plenum Press, 1972, p. 511.
7. VELASCO, ME, TALEISNIK, S: Release of gonadotropins induced by amygdaloid stimulation in the rat. Endocrinology 84: 132, 1969.
8. GORSKI, RA: Gonadal hormones and the perinatal development of neuroendocrine function, in Frontiers in Neuroendocrinology 1971, edited by Ganong, WF, Martini, L. New York, Oxford University Press, 1971, p. 237.
9. RAISMAN, G, FIELD, PM: Sexual dimorphism in the preoptic area of the rat. Science 173: 731, 1971.
10. BARRACLOUGH, CA, YRARRAZAVAL, S, HATTON, R: A possible hypothalamic site of action of progesterone in the facilitation of ovulation in the rat. Endocrinology 75: 838, 1964.
11. BROWN-GRANT, K, RAISMAN, G: Reproductive functions in the rat following selective destruction of afferent fibres to the hypothalamus from the limbic system. Brain Res 46: 23, 1972.
12. HARRIS, GW: Sex hormones, brain development and brain function. Endocrinology 75: 627, 1964.
13. RAISMAN, G, FIELD, PM: Sexual dimorphism in the neuropil of the preoptic area of the rat and its dependence on neonatal androgen. Brain Res 54: 1, 1973.
14. BROWN-GRANT, K: Recent studies on the sexual differentiation of the brain, in Proceedings of the Sir Joseph Barcroft Centennial Symposium on Foetal and Neonatal Physiology, edited by Comline, RS, Dawes, GS, Nathanielsz, PW, Cross, KW. London, Cambridge University, 1972, p. 527.

DISCUSSION

DR. DOMINICK PURPURA (Bronx, New York): I would like to congratulate Dr. Raisman on what is certainly the first paper of its kind in the world literature concerning the question of differences between fine structure in relation to sex and the plasticity that develops presumably in these early stages. There are cycles in the historical development of ideas. Thirty-five years ago, the brain was considered capable of being modified by various perturbations of the intrinsic and extrinsic milieu. After Sperry's work came a period of extreme specificity, where we still are, although there is recent evidence of dopaminergic and catecholaminergic systems that have a great deal of plasticity.

Dr. Raisman shows the possibility of reorganization of neuropil during the first few days. Speaking now as a physiologist, if I may switch hats from anatomy to physiology, I'll say that it is very difficult for me to attribute functional significance to a change in the distribution of synapses from spine to shaft. I presume they may be excitatory, although they might be inhibitory. Nobody can really know without impaling such cells in order to study them in the rat or another animal. It is very difficult, with small neurons of this kind, to comprehend the significance unless Dr. Raisman can tell us something about total numbers of synapses. This may be impossible because they would have to be estimated in serial sections for the numbers to mean anything. But without some idea of the numbers and some knowledge of what each element is really doing, I cannot evaluate the effect of doubling or halving the number of spine synapses. Until there are such data, I will not get too involved with questions of nonspecificity and specificity.

DR. GEOFFREY RAISMAN (Oxford, England): I have no evidence, and I know of none, on the possible physiological significance of these different types of synapses in this particular area. Conceivably, one could argue that one type was excitatory. What evidence there is on spine synapses suggests that in most areas where they have been observed, they are an excitatory mechanism.

For the synapses on dendritic shafts, I think we must be completely open as to what they may be. It is possible that the shift in synaptic distribution represents some kind of shift between excitation and inhibition. I think the difference between the male and the female, insofar as we can see it, is a quantitative one. This is not something absolutely present in one and absent in the other. As for gonadotrophin release, the difference between the two sexes is rather curious in that, whereas both have gonadotrophin control mechanisms, only the female shows the explosive burst of activity which occurs in the preoptic area and is associated with ovulation. The female seems to have some kind of trigger which tips it over into this self-regenerating nervous activity. I have no more than the morphological data. But if one tried to think how it could possibly have a meaning, one would say that perhaps the female's preoptic area is endowed with a rather more potent excitatory mechanism that somehow manages, during this critical period in its cycle, to result in this burst of activity.

The second point which I also cannot answer concerns the total number of synapses. I can only say that the cross-sectional area within which we count is located at a fixed anteroposterior level, and that we can estimate the total number of synapses at that level. However, since we cannot and have not worked from front to back to determine the exact extent of this tissue, at best we can give the total numbers only at a particular level in the brain.

DR. DONALD REIS (New York, New York): Strumwasser, in studying the cyclical activity of neurons in Aplysia, has found in the invertebrate, cells that fire with a rhythmicity during a 24-hour cycle. These cells can be removed from the animal, kept in culture and will still show cycling behavior. In his model, which holds up at least on the basis of a simulated cell, one of the most important variables is cell surface which somehow controls the ion fluxes and then somehow is involved in a self-regenerating cycle, allowing rhythmic discharge. So perhaps one of the functions of the difference you find in spine and shaft is merely related to the cell surface itself which may ultimately have some relationship to rhythmic release of gonadotrophin.

DR. RAISMAN: Yes, I agree.

DR. SEYMOUR S. KETY (Boston, Massachusetts): Dr. Raisman's beautiful demonstration of the differences in synapses correlated with cycling brings the time much closer when we can begin to ask appropriate questions regarding the relationship between the injection or the availability of a chemical substance, testosterone, and the differentiation of sexual or cyclic behavior. Now, at least, we have one way station, the preoptic area and the morphological changes which he has seen there. Does this information furnish clues as to the possible mechanism by which testosterone may be affecting these synapses? Do we know enough about the ability of testosterone to induce particular enzymes to affect certain types of receptor formation? In general, what clues are sufficiently heuristic to prompt a focusing of attention upon that particular area from the biochemical point of view?

DR. RAISMAN: There are some highly suggestive anatomical features which I did not mention, partly because we do not know whether or not they are dimorphic in the sexes. I am speaking of the dendrites in this region which are a very peculiar varicose kind and which grow out at right angles to the fibers of the stria terminalis. There is a very marked rectilinear latticework reminiscent, for instance, of the lattice formed by parallel fibers in Purkinje cell dendrites in cerebellum. This may suggest that in some way the dendrites are growing out under the influence of, or are modulated by the incoming axons.

Also of interest in the biochemistry of this region is the presence of a very specific ascending norepinephrine-containing fiber pathway, which comes up through the region of the medial forebrain bundle and meets the stria terminalis. Its principal meeting place is in the bed nucleus of the stria terminalis, not in our region.

The bed nucleus of the stria terminalis is separated from our region by a small and rather characteristic group of cells which have not been described before and which we called the round nucleus. I do not know what it does, but I know what it does not do. It doesn't have a norepinephrine projection because the norepinephrine fibers circumvent this and run very specifically into our region. This appears to mean that the stria terminalis fibers, wherever they go, seem to meet an upcoming contingent of norepinephrine fibers, and one of the places they do this specifically is in our area. All I can say about them is that this could give us some clues as to where to proceed next.

DR. MAURICE RAPPOPORT (Chicago, Illinois): Are there morphological changes in adult peripheral tissues as well as in neonatal rats?

DR. RAISMAN: Of course, if the male is castrated, it has no testes as an adult, and phallic development is impaired. As for the female, if the androgen is given postnatally on day 4, there are, as far as we can see, well developed female external genitalia. If the androgen is given prenatally, however, there are somatic changes toward masculinization.

Chapter 4

THE HYPOTHALAMIC "SAVAGE" SYNDROME[1]

MURRAY GLUSMAN

Experimental studies of aggressive behavior in laboratory animals fall into two broad categories: 1) in which the organism is intact, and aggression is produced by some environmental modification or stimulus, and 2) in which the organism itself, especially its central nervous system, is modified, and aggressive behavior is produced by a stimulus consisting of some alteration of either the external or internal environment.

Investigators concerned with the laboratory analysis of aggressive and emotional behavior have developed a variety of techniques for eliciting aggression in laboratory animals.

Shock-induced Aggression

Pain is an extremely effective stimulus for eliciting aggression. Thus, O'Kelly and Steckle in 1939 (1) made the interesting observation that foot shock delivered to paired rats elicited fighting. Since then, shock-induced aggression has been studied intensively, and found to be a highly reliable and useful procedure for eliciting aggression in many species: mice (2), rats (3, 4), hamsters (3), squirrel monkeys (5) and cats (6).

Other types of painful stimuli are also effective in eliciting aggression, *e.g.*, heat, pinching the tail, vigorous tactile stimulation or subjecting one animal to the attack of another (3).

Isolation-induced Aggression

Based on observations in mice by Allee (7, 8), Scott (9) and others (10–12), isolation-induced aggression has been developed into a useful experimental technique for studying aggressive behavior. Yen and co-workers (13), Valzelli (14, 15) and others have made extensive use of isolation-induced aggression in mice to study the effects of pharmacological agents on aggressive behavior.

Extinction-induced Aggression

The behavioral technique of extinction-induced aggression provides still another means of eliciting aggression in laboratory animals. This

[1] This work was supported by National Institutes of Health Grant MY-3660 and National Institute of Mental Health Grant MH-10315.

phenomenon, which calls to mind the frustration-aggression hypothesis of Dollard and his associates (16), was described by Azrin and his co-workers (17, 18), who found that pigeons conditioned to peck a response key for food reinforcement attacked a nearby pigeon and even a stuffed model of a pigeon during periods of extinction. Thompson and Bloom (19) reported similar findings in rats, Hutchinson and his associates (20) observed it in monkeys and Kelly and Hake (21) described extinction-induced increases in an aggressive response in human subjects. Flory (22) noted in pigeons that even the transition from a fixed-ratio schedule of reward from 25 to 100 consistently produced attacks on nearby stuffed pigeons.

Shock-induced aggression, isolation-induced aggression and extinction-induced aggression are very valuable tools for the study of aggression because they are simple, applicable to small laboratory animals, such as mice and rats, and very reliable. Shock-induced aggression and isolation-induced aggression are particularly convenient procedures for pharmacologists concerned with studying the effects of drugs on aggressive behavior, or with screening large numbers of psychopharmacological compounds for therapeutic activity. They are also excellent procedures for neurochemists interested in the relationship between brain chemistry and aggressive behavior, because elaborate preparations are not necessary, and with a comparatively small expenditure of time and effort large numbers of animals may be prepared for study.

Because extinction-induced aggression is studied most effectively in the operant conditioning laboratory, it requires the investment of a considerable amount of time, effort and equipment in each experimental animal; hence the number of animals a given investigator can conveniently study is limited. Nevertheless, operant techniques are very well suited for the fine grained experimental analysis of many aspects of behavior, and the application of operant procedures to the study of aggressive behavior via a phenomenon such as extinction-induced aggression will undoubtedly be very productive.

The procedures discussed above have all been developed comparatively recently and all have an important advantage in that the behavior displayed by the subjects is behavior carried out by intact, conscious and unrestrained animals. The behavior is produced as a result of manipulating the organism's external milieu, or environment, not its internal milieu, e.g., brain or central nervous system (CNS). Counterbalancing the advantages of studying "natural" displays of aggressive behavior in intact animals are the limitations automatically imposed on the information that can be gained concerning the relationship of the body to aggressive behavior—in short, the physiological, biochemical and neurobiological aspects of aggression.

But aggressive behavior, like all other behavior, is totally dependent on the functioning of the central nervous system. It is there that one must look for the mechanisms that make aggressive behavior possible, integrate its patterns, determine its development, regulate its onset and termination, modulate its intensity, modify its thresholds and relate it to sensory input, sex hormones, brain chemistry and a host of other factors. Clarifying these phenomena requires investigation of the neuroanatomical, neurophysiological and neurochemical aspects of aggressive behavior. Unfortunately, investigations of this nature, by and large, cannot be carried out without physical intervention into the CNS, whether on a gross surgical level with ablations and electrolytic lesions, or on a less damaging level with the insertion of cannulas (for introducing chemicals directly into the brain or for perfusion studies), or the insertion of stimulating electrodes, or macro- or microrecording electrodes.

NEURAL BASIS OF AGGRESSIVE BEHAVIOR

Determining the neural basis of aggressive behavior is a complex task which has challenged investigators since 1892 when Goltz reported his now classic observations on chronic decorticate dogs (23). Goltz decorticated three dogs, managing to keep them alive for prolonged periods—1 for 51 days, 1 for 92 days and 1 for more than 18 months; he noted that the decorticate dog shows signs of rage, such as barking, growling and biting, in response to innocuous or trivial stimuli. Confirmation of these findings came some years later, when Dusser de Barenne (24) observed similar behavior in two chronic decorticate cats; and shortly thereafter, Rothmann (25) replicated Goltz's findings in a chronic decorticate dog. Some phenomena associated with rage had been observed by Woodworth and Sherrington (26) in decerebrate cats. These responses, called "pseudoaffective reflexes," were elicited only by strong afferent nerve stimulation, and observed against a background of decerebrate rigidity. They seemed to be short lived fragments of emotional behavior occurring singly or in small combinations, but never as a complete pattern of response.

In the 1920's Cannon (27), who was much interested in the physiological responses associated with emotional excitement, sought a way of consistently producing a full-blown picture of great emotional excitement in the laboratory animal. Aware of the intense behavior of Goltz's decorticate preparation, and the weak "pseudoaffective" responses of Sherrington's decerebrate animals, Cannon and Britton (28) reasoned that emotional responses were related to the thalamus and held in check by the inhibitory forces of the forebrain. Hence, "removal of the cortex in an acute experiment might, therefore, permit the activity of these lower centers to appear, and to prevail over the rigidity which usually masks them when the midbrain is transected. Typical and stereotyped behavior should then occur, such as may be natural in attack or defense (p. 285)." They proceeded to remove the cortex in cats, separating it from the thalamus by means of a stylet inserted through the orbit; and they succeeded in obtaining an acute preparation that manifested episodically, intense displays of great emotional excitement involving biting, clawing and struggling for which they coined the term "sham rage" (p. 287).

Phillip Bard in 1928 (29) demonstrated that the posterior hypothalamus was of the utmost importance in the integration of aggressive behavior. Carrying out a series of systematic ablations in cats, he was able to elicit Cannon's "rage" responses until the ablations passed behind the posterior hypothalamus. Caudal to the hypothalamus, decerebrate rigidity was produced, but with the posterior hypothalamus intact he obtained "sham rage." Still more precise localization was provided by Wheatley (30), who demonstrated that discrete lesions of the hypothalamus involving the ventromedial nucleus bilaterally made the animals permanently "savage."

Complementing the ablation studies was the work of Ranson and his group (31–33), Hess and his associates (34–38) and Masserman (39, 40), who demonstrated that rage reactions could be produced by electrically stimulating points in the hypothalamus.

The Bard and Mountcastle Hypothesis

In 1948, at a meeting of this Association on the frontal lobes, Bard and Mountcastle (41), on the basis of a series of systematic cortical ablations in cats, proposed a comprehensive formulation concerning the genesis of "sham rage." They postulated that inhibitory influences from various portions of the brain—the transitional cortex of the midline, the neocortex and the amygdala—funneled through the amygdala to the region of the ventromedial nuclei of the hypothalamus (HVM) to exert a suppressing action on brain stem mechanisms concerned in the expression of anger. Neocortical influences were considered important for the accuracy and timing of the "rage" behavior, and they suggested that the neocortex also exerts facilitating influences which do not pass through the amygdaloid "funnel." The important suppressor role assigned to HVM at the end of the "inhibitory funnel" was based on Wheatley's demonstration, mentioned above, that bilateral localized destruction of HVM in the cat results in the development of permanent "savage" behavior.

The Bard and Mountcastle hypothesis is important because it proposes a comprehensive formulation of the relationship of the brain to aggressive behavior. Despite its considerable interest, however, it is based on an inadequate theoretical foundation; consequently, as will be noted below, it fails to explain some critical findings.

In essence, the Bard and Mountcastle hypothesis interprets the development of "rage" or placidity following a given lesion in terms of the net effect of the lesion on a balance of inhibitory and excitatory controlling influences operating in the CNS hierarchy. Implicit in the hypothesis are the assumptions that the function of a given region is antithetically related to the effects observed when the region is destroyed, and that the occurrence of exaggerated activity after a lesion is an indication of release of lower centers from tonic restraining influences normally exercised either by the region destroyed or by related higher centers.

The Bard and Mountcastle hypothesis is based on Jackson's (42) classical but oversimplified approach to the analysis of CNS function, which treats a lesion in an idealized fashion, purely as a means of interfering with inhibitory control, excitatory influences or both; it does not take cognizance of the fact that a lesion not only frees a lower center of higher control, it drastically alters the physical and chemical environment of adjacent and inter-related neural regions. And it is entirely possible that under some circumstances, or perhaps in some locations, the environmental alterations themselves may create distortions of activity which become the most prominent effects of the lesion; in which case, they are apt to be attributed erroneously to functional deficits created by the lesion or to "release" effects of the lesion.

Paradoxically Similar Effects from Stimulating or Destroying HVM

Our concern with the shortcomings of the idealized analysis presented by the Bard and Mountcastle hypothesis, and our interest in the effects of lesions other than those attributable to interference with facilitating or inhibiting pathways, stems from the necessity to explain certain phenomena manifested by "rage" preparations. For example, we have observed that paradoxically similar behavioral effects may be produced either by stimulating or destroying the ventromedial nuclei of the hypothalamus in the cat (43, 44). Evidence was obtained as follows.

1. Aggressive Response Elicited by Stimulation of HVM

Agonistic responses (fight and flight reactions) elicited by hypothalamic stimulation were studied in 23 conscious, unrestrained cats with electrodes permanently implanted in the hypothalamus (43). The electrodes were stainless steel wires, 0.25 mm. in diameter, insulated with Formvar, except for 1 mm. left bare at the tips, and implanted in pairs with the tips staggered and 1.5 mm. apart. Responses were elicited by electrical stimulation with biphasic square wave pulses at a frequency of 100 Hz. and with a pulse duration of 2.5 milliseconds. To identify electrode sites the hypothalamus was cut in serial coronal sections; every 10th section was stained for cells, and every 11th for myelin sheaths.

Electrical stimulation via the implanted electrodes in these animals elicited dramatic patterns of flight or attack (fight). The flight responses often included well directed efforts to escape; thus some animals rapidly searched every corner of the observation cage for an exit, and when an opening was presented, by leaving the cage door slightly ajar, they promptly squeezed through, leaping rapidly from the cage. Some showed rapid flight but without directed search. In still others flight was preceded by a most dramatic posture—with back arched, ears flattened, hair on end, pupils widely dilated and the entire body cringing backward—as is sometimes seen when a cat is cornered and menaced by a large dog (Fig. 4.1).

Several types of attack responses may be elicited from the hypothalamus: directed attack with extensive autonomic reactions, undirected at-

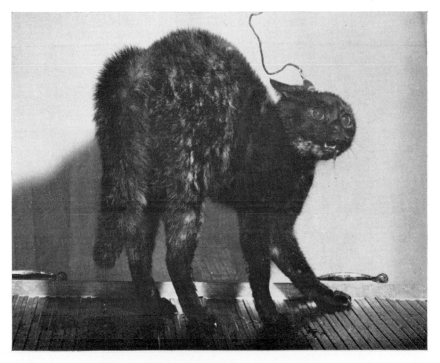

Fig. 4.1. Stimulation of hypothalamic flight point. Occasional attitude preceding flight. Posture resembles cat cornered by menacing dog.

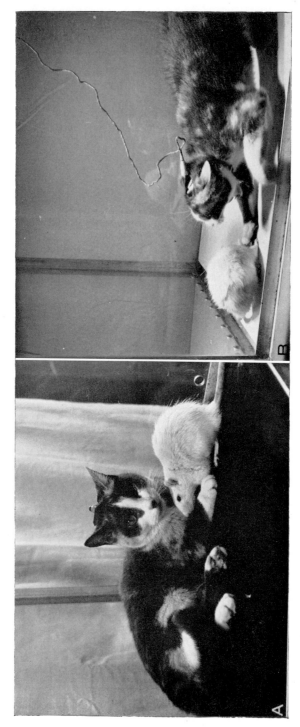

Fig. 4.2. Directed attack elicited by hypothalamic stimulation. A, cat with rat, at rest prior to stimulation. B, directed attack during hypothalamic stimulation.

tack with autonomic display and a form of stalking attack elicited by Wasman and Flynn (45) from the lateral hypothalamus, and resembling feline predatory behavior. We concerned ourselves only with directed attack because our interest was in the neural basis of aggressive behavior. Undirected attack is often confused with flight, and stalking attack is perhaps more closely related to feline hunting and feeding behavior than it is to the agonistic behavior of fight or flight or aggression and defense.

The directed attack responses were quite characteristic; they began with baring of the teeth, snarling, unsheathing of the claws and flattening of the ears, and culminated in an exquisitely directed attack at the observer. A laboratory rat sharing the cage with the cat was generally not molested (Fig. 4.2A) until an attack response was elicited by the electrical stimulus, and then the response included extremely rapid and skillful pursuit of the rat about the cage, terminating in a savage, lethal, clawing and biting attack on the rat (Fig. 4.2B).

Pupillary dilation, piloerection, salivation, accelerated respiration, urination and defecation accompanied both the flight and the attack responses but were generally more intense for the latter. Both attack and flight responses were closely bound to the stimulus, beginning 1 or 2 seconds after its onset and subsiding rather abruptly upon termination of the stimulus. Sharp and consistent thresholds were readily demonstrable for the directed attack responses; in contrast, the flight responses were graded so that as the stimulus intensity was increased, flight simply became more active. With strong stimulation both the flight and the attack responses were converted into frenzied, panicky flight.

Analysis of the histological data from the 23 animals which were implanted indicated that directed attack responses were elicited from a relatively restricted hypothalamic region which included the ventromedial nucleus of the hypothalamus; flight was elicited from a larger diffuse surrounding region.

The data from this study are summarized in Figure 4.3A on diagrams from the stereotaxic atlas of Jasper and Ajmone-Marsan (46). Responses were elicited from 67 electrode placements.[2] Directed attack was obtained from 26 placements (solid circles), flight was elicted from 29 (hollow circles) and equivocal or inconsistent agonistic responses (half-filled circles) were obtained from 12 points. Of the 11 placements shown impinging upon or penetrating HVM, 9 consistently produced directed attack, 1 produced flight and 1 equivocal responses. Figure 4.3B, which shows an electrode track touching the dorsal border of HVM, illustrates one of the

---

[2] Actually, 68 placements are shown in Fig. 4.3A, but no responses were elicited from one of them (indicated by x inside a hollow circle, lateral to the fornix at Fr. 12.5). The electrode in this location was evidently defective.

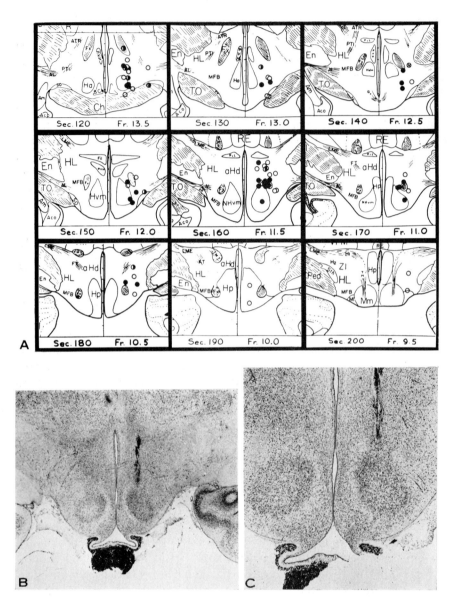

Fig. 4.3. A, electrode sites from which directed attack (solid circles) and flight (hollow circles) were elicited in 23 implanted cats. Half-filled circles indicate inconsistent or equivocal agonistic responses. Diagrams from Jasper and Ajmone-Marsan's stereotaxic atlas (1954). B, electrode track touching superior border of HVM; response elicited was directed attack. C, same as animal in B, enlarged adjacent section.

TABLE 4.1

Relationship of directed attack and flight placements to HVM and its immediate vicinity

Response Elicited	Electrode Site		Totals
	Within 0.5 mm. of HVM	Outside 0.5-mm. zone	
Directed attack.................	15	11	26
Flight.........................	1	28	29
Inconsistent....................	1	11	12
Total placements................	17	50	67

placements from which well directed aggressive behavior was elicited. Figure 4.3C is from the same animal as Figure 4.3B, but at somewhat greater magnification.

If as an arbitrary measure of proximity a 0.5-mm. zone surrounding the nucleus is considered the "vicinity" of HVM, virtually all the flight and equivocal or inconsistent response placements of Figure 4.3A (39 of 41) fall outside the 0.5-mm. zone, whereas most of the placements from which directed attack was obtained (15 of 26) fall inside the zone (Table 4.1).

Other investigators (47–49) have obtained similar results. The importance of the perifornical region in electrically elicited affective-defense responses was stressed by Hess (35), but the perifornical region may be regarded as including the ventromedial hypothalamus. Aggressive responses, elicited by electrical stimulation, are not limited to the ventromedial nuclei; they can be elicited from other regions of the brain, including the mesencephalic central gray (50, 51) and the amygdaloid nuclei. But what is important is the clear demonstration that stimulation of HVM elicits aggressive behavior, because destruction of this region does not produce a loss of aggressivity or placidity—it produces a paradoxically similar behavioral effect.

2. *"Savage" Behavior Produced by Destruction of HVM*

Wheatley (30) reported that destruction of the area of HVM resulted in "the development of a savage type of behavior (p. 313)." He investigated the behavioral effects of bilateral hypothalamic lesions in 42 cats and noted that 13 of his animals remained friendly, 8 became slightly irritable, 7 definitely "savage," 10 "very savage" and 4 were alternately friendly and aggressive. The animals with marked behavioral changes were those in which the lesions involved HVM. In fact, with one exception, (an animal in which HVM was completely destroyed on the right and only 60 percent on the left) the "savage" animals all showed complete destruction of HVM bilaterally.

In an investigation, described below, of the effects of midbrain lesions on "savage" behavior produced by hypothalamic lesions in the cat, we had ample opportunity to confirm Wheatley's original observation that bilateral destruction of HVM results in the development of permanent "savage" behavior.

3. Effects of Stimulating and Destroying HVM in the Same Animals

The findings discussed in sections 1 and 2 above leave open the possibility that the effects produced by stimulating the hypothalamus and those produced by the lesions were obtained from closely related but not necessarily identical hypothalamic sites. Remote though this possibility seemed, it nevertheless was considered worth examining; hence the following study was carried out (Glusman, previously unpublished data). In five animals electrodes were implanted bilaterally in the region of HVM. In three of these animals well directed aggressive behavior was elicited by stimulating either side of the hypothalamus. Lesions were then created at the tips of the stimulating electrodes on both sides of the brain, and the animals eventually became "savage." The electrodes in these preparations were cemented in place, hence the points stimulated and then destroyed were identical. Histological data verified the location of the electrodes in these three animals in the vicinity of HVM bilaterally. Figure 4.4 shows the location of the regions stimulated and then destroyed in one of the three. In the remaining two animals aggressive behavior was elicited from one side of the brain only and the lesions did not produce "savage" behavior. Our slides showed that the electrodes had been asymmetrically placed in these animals and HVM had not been implanted bilaterally.

4. Effects of Procaine Infiltration of HVM

Similar effects from stimulation or destruction of HVM could be readily explained if the electrical stimulus merely blocked the function of the nucleus and its environs temporarily. The "functional ablation" caused by the stimulus and the structural ablation of the lesion would then act in the same fashion and produce "rage" via "release" of brain stem mechanisms from HVM's suppressing role. If this explanation were valid, blocking HVM with procaine would produce effects identical to those obtained by electrical stimulation.

This possibility was tested (Glusman, previously unreported data) with animals in the stereotaxic apparatus under very light ether. Electrodes were lowered into the region of HVM bilaterally and stimulation of each

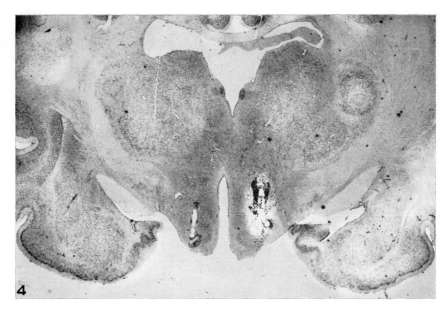

Fig. 4.4. Directed attack and "savage" behavior elicited from same hypothalamic sites. Lesions indicate locations of implanted electrodes. Stimulation of either site at first produced directed attack. Bilateral lesions via same electrodes produced "savage" syndrome.

side of the brain produced intense responses—maximal pupillary dilation, piloerection, unsheathing of the claws, flattening of the ears and rhythmic snarling. The electrodes were withdrawn and 3.0 μl. of 2 percent procaine were injected via a length of fine (27 gauge) hypodermic tubing into the points previously stimulated; none of the effects noted above were obtained. When the injection tubing was withdrawn, and the stimulating electrodes were returned to their original locations, it was found that the responses to electrical stimulation were effectively blocked for approximately 2½ hours, and as the effects of the procaine wore off, the responses returned gradually and almost to their initial intensity. Figure 4.5 shows the regions stimulated and then infiltrated with procaine in one of these experiments. The small dilations at the ventral extremities of the tracks made by the electrodes and injection tubing were caused by small electrolytic lesions made to locate the tips of the stimulating electrodes.

Clearly then the development of "savage" behavior after bilateral destruction of HVM is not a simple matter of "release," and it cannot automatically be assumed from the effects of the lesions that HVM normally exerts tonic restraining influences over brain stem mechanisms concerned with "rage."

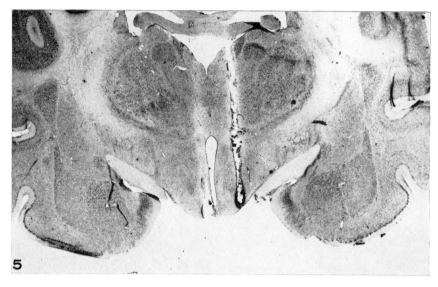

Fig. 4.5. Hypothalamic sites stimulated to produce affective responses and then injected with procaine to block responses. Dilations at ventral extremities of cannula and
electrode tracks were created by "marking" lesions to locate electrode tips.

5. Some General Observations concerning HVM "Savage" Cats

Our observations of animals with bilateral HVM lesions (44) may provide us with clues concerning the nature of the "savage" state and the
paradoxically similar behavioral effects of stimulating or destroying HVM.
First, it is probably more accurate to describe animals with bilateral HVM
lesions as displaying a unique state of hyperirritability, in which slight
stimulation elicits aggressive behavior, than it is to refer to them as "savage." These preparations never launch an unprovoked attack and they
never show spontaneous outbursts of aggressive behavior. Unless disturbed,
they are difficult to distinguish from normal resting cats, but they are
readily provoked by slight stimulation into highly aggressive reactions.
Second, this hyperirritable state does not appear immediately after destruction of the nuclei; it generally develops gradually, after a delay of 2 weeks
to 2 months, or even longer, after operation. Immediately after operation,
and for a variable period thereafter, aggressive behavior in response to
provocation is often reduced and elicited with difficulty; eventually, however, the hyperirritability gradually develops.

The prolonged delay in the development of the hyperirritability after
the lesions and the fact that the symptoms, once they develop, are in the
same direction or have the same sign as those produced by stimulation—

i.e., in both instances aggressivity is increased—are phenomena which are not explicable in terms of any hypothesis based on a simple net balance of excitatory and inhibitory influences. Clearly, other phenomena are involved and other explanations must be considered, as for example, denervation supersensitivity.

Denervation Supersensitivity as a Possible Explanation for the HVM Syndrome

Cannon and his co-workers (52, 53) formulated a postulate concerning the supersensitivity of denervated structures (53) which states: "When in a functional chain of neurons one of the elements is severed, the ensuing total or partial denervation of some of the subsequent elements in the chain causes a supersensitivity of all the distal elements, including those not denervated, and effectors if present, to the excitatory or inhibitory action of chemical agents and nerve impulses; the supersensitivity is greater for the links which immediately follow the cut neurons and decreases progressively for more distant elements (p. 186)." Cannon's observations dealt largely with experiments involving structures outside the central nervous system, *e.g.,* muscles, glands, blood vessels and sympathetic ganglia. However, Stavraky (54), Sharpless (55, 56) and others have reported evidence indicating that denervation supersensitivity could be demonstrated in the central nervous system. Since Hunsperger (50, 51) demonstrated the existence of a separate zone in the midbrain central gray from which "affective defense" reactions climaxed by directed attack could be elicited by electrical stimulation, we speculated that electrical stimulation of HVM excites or activates a chain of neurons involved in the mediation of aggressive behavior and that bilateral destruction of HVM, perhaps, leads to the development of a state of supersensitivity—reflected behaviorally as the "savage" state—in the remaining links which include the midbrain central gray. In line with this formulation we undertook an investigation of the effect of destroying the hypothetically supersensitive mesencephalic links on the "savage" behavior of the HVM preparation.

A necessary preliminary to this study was the task of devising some means of quantifying and recording "savage" behavior, hence a rating scale (Fig. 4.6) was developed for this purpose (57).

In utilizing the scale, observations were made in accordance with a fixed schedule which called first for the observer's rating of the animal from a distance (operant condition) and then for successive ratings under seven increasingly intense degrees of gross stimulation. The behavior of the cat under each of the eight stimulus conditions was recorded on the scale by noting the presence or absence of 16 types of activity arranged in

ANIMAL BEHAVIOR RATING SCALE FOR AGONISTIC BEHAVIOR*

Form A -- CATS

Score_____

SUBJECT_____

OBSERVER_____

OCCASION_____

DATE_____

	(6) Operant	(5) Approach	(4) Whis-tling	(3) Blowing	(3) Brushing Back	(3) Petting	(2) Brushing Belly	(1) Prod-ding
1. Alerted								
Watchful								
Restless								
Flinching								
Retreating								
Startled								
2. Horripilated								
Flattening of ears								
Twitching tail								
Fleeing								
3. Protesting								
Growling								
Snarling								
4. Feinting w. forepaw or clawing								
5. Feinting w. head or biting								
6. Springing								

* Instructions to observer: Enter 1 for occurrence of behavior, 0 for non-occurrence

Fig. 4.6. Facsimile of scale devised to rate agonistic behavior in cats.

order of increasing magnitude of agonistic response. Weights proportional to the intensity of the response and inversely proportional to the intensity of stimulation were assigned to each row and column, respectively. A score was computed for each animal, on each occasion of observation, by adding up all the significant responses, properly weighted, by rows and columns. The larger the total score, the greater the magnitude of agonistic behavior displayed.

A total of 15 laboratory cats was observed repeatedly at intervals of a few days, over the course of a 2-month observation period, by two observers who made independent records of their observations. Reliability was examined by a two-way analysis of variance applied to the 15 pairs of initial ratings. The results are shown in Table 4.2.

The difference between the two observers is insignificant. The intraclass correlation of 0.964 indicates that less than 4 percent of the variance of a score is attributable to residual error variance. In Figure 4.7, the scores reported represent the means for two observers. Figure 4.7 illustrates the

TABLE 4.2

Analysis of variance of scores on animal behavior rating scale

Source of Variation	Sum of Squares	df	Mean Squares
Animals........................	145466.87	14	10390.490
Observers......................	34.13	1	34.13 ($F = 0.181$)
Residual.......................	2632.87	14	188.062
Total.........................	148133.87	29	

$$R_{\text{intraclass}} = \frac{MS_{\text{an}} - MS_{\text{res}}}{MS_{\text{an}} + MS_{\text{res}}} = 0.964$$

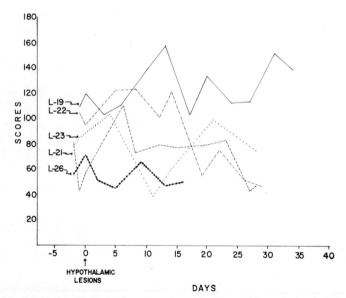

Fig. 4.7. Agonistic ratings in five controls with bilateral hypothalamic lesions. Animals did not become "savage."

scores for five control animals before and after the placement of hypothalamic lesions which did not destroy HVM bilaterally; these animals did
not become "savage" and the scores remained relatively low. The scores
for two experimental animals, L-20 and L-25, that did become "savage"
are shown in Figure 4.8A. The scores for L-25 climbed to approximately

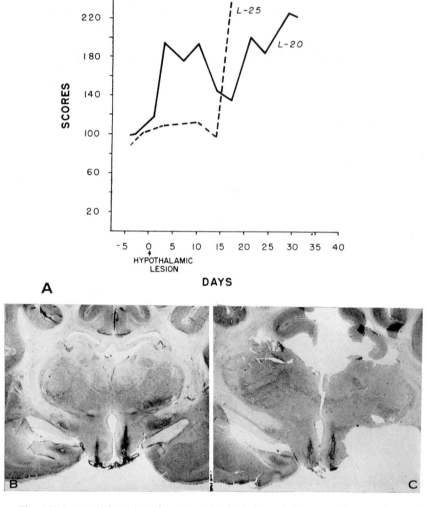

Fig. 4.8. A, agonistic ratings for two animals, L-20 and L-25, that became "savage"
following placement of lesions in HVM. B, hypothalamic lesions in L-20 involving HVM
bilaterally. C, Bilateral HVM lesions in L-25.

250 some 2 to 3 weeks postoperatively, whereas those for L-20 rose to 230 approximately 1 month after operation. The hypothalamic lesions in L-20 and L-25 are shown in Figure 4.8, B and C.

In general we found our rating scale to be a simple and useful means of quantifying agonistic behavior in the HVM preparations. The following study was then carried out.

Effect of Secondary Midbrain Lesions

A total of 12 HVM "savage" preparations was employed to study the effects of midbrain lesions on the HVM "savage" syndrome. In this investigation we were interested in observing not only the effects of secondary lesions in the mesencephalic central gray, for the reasons mentioned above, but the effects of lesions elsewhere in the midbrain (44).

In 10 "savage" preparations bilateral lesions were placed at a secondary operation in the rostral mesencephalon at the level of the superior colliculi; in one HVM "savage" animal the secondary lesions were placed in the gyrus suprasylvius medius and subjacent white matter; and in another, very large secondary lesions, described below, were placed in the rostral mesencephalon and caudal thalamus. The locations of the lesions and their effects were as follows.

Central Gray and Environs

Secondary lesions were placed bilaterally in the central gray and adjacent regions in three HVM "savage" animals. All three promptly became docile, but after 4 to 6 weeks the "savage" behavior gradually returned. The secondary lesions in two of these animals, L-2 and L-18, are shown in Figure 4.9, B and C; the primary hypothalamic lesions, which initially made these animals "savage," are not illustrated. The agonistic ratings for L-2 and L-18 (Fig. 4.9A) show the abrupt reduction in "savage" behavior in both animals immediately after the creation of the secondary lesions and then the increase in scores as the "savage" behavior returned 4 to 6 weeks later.

The central gray lesions in the third animal, L-24 (Fig. 4.10A), were very large, completely involving the central gray and a sizeable surrounding zone. Necrotic debris from the lesions occluded the aqueduct, resulting in the development of an obstructive hydrocephalus which accounts for the molding of the tectum in Figure 4.10C and the dilation of the 3rd ventricle with thinning of its walls (Fig. 4.10B). After the initial HVM lesions in this animal (Fig. 4.10B), the agonistic ratings (Fig. 4.10A) climbed to a very high level in 3 weeks and the animal became very "savage." The ratings dropped abruptly, immediately after the central gray lesion, and the animal became docile; but then the scores began to climb again and in 30

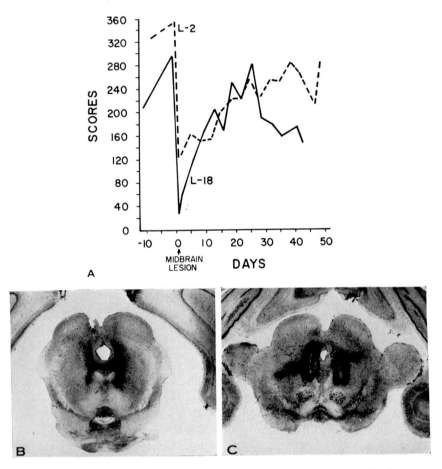

Fig. 4.9. A, agonistic ratings for two HVM "savage" animals, L-2 and L-18, that were subjected to secondary lesions of mesencephalic central gray and environs. B, location of the secondary lesions in L-2. C, Secondary mesencephalic lesions in L-18.

days the animal was again showing "savage" behavior, despite the development of the obstructive hydrocephalus which so impaired the health of the animal that it had to be sacrificed.

Lateral Tectum and Dorsal Tegmentum

In three animals secondary lesions, sparing the central gray, were placed in the lateral tectum and dorsal tegmentum. One of these animals (Fig. 4.11A, scores not illustrated), with lesions extending ventrally to the ventral plane of the iter, showed no taming. A second (Fig. 4.11B), with lesions extending slightly more ventrally to the level of the third nerve nucleus, became transiently docile for approximately 2 weeks. The third animal, with lesions somewhat more lateral than those in Figure 4.11, A and B, showed more prolonged docility; "savage" responses in this animal began to return after 6 weeks but were still attenuated at sacrifice almost 3 months postoperatively (not illustrated).

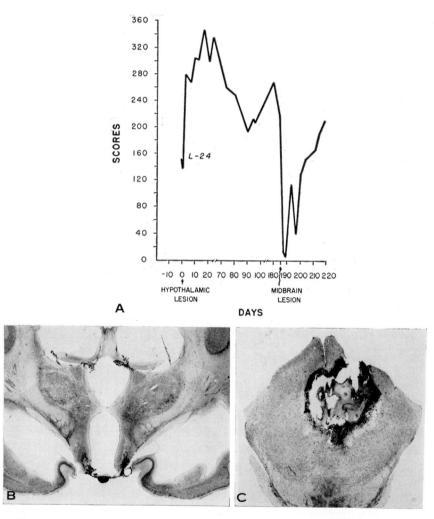

Fig. 4.10. A, agonistic ratings for L-24 prior to initial placement of HVM lesions, then as it became "savage;" transient taming after massive central gray lesion; and finally gradual increase in scores with return of "savage" behavior. B, bilateral HVM lesions in L-24. Dilation of ventricles attributable to obstructive hydrocephalus as a result of the secondary central gray lesions. C, Massive lesions destroying central gray in L-24.

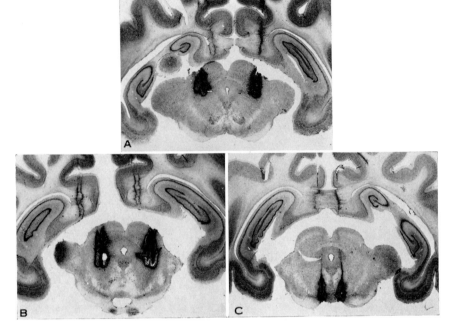

Fig. 4.11. A, secondary mesencephalic lesions of lateral tectum and dorsal tegmentum in L-33; produced no taming. B, secondary lesions in L-35 similar to those in A but extending more ventrally; produced transient docility for 2 weeks. C, secondary lesions of rubral region extending to base of mesencephalon bilaterally in L-27; no taming.

Rubral Region

The secondary lesions were placed bilaterally in the rubral region in one animal (Fig. 4.11C). No taming was observed.

Lemniscal Region

In three animals the secondary lesions were placed in the lemniscal region of the lateral tegmentum. The effects were quite striking. One of the animals showed prolonged docility followed by gradual return of the "savage" responses which, however, were still attenuated when the animal was sacrificed 11 weeks postoperatively. The remaining two animals showed an apparently permanent reduction or abolition of the "savage" state. The agonistic ratings and the location of the secondary lesions in one of these two animals, L-42, are shown in Figure 4.12, A and B. The lesions in L-42 involved the lemniscal region of the lateral tegmentum and were not very large (compared to the massive central gray lesions in Figure 4.10C which had only a temporary effect); nevertheless, the animal

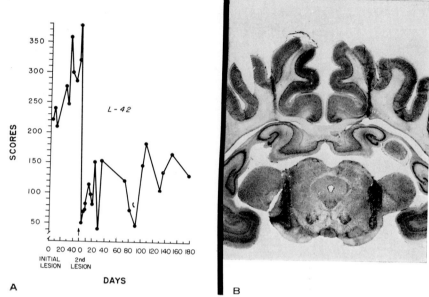

Fig. 4.12. A, agonistic ratings in L-42 during gradual development of "savage" behavior following the initial hypothalamic lesions. Abrupt drop in ratings occurred following placement of bilateral secondary lesions in lemniscal region of lateral tegmentum. Ratings show persistence of taming for 6 months until sacrifice. B, lateral tegmental lesions responsible for the taming in L-42.

became tame immediately after placement of the secondary lesions and remained docile for 6 months when it was eventually sacrificed.

Cerebral Cortex

In one "savage" animal control secondary lesions (not illustrated) were placed in the gyrus suprasylvius medius and subjacent white matter; there was no reduction in "savage" behavior.

Mesodiencephalic Junction

An unplanned but excellent control was provided by a "savage" animal in which massive bilateral lesions, intended elsewhere, were erroneously placed at the mesodiencephalic junction. The lesions extended from the rostral limits of the superior colliculi through the pretectal region and the nucleus of the posterior commissure into the caudal thalamus and center median nucleus. Medially, the lesion extended into the lateral margins of the central gray, and ventrally, at the rostral margins of the superior colliculi, to the level of the third nerve nuclei. Figure 4.13B shows a rostral section of the lesions, involving the center median nuclei, and Figure

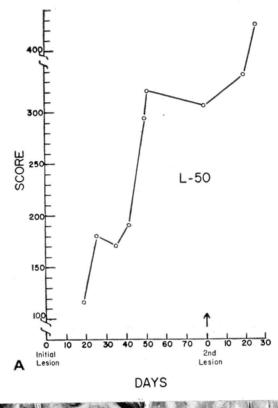

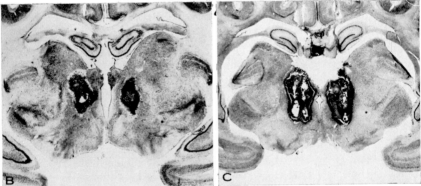

Fig. 4.13. A, agonistic ratings showing lack of taming by the secondary lesions in L-50. B, section through the rostral portions of the massive lesions at mesodiencephalic junction in L-50. Lesions involve center median nuclei. C, section through a more caudal portion of the same lesion showing massive destruction at the level of the pretectal region.

4.13C, a more caudal section, illustrating the massive destruction at the level of the pretectal region and the nucleus of the posterior commissure. The scores for this animal, L-50, are shown in Figure 4.13A. It may be noted that the full-blown "savage" state in this animal did not develop until approximately 2 months after the creation of the initial hypothalamic lesions. Even more striking, the secondary lesions, despite their massive size, had no effect on the "savage" behavior of this animal. There was severe visual impairment after the secondary lesions; the animal was virtually blind, but it remained "savage" nevertheless (Fig. 4.13A).

Thus, the secondary lesions modified the "savage" syndrome in 8 of the 12 animals. Taming effects were produced from two regions: the central gray and its environs, and the lemniscal region of the lateral tegmentum. The effects from the region of the central gray were temporary and followed by a more or less complete return of the "savage" syndrome. The most prolonged taming effects were produced by lesions of the lemniscal region of the lateral tegmentum. Permanent abolition of the "savage" syndrome seems probable by such lesions.

Two important findings emerged from this study. First, destruction of the region of the mesencephalic central gray—the zone from which Hunsperger (50, 51) elicited aggressive responses—produced only a temporary loss of aggressive behavior in the HVM preparations with eventual return of the "savage" syndrome in 4 to 6 weeks. This is consonant with the denervation supersensitivity hypothesis, discussed above, in which the midbrain central gray region is viewed as a link in a chain of neural structures which mediate aggressive behavior. Destruction of a link, e.g., HVM, denervates more distal elements in the chain which included the region of the mesencephalic central gray, resulting initially in a reduction of aggressive behavior. Then, as denervation supersensitivity develops in the remaining links of the chain, exaggerated aggressive behavior reappears. Destruction of the mesencephalic central gray zone after the destruction of HVM—as in the study above—repeats the process with the same result; there is an initial reduction of aggressive behavior followed by the delayed return of the "savage" syndrome as denervation supersensitivity develops in still more distal elements in the chain.

Although the results obtained in this study are explicable in terms of the denervation supersensitivity hypothesis, direct evidence that denervation supersensitivity does occur following HVM lesions or central gray lesions is still lacking.

The second finding was the somewhat unexpected and surprising observation that bilateral lesions in the lemniscal region of the rostral mesencephalon abolished the HVM "savage" syndrome, evidently permanently. Sprague and his co-workers (58) noted a profound impairment of affective behavior in cats among the consequences of massive lesions of the lateral mesencephalic tegmentum. By contrast, the lateral tegmental lesions in our animals were quite small (Fig. 4.12B); no grossly observable behavioral or neurological impairment was produced; nevertheless, the HVM "savage" syndrome was abolished.

Midbrain Lesions and Electrical Stimulation of Hypothalamus

The dramatic "taming" effect of lateral tegmental (LT) lesions on the "savage" behavior of animals with HVM lesions raised a question concerning the effect of LT lesions on agonistic responses produced not by destruction of HVM, but by electrical stimulation of the intact hypothalamus.

To answer this question the following procedure was carried out in 10 cats (Glusman, previously unpublished observations). With the animals in the stereotaxic apparatus under very light ether anesthesia, electrodes were lowered into the region of HVM, and upon stimulation the usual intense responses were elicited: mydriasis, piloerection, unsheathing of the claws, flattening of the ears, snarling and struggling. With the stimulating electrodes left in place, large lesions were placed, bilaterally, in the lemniscal region of the rostral midbrain in two animals. No effect was produced by the lesions either on the character of the responses elicited from the hypothalamus or on the thresholds for these responses. In two other animals lesions were placed bilaterally, first in the lemniscal region and then in the region of the central gray. The lemniscal lesions were again without effect, but the central gray lesions attenuated the hypothalamic responses; furthermore, it was noted that by enlarging these lesions to include the neighboring tegmentum, the hypothalamic responses could be blocked almost completely. Finally, in six animals, lesions were placed in the region of the central gray alone. Again it was found that when the central gray was destroyed the responses were attenuated, and when the lesions were progressively enlarged to include the neighboring tegmentum, the responses were almost completely blocked. Furthermore, it was observed that when the central gray and its environs were destroyed on the same side of the brain as the hypothalamic stimulus, the responses were attenuated to a much greater degree than when the lesions were created in the contralateral central gray region.

These observations, taken in conjunction with the findings of our study, described above, of the effect of midbrain lesions on the HVM "savage" syndrome, point to separate afferent and efferent arms in the brain stem pathways subserving agonistic behavior. Emotional behavior in the normal animal (58) and in the HVM "savage" preparation seems to depend to a considerable extent on afferent input via the long sensory pathways in the lemniscal region of the brain stem. The region of HVM and the zone of the mesencephalic central gray are part of the efferent limb of the pathways involved in agonistic behavior. From the experiments just described it would seem that the responses elicited by stimulating HVM and the descending, efferent limb of the circuit are not impaired by massive interference with the afferent limb of the circuit in the mesencephalon. Finally, the ability to block the responses elicited from the hypothalamus by destroying the region of the central gray provided important confirmation for results reported by Hunsperger (50, 51).

Aversive Thresholds in the "Savage" Syndrome

In searching for an explanation for the "savage" syndrome, we considered the possibility that disordered pain thresholds bore an important, perhaps causal, relationship to the unusual behavior. It was pointed out at the outset of this paper that pain is one of the most effective and reliable stimuli for eliciting aggression, so effective that pain-induced or shock-induced aggression has become a standard tool for studying aggression in many laboratories. In our work with HVM preparations we observed that the animals are generally at peace and at rest, and often quite hypoactive, unless disturbed by some stimulus, in which case they reacted with hissing, clawing and biting attack. Of the various kinds of stimuli we employed in studying these animals, *e.g.*, light flash, auditory stimulation, approach, threat or tactile stimulation, we noted that tactile stimulation was one of the most provocative and reliable means of eliciting aggressive behavior in the HVM preparation. This led us to speculate that the hypothalamic lesions in some way distorted sensation so that a normally innocuous tactile stimulus was perceived as painful, much as an incautious bather, overexposed to the sun, perceives tactile stimulation as painful. In short, we wondered whether in some manner the central problem in the HVM preparation was not really an alteration in disposition which rendered the animal vicious or "savage" but an alteration in sensitivity to stimulation, so that ordinarily innocuous stimuli were perceived as painful. In other words, the question to be investigated was: Did the animals, as a result of the lesions, become hyperesthetic or hyperalgesic with the chief effect of the lesions being a reduction of pain thresholds?

There was some additional suggestive evidence in support of this possibility. In a study of the effect of brain stem lesions on pain thresholds in the cat we found that lesions in the lateral tegmentum of the midbrain greatly elevated aversive or pain thresholds (59). Since the lesions in Figure 4.14 which elevated pain thresholds were quite similar to those in Figure 4.12B which abolished the "savage" syndrome in the HVM preparations,

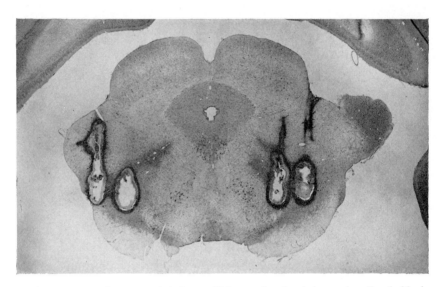

Fig. 4.14. Lateral tegmental lesions which greatly elevated aversive thresholds in study by Kelly and Glusman (see Reference 59.)

it seemed reasonable to speculate that the "taming" effect of the LT lesions was attributable to an elevation of pain thresholds or hypalgesia produced by such lesions. Thus, the LT "taming" lesions were perhaps doing nothing more than restoring to near normal levels pain thresholds which had in some manner been lowered by the HVM lesions.

To test the hypothesis that the development of aggressive behavior following HVM lesions was attributable to a reduction in thresholds for aversive stimulation, an investigation was carried out (Glusman and Fields, previously unpublished data) in which "savage" behavior and pain thresholds were concurrently measured in cats before the ventromedial nuclei were destroyed and for several months afterward as the "savage" syndrome developed.

"Savage" behavior was measured by means of our agonistic rating scale (Fig. 4.6). To determine pain thresholds, a discrete trial titration procedure was utilized (59, 60). Disc electrodes were strapped to the skin of the lower lateral abdominal regions and electrical stimulation was carried out with the aid of a constant current stimulator which delivered 10-millisecond biphasic pulses at 50 Hz. with intensities ranging from 0 to 3.8 ma. in 0.2-ma. steps (Fig. 4.15, A and B). Stimulation was programmed so that a shock of given intensity was presented for a period of 10 seconds or until the animal responded by pressing a lever. A shock-free interval lasting 20 seconds followed regardless of whether the shock had been terminated by

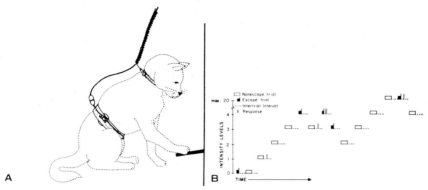

Fig. 4.15. A, diagrammatic representation of cat during behavioral titration to determine its aversive thresholds. Stimulating electrodes are strapped to the animal. Lever press controls intensity of stimulus. B, discrete trial titration; schematic sequence of events in the procedure employed to measure aversive thresholds in the animals pre- and postoperatively.

a response or the expiration of the 10-second shock period. If the animal failed to respond with a lever press, the next shock was increased by 0.2 ma.; if it terminated the shock by a response, the next shock was decreased by 0.2 ma. Each test session consisted of 100 shock presentations, with intensities starting at 0.0 ma. and ranging upward to limits established by the animal.

"Behavioral titration" may be viewed, psychophysically, as a method of limits procedure, hence the average shock level separating intensities which evoked responding from those that did not was taken as the aversive threshold. Thresholds were determined for at least 20 days before bilateral placement of lesions in HVM and then each weekday postoperatively.

Agonistic behavior was scored by means of our rating scale on at least three occasions preoperatively and then twice a week postoperatively.

The experimental group consisted of four cats that became "savage" after the hypothalamic lesions; several animals with hypothalamic lesions that did not produce savage behavior served as controls.

The data obtained in this study indicated that aversive thresholds were not reduced in the HVM syndrome; if anything, they were elevated.

Figure 4.16A presents the results obtained in one of the experimental animals, T-41. This animal became "savage" postoperatively, and its agonistic ratings rose from a fairly stable preoperative base line of approximately 50 to more than 200 some 50 days after placement of the lesions. Thereafter, the ratings dropped somewhat, but 3 months postoperatively they were still near 200. The aversive thresholds, measured

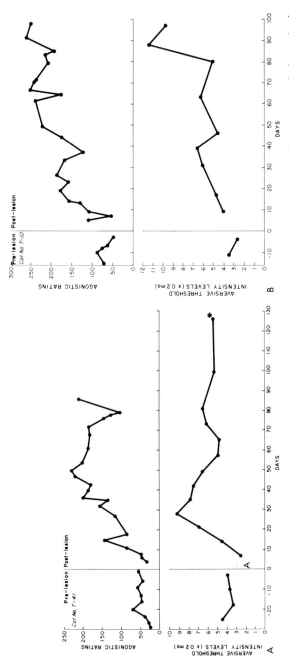

Fig. 4.16. A through D. Agonistic ratings (upper portion of each illustration) and aversive thresholds (lower portion) determined pre- and postoperatively in four HVM "savage" cats. Agonistic ratings in all four animals increase as syndrome develops. Aversive thresholds, measured concurrently, also show tendency to increase.

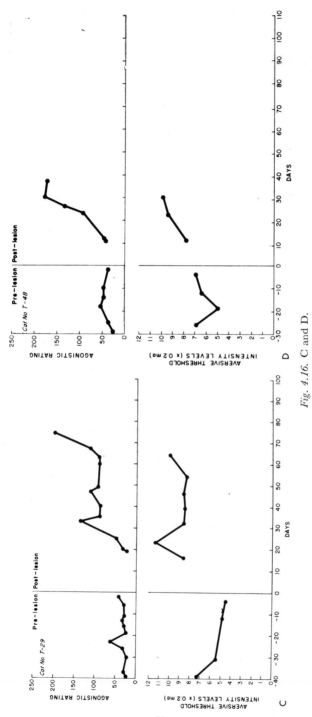

Fig. 4.16. C and D.

81

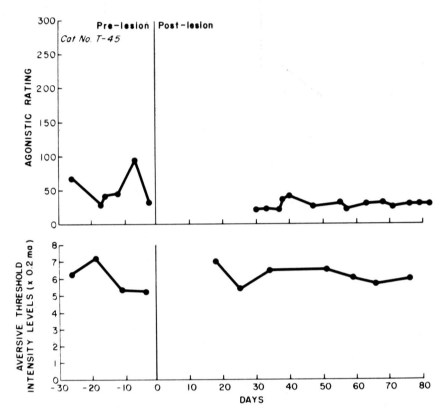

Fig. 4.17. Agonistic ratings and aversive thresholds in control animal, T-45, with hypothalamic lesions. Animal did not become "savage;" agonistic ratings and aversive thresholds remain at the same levels pre- and postoperatively.

concurrently with the agonistic ratings, showed a steady rise postoperatively from a rather stable preoperative base line to a maximum approximately 30 days postoperatively. Thereafter, they declined gradually to a new level, near, but still above, the preoperative base line.

The remaining three experimental animals, T-10 (Fig. 4.16B), T-29 (Fig. 4.16C) and T-48 (Fig. 4.16D), showed essentially similar results.

Data for one of the controls, T-45, are illustrated in Figure 4.17. This animal did not become "savage" postoperatively, and Figure 4.17 indicates that the agonistic ratings and aversive thresholds for this animal remained essentially the same postoperatively as they had been preoperatively.

This study, therefore, indicated that the "savage" syndrome could not be attributed to a simple reduction of pain thresholds, because, if anything, pain thresholds in the "savage" cats were increased. In mice and rats, however, Turner and his associates (61) found that shock thresholds for flinch and jump responses were reduced by bilateral, ventromedial hypothalamic lesions (produced with gold thioglucose in the mice, and electrolytically in the rats). Turner and his associates administered shock to the feet of their animals via an electrified metal grid and measured current intensities required to produce flinch responses or jerk, jump or vocalization. Inasmuch as the thresholds measured by this procedure involve not only sensory stimulation but also motor reflexes, *e.g.,* flinching, jerking and jumping, the possibility was not excluded that the lowered thresholds reflected hyperreflexia produced by the experimental interventions and not an actual reduction of pain thresholds. This difficulty was avoided in the behavioral titration procedure used in our study because threshold criteria were based not on simple withdrawal reflexes but on a complex, trained operant, the lever-press response, which is not easily affected by a factor such as hyperreflexia.

It is difficult to determine the significance of species differences in comparing data from our study in cats with that by Turner and his associates (61) in mice and rats, but clearly there are species differences. The mice and rats did not develop a syndrome comparable to the "savage" syndrome in the cat; Turner and his associates (61) noted instead: "The experimental groups, both mice and rats, emitted strong escape tendencies before the onset of shock and in response to shock. Repeated attempts were made to jump or climb out of the test apparatus (p. 242)." It is quite possible that the general state of excitability or jitteryness of the animals contributed to the reduced "flinch-jump" thresholds found in the study of Turner and his associates (61).

SPROUTING AS A POSSIBLE EXPLANATION FOR THE HVM SYNDROME

Still another phenomenon must be considered as a possible explanation for the paradoxically similar behavioral effects observed on stimulating or destroying HVM in the cat. Regenerative phenomena occur following the destruction of nervous tissue not only in the peripheral nervous system but in the central nervous system as well. Ramón y Cajal (62) described such phenomena in considerable detail, including the sprouting of new processes from the axons, dendrites and soma of central neurons in response to trauma and damage, and he reviewed a very extensive literature devoted to the topic in the early years of this century. But the early investigators concerned with the problem of CNS regeneration were hampered by a lack of appropriate histological staining techniques for demonstrating the fine processes and delicate terminals associated with sprouting and regeneration. With the development of improved histological techniques (62, 63), the utilization of electron microscopy (64–66) and the development of histofluorescence techniques for the visualization of catecholamine-containing fibers (67), it has become possible to study sprouting in the CNS and the morphological sequelas of CNS damage more readily. Thus, histological evidence was obtained by Liu and Chambers (68) that intraspinal sprouting occurs in the cat—with the formation of new collaterals and preterminals from the intraspinal processes of intact dorsal roots—in response to partial denervation of the spinal cord by section of a series of dorsal roots. McCouch and his co-workers (69) suggested that sprouting produces functional connections following spinal cord injury and that the excessive activity of such connections may be a cause of spasticity.

Sprouting has been described in various regions of the mammalian brain: the septal nuclei of the rat after partial denervation (66, 70), the optic tract projections in the brain stem of the rat after removal of occipital cortex (71) and the mesencephalon of the rat after electrolytic destruction of the substantia nigra and part of the ventromedial midbrain tegmentum (72). Furthermore, there is increasing evidence that sprouting after brain lesions may give rise to permanently functional connections (73). An important feature of the phenomena associated with sprouting is that they are delayed phenomena; it takes time for sprouts to develop. Thus, Katzman and his associates (72) found that sprouts developed 1 to 7 weeks after the mesencephalic lesions in their animals. It is conceivable, therefore, that the delayed development of the HVM syndrome may be attributable to the time required for the development of exaggerated activity associated with sprouting, and that sprouting may be the cause of the paradoxically similar effects obtained by stimulating or destroying HVM.

Difficulties in Interpreting the Effects of Lesions

This report has been concerned with some contributions from our laboratory to the study of neural mechanisms involved in aggressive behavior. Special attention was devoted to the apparent paradox that aggressive behavior in the cat can be produced either by stimulating or destroying HVM because it underscores the difficulty of trying to explain the effects of lesions solely in terms of some alteration in a regulatory balance of postulated excitatory and inhibitory forces exerted by higher neural centers on lower centers. The basic formulation from which such regulatory and "release" hypotheses derive was that proposed by Jackson (42) almost a century ago. Jackson viewed the central nervous system as a hierarchy of levels of organization with the highest and least organized levels controlling and regulating the lowest and most organized levels. Damage to the higher levels, he speculated, impaired control over some lower levels "releasing" them to act in an unopposed and unregulated fashion. Jackson's views influenced Cannon's notions on the genesis of "sham rage" in decorticate cats; they influenced Bard and Mountcastle, and they have had an enormous influence on thinking in modern clinical neurology.

Disturbance of the Chemical Milieu (Blood-brain Barrier, Neurotransmitters)

Clearly, we must take into consideration the fact that a brain lesion in an experimental animal is not merely a convenient means of manipulating an elaborate system of hierarchically ordered facilitation and inhibition. Obviously, a lesion creates a considerable amount of havoc in the nervous system, altering, as was mentioned earlier, the physical and chemical environment of the affected region and of interrelated neural regions as well. Thus, it is well known that many substances, such as electrolytes, colloids, various vital dyes and large, complex molecules, are unable to pass into the CNS from the blood stream because of the blood-brain barrier (74, 75). Even adrenaline is unable to cross the blood-brain barrier, except to a very minor degree in the hypothalamus, as Weil-Malherbe and his co-workers (76) demonstrated with ^{3}H-adrenaline. But injury to the brain, even a stab wound with a heated needle, breaks down the barrier for the injured area and a variably sized surrounding region, as Bakay (74) demonstrated in his studies with ^{32}P and earlier investigators found with vital dyes such as trypan blue. Impairment of the barrier is greatest for the first few hours after injury; and thereafter permeability gradually decreases, but a significant difference in permeability is still demonstrable 6 weeks after a stab wound with a hot needle (74). One would certainly expect that with a more massive brain injury such as that involved in producing a "sham rage" preparation by decortication, considerable damage is done to the blood-brain barrier. In view of the findings by Reis and his associates (77, 78) that noradrenaline-containing neurons are involved in the "sham rage" of acutely decerebrated cats (prepared by section above the colliculi, leaving the posterior hypothalamus intact) it is not unreasonable to consider the possibility that catecholamines and other constituents of the blood stream, provided with sudden access to the hypothalamus by the surgical trauma, may play a role in the genesis of "sham rage" reactions.

In this connection it is interesting to note in the study by Reis and his co-workers (77) that the adrenals of the animals manifesting "sham rage" were depleted of noradrenaline and adrenaline, probably as a result of release into the blood stream during increased sympathetic activity. Thus, via the adrenals, increased supplies of catecholamines may be made available to the brain stem, by way of the damaged blood-brain barrier, for a possible role in enhancing and sustaining the "sham rage" responses.

Brain Lesions and Dopamine

Still another phenomenon associated with acute lesions of the CNS should be mentioned. Andén and his co-workers (79) found in rats that hemisection of the forebrain through the caudal hypothalamus produced a rapid, selective increase in dopamine levels of the brain rostral to the lesion. The increase in dopamine became evident 15 minutes postoperatively and persisted for approximately 24 hours before dropping sharply to very low values at 7 days and disappearing as nerve degeneration occurred. Noradrenaline levels were not similarly affected.

These findings have been confirmed by other studies (80, 81). Cerebral hemisection involves axotomy of the ascending dopamine fibers which results in a markedly increased rate of tyrosine hydroxylation in the forebrain. Carlsson and his associates (80) have suggested that the interruption of nervous impulses in the dopamine fibers by axotomy leads to diminished release of dopamine into the synaptic cleft with depletion of dopamine at the receptor sites. Decreased receptor activation then, by some feedback regulatory system, causes an increased rate of tyrosine hydroxylation and an increase in dopamine.

Because of the recency of these findings, the functional significance of the changes in dopamine after axotomy is not clear. Dopamine, however, is an extremely important catecholamine with considerable behavioral significance and with a very important role in neurotransmission. The unexpected increase in dopamine and the increased rate of tyrosine hydroxylation provide a good example of the effect of a lesion in distorting the chemical environment of adjacent and related neural regions.

It seems evident, therefore, that damage to the CNS generates some phenomena which are of rapid onset and of limited duration (*e.g.,* alterations of the blood-brain barrier and disturbances in the concentration and metabolism of neurotransmitters) as well as some phenomena that have a delayed onset and are of prolonged duration (*e.g.,* denervation supersensitivity and sprouting). It is suggested that functional disturbances created by these phenomena may complicate and distort the effects of a lesion to such an extent that attempts to interpret the functional significance of the lesion within the restricted framework and limited options of Jacksonian theory will lead to erroneous or paradoxical results such as those described above in connection with the HVM syndrome.

ACKNOWLEDGMENTS

The author expresses his very deep appreciation to several associates who contributed most actively to various aspects of the work described above. Special thanks are due to Drs. Eugene Burdock, Lanny Fields, Dennis Kelly, Joseph Ransohoff, Leon Roizin and William Won.

REFERENCES

1. O'KELLY, LW, STECKLE, LC: A note on long enduring emotional responses in the rat. J Psychol 8: 125, 1939.
2. TEDESCHI, RE, TEDESCHI, DH, MUCHA, A, COOK, L, MATTIS, PA, FELLOWS, EJ: Effects of various centrally acting drugs on fighting behavior of mice. J Pharmacol Exp Therap 125: 28, 1959.
3. ULRICH, RE, AZRIN, NH: Reflexive fighting in response to aversive stimulation. J Exp Anal Behav 5: 511, 1962.
4. ULRICH, R, SYMANNEK, B: Pain as a stimulus for aggression, in Biology of Aggressive Behavior, edited by Garattini, S, Sigg, EB. New York, John Wiley & Sons, 1969.
5. AZRIN, NH, HUTCHISON, RR, HAKE, DF: Pain-induced fighting in the squirrel monkey. J Exp Anal Behav 6: 620, 1963.
6. ULRICH, RE, WOLFF, PC, AZRIN, NH: Shock as an elicitor of intra- and inter-species fighting behavior. Anim Behav 12: 14, 1964.
7. ALLEE, WC: Group organization among vertebrates. Sciences 95: 289, 1942.
8. ALLEE, WC: Social dominance and subordination among vertebrates. Biol Symposia 8: 139, 1942.
9. SCOTT, JP: Incomplete adjustment caused by frustration of untrained fighting mice. J Comp Psychol 39: 379, 1946.
10. GINSBURG, B, ALLEE, WC: Some effects of conditioning on social dominance and subordination in inbred strains of mice. Physiol Zool 15: 485, 1942.
11. SCOTT, JP, FREDERICKSON, E: The causes of fighting in mice and rats. Physiol Zool 24: 273, 1951.
12. SCOTT, JP, MARSTON, MV: Nonadaptive behavior resulting from a series of defeats in fighting mice. J Abnorm Soc Psychol 48: 417, 1953.
13. YEN, CY, STANGER, RL, MILLMAN, N: Ataractic suppression of isolation-induced aggressive behavior. Arch Int Pharmacodyn Ther 123: 179, 1959.
14. VALZELLI, L: Drugs and aggressiveness, in Advances in Pharmacology, edited by Garattini, S, Shore, PA. New York, Academic Press, 1967.
15. VALZELLI, L: Aggressive behavior induced by isolation, in Biology of Aggressive Behavior, edited by Garattini, S, Sigg, EB. New York, John Wiley & Sons, 1969.
16. DOLLARD, J, MILLER, NE, DOOB, LW, MOWRER, OH, SEARS, RR (eds): Frustration and Aggression. New Haven, Yale University Press, 1939.
17. AZRIN, NH, HUTCHINSON, RR: HAKE, DF: Extinction-induced aggression. Am Psychol 20: 583, 1965.
18. AZRIN, NH, HUTCHINSON, RR, HAKE, DF: Extinction-induced aggression. J Exp Anal Behav 9: 191, 1966.
19. THOMPSON, T, BLOOM, W.: Aggressive behavior and extinction-induced response-rate increase. Psychonom Sci 5: 335, 1966.
20. HUTCHINSON, RR, AZRIN, NH, HUNT, G: Attack produced by intermittent reinforcement of a concurrent operant response. J Exp Anal Behav 11: 489, 1968.

21. KELLY, JF, HAKE, DF: An extinction-induced increase in aggressive response with humans. J Exp Anal Behav 14: 153, 1970.

22. FLORY, RK: Attack behavior in a multiple fixed-ratio schedule of reinforcement. Psychonom Sci 16: 156, 1969.

23. GOLTZ, F: Der Hund ohne Grosshirn. Pflügers Arch Gesamte Physiol Menschen Tiere 51: 570, 1892.

24. DUSSER, DE BARENNE, JG: Recherches experimentales sur les fonctions du systeme nerveux central, faties en particulier sur deux chat dont le neopallidum avait ete enleve. Arch Neer Physiol 4: 31, 1920.

25. ROTHMANN, H: Zusammenfassender Bericht über den Rothmannschen grosshirnlosen Hund nach klinischer und anatomischer Untersuchung. Z Gesamte Neurol Psychiatr 87: 247, 1923.

26. WOODWORTH, RS, SHERRINGTON, CS: A pseudoaffective reflex and its spinal path. J Physiol 31: 234, 1904.

27. CANNON, WB: Bodily Changes in Pain, Fear, Hunger and Rage. (2nd ed). Boston, Charles T. Branford, 1953. (Originally published: New York, Appleton-Century-Crofts, 1929.)

28. CANNON, WB, BRITTON, SW: Studies on the conditions of activity in endocrine glands. XV. Pseudoaffective medulliadrenal secretion. Am J Physiol 72: 283, 1925.

29. BARD, P: A diencephalic mechanism for the expression of rage with special reference to the sympathetic nervous system. Am J Physiol 84: 490, 1928.

30. WHEATLEY, MD: The hypothalamus and affective behavior in cats: A study of the effects of experimental lesions, with anatomic correlations. Arch Neurol Psychiatr 52: 296, 1944.

31. RANSOM, SW: The hypothalamus: Its significance for visceral innervation and emotional expression. Trans Stud Coll Physicians Phila 2: 222, 1934.

32. RANSON, SW: Some functions of the hypothalamus. Harvey Lect 32: 92, 1937.

33. KABAT, H, ANSON, BJ, MAGOUN, HW, RANSON, SW: Stimulation of the hypothalamus with special reference to its effect on gastro-intestinal motility. Am J Physiol 112: 214, 1935.

34. HESS, WR: Das Zwischenhirn: Syndrome, Lokalisationen, Funktionen. Basel, Schwabe, 1949.

35. HESS, WR: Diencephalon: Autonomic and Extrapyramidal Functions. New York, Grune & Stratton, 1954.

36. HESS, WR: The Functional Organization of the Diencephalon. New York, Grune & Stratton, 1957.

37. HESS, WR, BRÜEGGER, M: Das subjortikale Zentrum der affekitiven Abwehrreaktion. Helv Physiol Pharmacol Acta 1: 33, 1943.

38. HESS, WR, AKERT, K: Experimental data on role of hypothalamus in mechanisms of emotional behavior. Am Med Assoc Arch Neurol Psychiatr 73: 127, 1955.

39. MASSERMAN, JH: Is the hyopthalamus a center of emotion? Psychosom Med 3: 3, 1941.

40. MASSERMAN, JH: Behavior and Neurosis: An Experimental Psychoanalytic Approach to Psychobiologic Principles. Chicago, University of Chicago Press, 1943.

41. BARD, P, MOUNTCASTLE, VB: Some forebrain mechanisms involved in expression of rage with special reference to suppression of angry behavior. Res Publ Assoc Nerv Ment Dis 27: 362, 1948.

42. JACKSON, JH: On some implications of dissolution of the nervous system, in Selected Writings of John Hughlings Jackson, edited by Taylor, J. New York, Basic Books, 1958. (Medical press and circular 2: 411, 1882.)

43. GLUSMAN, M, ROIZIN, L: Role of the hypothalamus in the organization of agonistic behavior in the cat. Trans Am Neurol Assoc 177, 1960.

44. Glusman, M, Won, W, Burdock, EI, Ransohoff, J: Effects of midbrain lesions on "savage" behavior induced by hypothalamic lesions in the cat. Trans Am Neurol Assoc 216, 1961.

45. Wasman, M, Flynn, JP: Directed attack elicited from hypothalamus. Arch Neurol 6: 220, 1962.

46. Jasper, HH, Ajmone-Marsan, C: A Stereotaxic Atlas of the Diencephalon of the Cat. Ottawa, National Research Council of Canada, 1954.

47. Nakao, H.: Emotional behavior produced by hypothalamic stimulation. Am J Physiol 194: 411, 1958.

48. Yasukochi, G.: Emotional responses elicited by electrical stimulation of the hypothalamus in cat. Folia Psychiatr Neurol Jap 14: 260, 1960.

49. Romaniuk, A: Representation of aggression and flight reactions in the hypothalamus of the cat. Acta Biol Exp 25: 177, 1965.

50. Hunsperger, RW: Role of substantia grisea centralis mesencephali in electrically-induced rage reactions, in Progress in Neurobiology, edited by Kappers, JA. Amsterdam, Elsevier Press, 1956.

51. Hunsperger, RW: Affektreaktionen auf elektrische Reizung im Hirnstamm der Katze. Helv Physiol Pharmacol Acta 14: 70, 1956.

52. Cannon, WB, Rosenblueth, A, Garciá Ramos, J: Sensibilizatión de las neuronas espinales por denervacion parcial. Arch Inst Cardiol Mex 15: 327, 1945.

53. Cannon, WB, Rosenblueth, A: The Supersensitivity of Denervated Structures. New York, Macmillan, 1949.

54. Stavraky, GW: Supersensitivity following Lesions of the Nervous System. Toronto, University of Toronto Press, 1961.

55. Sharpless, SK: Reorganization of function in the nervous system—use and disuse. Annu Rev Physiol 26: 357, 1964.

56. Sharpless, SK: Isolated and deafferented neurons: Disuse supersensitivity, in Basic Mechanisms of the Epilepsies, edited by Jasper, HH, Ward, AA, Jr, Pope, A. Boston, Little, Brown, 1969.

57. Burdock, EI, Glusman, M, Zener, J: An animal behavior rating scale for quantification of savage behavior in cats. Fed Proc 20: 327, 1961.

58. Sprague, JM, Chambers, WW, Stellar, E.: Attentive, affective and adaptive behavtion of savage behavior in cats. Fed Proc 20: suppl. 1, 327, 1961.

59. Kelly, DD, Glusman, M: Aversive thresholds following midbrain lesions. J Comp Physiol Psychol 66: 25, 1968.

60. Halpern, L, Alleva, F: Drug induced changes in thresholds for aversive stimulation in chronically implanted monkeys. Fed Proc 23: (Part 1), 284, 1964.

61. Turner, SG, Sechzer, JA, Liebelt, RA: Sensitivity to electric shock after ventromedial hypothalamic lesions. Exp Neurol 19: 236, 1967.

62. Ramon Y Cajal, S: Degeneration and Regeneration of the Nervous System, translated and edited by May, RM. New York, Hafner, 1959.

63. Nauta, WJH, Gygax, PA: Silver impregnation of degenerating axons in the central nervous system: A modified technique. Stain Technol 29: 91, 1954.

64. Lampert, P, Cressman, M.: Axonal regeneration in the dorsal columns of the spinal cord of adult rats. An electron microscopic study. Lab Invest 13: 825, 1964.

65. Bernstein, JJ, Bernstein, ME: Ultrastructure of normal regeneration and loss of regenerative capacity following teflon blockage in goldfish spinal cord. Exp Neurol 24: 538, 1969.

66. Raisman, G: Neuronal plasticity in the septal nuclei of the adult rat. Brain Res 14: 25, 1969.

67. Falck, B., Hillarp, NÅ, Thieme, G, Torp, A: Fluorescence of catecholamines and

related compounds condensed with formaldehyde. J Histochem Cytochem 10: 348, 1962.

68. LIU, CN, CHAMBERS, WW: Intraspinal sprouting of dorsal root axons. Development of new collaterals and preterminals following partial denervation of the spinal cord in the cat. Arch Neurol Psychiatr 79: 46, 1958.

69. MCCOUCH, GP, AUSTIN, GM, LIU, CN, LIU, CY: Sprouting as a cause of spasticity. J Neurophysiol 21: 205, 1958.

70. MOORE, BY, BJÖRKLUND, A, STENEVI, U: Plastic changes in the adrenergic innervation of the rat septal area in response to denervation. Brain Res 33: 13, 1971.

71. GOODMAN, DC, HOREL, JA: Sprouting of optic tract projections in the brain stem of the rat. J Comp Neurol 127: 71, 1966.

72. KATZMAN, R, BJÖRKLUND, A, OWMAN, CH, STENEVI, U, WEST, KA: Evidence for regenerative axon sprouting of central catecholamine neurons in the rat mesencephalon following electrolytic lesions. Brain Res 25: 579, 1971.

73. LYNCH, G, DEADWYLER, S, COTMAN, C: Postlesion axonal growth produces permanent functional connections. Science 180: 1364, 1973.

74. BAKAY, L: The Blood-brain Barrier. Springfield, Ill., Charles C Thomas, 1956.

75. DAVSON, H: The blood-brain barrier, in Advances in Experimental Medicine and Biology (Vol. 13), edited by Paoletti, R., Davison, AN. New York, Plenum Publishing Corp., 1971.

76. WEIL-MALHERBE, H, AXELROD, J, TOMCHICK, R: Blood-brain barrier for adrenaline. Science 129: 1226, 1959.

77. REIS, DJ, MIURA, M, WEINBREN, M, GUNNE, LM: Brain catecholamines: Relation to defense reaction evoked by acute brain stem transection in cat. Science 156: 1768, 1967.

78. GUNNE, LM: Brain catecholamines in the rage response evoked by intracerebral stimulation and ablation, in Biology of Aggressive Behavior, edited by Garattini, A, Sigg, EB. New York, John Wiley & Sons, 1969.

79. ANDÉN, NE, BÉDARD, P, FUXE, K, UNGERSTEDT, U: Early and selective increase in brain dopamine levels after axotomy. Experientia 28: 300, 1972.

80. CARLSSON, A, KEHR, W, LINDQVIST, M, MAGNUSSON, T, ATACK, CV: Regulation of monoamine metabolism in the central nervous system. Pharmacol Rev 24: 371, 1972.

81. STOCK, G, MAGNUSSON, T, ANDÉN, NE: Increase in brain dopamine after axotomy or treatment with gammahydroxybutyric acid due to elimination of the nerve impulse flow. Naunyn-Schmiedebergs Arch Pharmakol 278: 347, 1973.

DISCUSSION

DR. PAUL D. MACLEAN (Bethesda, Maryland): Dr. Glusman and his colleagues are certainly to be admired for their persistence in pursuing this important problem. It still remains a curious fact, however, that after all these years we do not really know the efferent pathways involved in the expression of angry behavior. We are all impressed when the cat or the monkey acts angry or fearful as soon as an electrode approaches the pallidohypothalamic pathway or the place where the pathway crosses the anterior hypothalamus. Hess was confused about which pathways might be involved. I would like to ask if your thinking has developed any further along these lines? The norepinephrine systems seem implicated in the expression of aggressive behavior. With histofluorescence work, one sees, in the anterior part of the hypothalamus, around the perifornical area, a bright fluorescence from the norepinephrine fibers. This, of course, would be the so-called intermediate zone of Hess.

DR. MURRY GLUSMAN (New York, New York): We do not have very detailed information on the efferent pathways involved in aggressive behavior. In a general way we know that the efferent pathways extend through and involve the mesencephalic central gray and the adjacent tegmentum because large lesions in this region block responses elicited by hypothalamic stimulation. As for the relationship of norepinephrine and the biogenic amines to aggressive behavior, I'm sure Don Reis's paper will cover what is known in this area.

DR. FRED PLUM (New York, New York): Some of the attack patterns are vividly apparent in human neuropathology. Two years ago, Reeves and I reported in the *Archives of Neurology* the case of a young woman with a ganglioglioma in the ventral medial hypothalamus which in its largest diameter was 8 mm. When she died of a pulmonary infarct, it was found that the total destruction was confined to the ventromedial nucleus. Meanwhile, for the last 6 months of her life, she showed the most extraordinary persistent hyperphagia and attack behavior whenever her continuous eating was interrupted. Any attempt to limit her caloric intake elicited bites, kicks and screams.

DR. PHILIP BARD (Baltimore, Maryland): While I could comment on many aspects of Dr. Glusman's very interesting paper, I would like to offer confirmation on the mesencephalic basis of aggressive behavior. In our studies of chronic decerebrate cats with a complete mesencephalic transection of the brain stem, with the hypothalamus and pituitary isolated in front of the transection in order to make long survival possible, some of the animals would regularly show aggressive or rage behavior on rather strong stimulation, not unlike Sherrington's early results. This shows that there is in the midbrain a mechanism capable of fashioning this type of behavior. A hypothalamic animal, however, with a much lower threshold, will show anger on rather slight stimulation. I think it is in line with Dr. Glusman's results that the mesencephalic creatures have the neural wherewithal to show this kind of behavior. Since a lesion in the hypothalamus and stimulation may do exactly the same thing, one may ask which is the worst procedure to use in studying this matter.

In my own experience, the most amazing thing I have seen was the state of placidity which Mountcastle and I obtained in cats from which only the neocortex was removed, with the midline cortex of the cingular gyrus and the amygdala and so forth left intact. Even with the most painful stimulus, those animals could not be made to show the slightest sign of anger, nor did they show any of the autonomic responses: no pupillary dilatation, no increase in cardiac rate, no increase in cardiac output, no sweating and not even a rise in blood sugar. These placid animals had all the hypothalamus and the whole limbic system intact, yet showed not the slightest reaction of aggression or rage. But removal of either the amygdala or the midline cortex which connects with the anterior thalamic nuclei immediately produced a very aggressive, nasty creature. As far as I know, this has never been explained. I think it has a bearing on Dr. Glusman's paper.

DR. E. A. WEINSTEIN (Bethesda, Maryland): What is the behavior of Wheatley cats when they are not savage?

DR. GLUSMAN: The animals we studied were really quite indistinguishable from normal animals unless they were stimulated in some way. A tactile stimuli, such as brushing or petting, seemed the most provocative. Otherwise they were, if anything, hypoactive and tended to become obese.

Chapter 5

ELECTROPHYSIOLOGICAL STUDIES IN AN ANIMAL MODEL OF AGGRESSIVE BEHAVIOR

**JEROME SUTIN, JAMES ROSE, LOCHE VAN ATTA
AND ROBERT THALMANN**

INTRODUCTION

Inasmuch as there are very few mammalian behaviors for which we have a reasonable understanding of the underlying neuronal mechanisms, it should come as no surprise that knowledge of neuronal activity related to aggressive behavior is in its early, descriptive phase. In order to study neural coding in a situation in which a sensory stimulus leads to agonistic behavior, we have chosen the unique behavior triggered by vaginal probing in the estrous cat. A large number of studies employing electrical stimulation and ablations have led neurobiologists interested in aggressive behavior to focus their attention upon the basal diencephalon and temporal lobes. This has prompted several laboratories to study input and output paths of the hypothalamus and the regions from which aggressive behavior can be elicited by electrical stimulation. Threat responses have been obtained from the amygdala (1–3) and stria terminalis (2, 4). Similar behavioral displays may also be obtained upon stimulation of the perifornical region of the hypothalamus (5). Magnus and Lammers (6) suggested that the threat behavior evoked by amygdaloid stimulation is attributable to the efferent projections of this structure upon the hypothalamus, particularly through the stria terminalis. Although such a role for the stria terminalis has some support in the experiments of de Molina and Hunsperger (7), Hilton and Zbrozyna (8) show that the ventral amygdalofugal path, and not the stria terminalis, is the more important link between the amygdala and hypothalamus as far as agonistic behavior is concerned. Although threat displays can be elicited from the amygdala, hypothalamus and midbrain central gray, stalking attack without a prior threat display is obtained primarily by stimulation of the lateral (9) or dorsomedial (10) hypothalamus and preoptic region. In addition, the latency of hypothalamically induced stalking attack can be modified by concomitant stimulation within the amygdala, thalamus or mesial cortex (11–13). A more extensive review of hypothalamic mechanisms in aggressive behavior is discussed by Glusman in Chapter 4.

When the distribution of stimulus sites in the hypothalamus that lead to attack behavior is compared with the extent of degeneration resulting from lesions involving the hypothalamic ventromedial nucleus (HVM) and surrounding tissue, or in regions which project to HVM, there is a striking correspondence. Roberts and Kiess (10) were able to elicit biting attack from a region immediately dorsal to HVM and extending superiorly toward the thalamus, which corresponds to a medial column of ascending degeneration found after tuberal lesions (14). The preoptic region is another site from which this behavior is elicited, and Chi (15) has shown that preoptic axons reach the central core of HVM. Projections of HVM upon the lateral hypothalamus are especially dense in the perifornical region, but also extend superiorly toward the subthalamus and ventrally into the region of the medial forebrain bundle. (When discussing efferent projections of HVM, we include degeneration resulting from destruction of pericapsular tissue about the nucleus; in the rat Millhouse (16) has found axons from HVM cells passing to the lateral hypothalamus.) Within this region there is an admixture of points which produce quiet biting attack and attack associated with threat displays (9). Stimulation of regions lying between the optic chiasm and the rostral pole of HVM results mainly in threat attack behavior, while a large number of sites yielding stalking attack are found between the levels of HVM and the mammillary bodies, a region in which degeneration can be demonstrated following tuberal lesions (14).

RESULTS

The female cat shows a hormone-dependent change in agonistic behavior following genital stimulation, and therefore provides an opportunity to study the organization of an intraspecific aggressive display. Because of the demonstrated role of the hypothalamus in both aggressive and reproductive behaviors, we chose initially to study the response of hypothalamic neurons to genital stimulation. Since the hypothalamus is concerned with diverse functions, we tried to classify the response properties of lateral hypothalamic neurons after stimulation of afferent pathways originating in the limbic system or in the HVM. The known projections of the amygdala, septum, preoptic region and some other limbic structures upon the hypothalamus (14, 15, 17–20) have led us to examine the effects of stimulation in these regions upon the behavior of lateral hypothalamic neurons as an initial step in the analysis (21). Our observations were made in locally anesthetized male and female cats. Stimulating electrodes were placed in the corticomedial amygdala and stria terminalis, basomedial amygdala and lateral amygdala; additional electrodes were placed in the septum, preoptic region, dorsal and ventral hippocampus and HVM. The effects of single and repetitive stimuli upon the responses of cells were

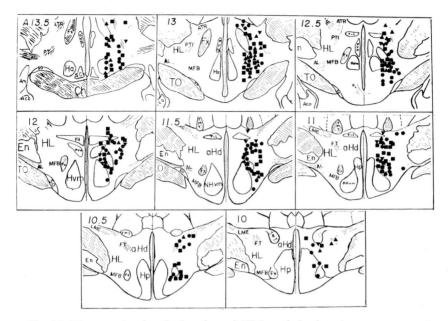

Fig. 5.1. Diagrams showing the locations of 225 hypothalamic units. ●, convergently driven units; ■, units driven from single stimulation sites; ▲, convergently suppressed units; ▼, units suppressed from single stimulation sites. Horsely-Clarke planes A 13.5 to A 10 are represented. From Van Atta and Sutin (21). aHd, dorsal hypothalamic area; AL, ansa lenticularis; Ch, optic chiasm; Fil, paraventricular nucleus; Fx, fornix; Ha, anterior hypothalamic area; Hdn, dorsal hypothalamic nucleus; HL, lateral hypothalamus; Hp, posterior hypothalamic area; MFB, medial forebrain bundle; NHvm, hypothalamic ventromedial nucleus; TO, optic tract.

examined throughout the rostro-caudal extent of the lateral hypothalamus. The regions from which these recordings were made are shown in Figure 5.1. Two general classes of responses were found in the lateral hypothalamus: excitation and suppression. Each class can be further subdivided according to whether the response was obtained from single or multiple stimulation sites. In Figure 5.1, the closed circles designate the location of cells driven (excited) from multiple stimulus sites and squares designate cells excited from a single site. Upright triangles depict the location of cells whose firing was suppressed from more than one stimulus site, whereas inverted triangles designate units suppressed by stimulation from a single site. Cells responding to limbic or HVM stimulation were distributed widely throughout the lateral hypothalamus, especially at anterior and tuberal levels. Although the region was sampled extensively, relatively few neurons in the posterior hypothalamus were affected. In the anterior hypothalamus and preoptic region, there was an admixture of

cells responding in both an excitatory and inhibitory manner. The perifornical region, however, contained only cells showing an excitatory response. Limbic and HVM stimulation drove cells in the midtuberal and
posterior fornical region, but in other parts of the hypothalamus both
driven and suppressed units were found. No responsive units were en-
countered in the region dorsolateral to the fornix at the level of the
rostral half of HVM, although this region was systematically explored.
This is a zone in which there is little degeneration following lesions
destroying HVM and adjacent tissue.

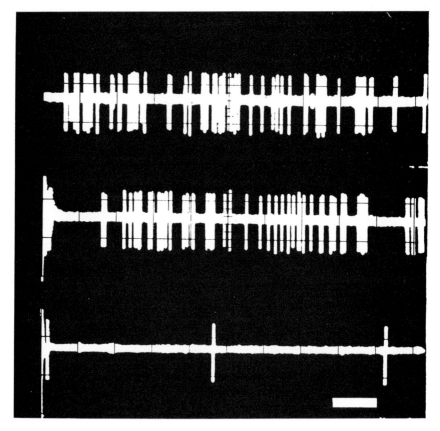

Fig. 5.2. Response of a lateral hypothalamic cell to 1-Hz. stimulation of the ventromedial nucleus. Top record, spontaneous activity; center and bottom records, effect of
HVM stimulation. The top and center records show 10 superimposed sweeps, whereas
the bottom record shows a single sweep. Note the driven action potential followed by
inhibition of 70-msec. duration. Because of the low spontaneous firing rate, the inhibition is apparent only upon superimposition of many sweeps or construction of a poststimulus histogram. Calibration = 50 msec. From Prescott and Sutin (unpublished data).

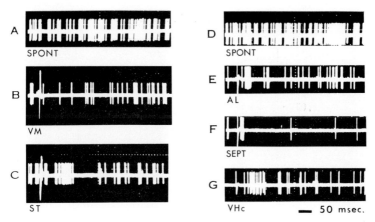

Fig. 5.3. Convergent inhibitory effects of stimulation of five different brain sites upon the same luteinizing hormone neuron. All of the records show 20 superimposed sweeps. A and D are samples of spontaneous activity for comparison with response to stimulation of HVM (B), stria terminalis (C), lateral amygdala (E), septum (F) and ventral hippocampus (G).

Cells that were excited made up 76 percent of the units studied. By "excited" we mean that the cell had action potentials fired at a fixed latency following the stimulus. The remaining 24 percent of the cells studied showed a suppression of discharge for 30 to several hundred milliseconds following the stimulus. Some illustrations of these response patterns and a poststimulus probability density histogram are shown in Figures 5.2, 5.3 and 5.4. Among the stimulus sites tested, HVM was most effective in influencing lateral hypothalamic cells. HVM and preoptic region yielded higher ratios of excitatory to inhibitory effects upon lateral hypothalamic cells than did stimulation of the amygdala, stria terminalis, septum or ventral hippocampus. A prominent feature of the lateral hypothalamic cells was the extensive convergence of afferent projections. About 45 percent of the cells studied responded to stimulation of two or more sites. Most typically all of the afferent pathways acting upon a cell produced the same type of response, *i.e.,* all excited or suppressed. In only a relatively small number of cells that were influenced from several stimulus sites did we find an admixture of excitatory and suppressive effects. The example shown in Figure 5.3 shows convergence from 5 stimulus sites on a single lateral hypothalamic neuron. Each record consists of 20 superimposed sweeps. A and D represent spontaneous discharge. B shows the response to HVM stimulation and C, the response to stria terminalis stimulation. Although both stimuli reduce the probability of firing of the cell, they do so in a different manner. HVM stimulation

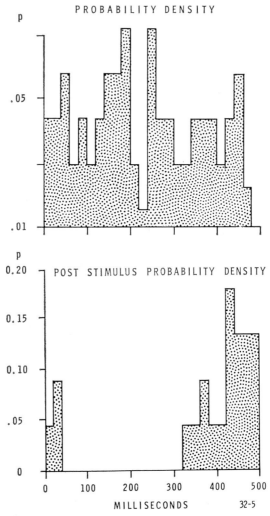

Fig. 5.4. Probability density of a lateral hypothalamic neuron during spontaneous firing and following 1/second of HVM stimulation. Note the prolonged suppression of firing produced by HVM stimulus. From Van Atta and Sutin (unpublished data).

produces a reduction in firing rate for 150 msec. with a gradual return toward the prestimulus spontaneous rate. When the stria terminalis is stimulated, suppression of spontaneous discharge does not begin for approximately 150 msec. following the stimulus. E, F and G represent stimulation of the lateral amygdala, septal nuclei and ventral hippocampus, respectively. Again, all resulted in decreased firing for a prolonged period

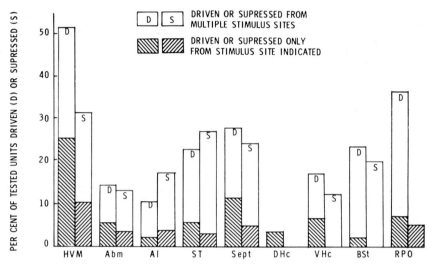

Fig. 5.5. Bar graph indicating the percentages of total units tested which were driven or suppressed by stimulation of the brain sites indicated. Single site stimulation effects are shown by the cross-hatched areas, whereas convergent effects are shown by the clear areas. Note the relatively small proportions of single site effects obtained from all sites of stimulation other than HVM. From Van Atta and Sutin (21). HVM, hypothalamic ventromedial nucleus; Abm, basomedial amygdaloid nucleus; Al, lateral amygdaloid nucleus; ST, stria terminalis-corticomedial amygdala; Sept, septal area; DHc, dorsal hippocampus; VHc, ventral hippocampus; BSt, bed nucleus of the stria terminalis; RPO, preoptic region.

following the stimulus, but lateral amygdaloid and septal stimulation led to brief periods of increased probability of discharge. These observations raise the possibility that at least some lateral hypothalamic neurons are capable of transmitting information in complex firing codes arising from phasic excitability changes initiated by inputs from various limbic system structures. However, it must be emphasized that the great majority of lateral hypothalamic cells respond in the same way irrespective of the afferent path stimulated (21).

The relative occurrence of excitatory and suppressive effects from the several stimulus sites employed in this study is shown in Figure 5.5. The following generalizations may be drawn from these data: 1) Convergence from two or more stimulus sites is commonplace in the lateral hypothalamus. 2) The HVM, stria terminalis, septum and preoptic area exert the most potent control over lateral hypothalamic neurons. 3) There is a preponderance of excitatory events in the lateral hypothalamus following ventromedial or preoptic stimulation.

All of the data presented thus far was obtained using single pulse stimulation. Although the spontaneous discharge rate of neurons in HVM and lateral hypothalamus is characteristically low with only a small percentage of the cells showing spontaneous firing rates of more than six per second, it is necessary to use stimulation rates of 50 Hz. or more in order to elicit aggressive behavior. With 50-Hz. stimulation of limbic structures or HVM, the responses in lateral hypothalamic neurons are in the same direction as those following 1-Hz. stimulation, but are of longer duration (22).

Having found that hypothalamic neurons can be classified into two main categories, we tried to determine whether genital stimulation, which evoked an aggressive response in anestrous cats, preferentially activated hypothalamic cells which were excited by limbic stimulation. The behavior of the estrous cat has been extensively studied by Bard (23), Michael (24) and Whalen (25), and only a brief summary is presented here. The anestrous cat will not permit intromission or artificial probing of the vagina and reacts to such attempts with vigorous attack behavior. The estrous cat, on the other hand, invites intromission by assuming an appropriate posture accompanied by treading movements of the hindlimbs. The sexually receptive female permits intromission for a 5- to 15-second interval. During intromission she emits a characteristic vocalization often described as an "angry cry." After the brief period during which intromission is tolerated, the female forcibly withdraws from the male and begins an "after-reaction" consisting of vigorous rolling, rubbing and grooming. During the after-reaction the female may strike out at the male and reacts to further attempts at mounting by striking or biting her partner. The after-reaction generally subsides in 5 to 7 minutes, but the female generally will not permit the male to mount again for a period of 15 to 20 minutes. Following this refractory period, the female will again become receptive and permit intromission. In the cat this entire behavioral repertoire is dependent solely upon estrogen, for unlike estrus in other species progesterone is not required. Since the anestrous animal always responds to vaginal probing in an agonistic manner, and the sexually receptive female changes in a matter of seconds from accepting to withdrawing from a vaginal probe, we felt that this system offered many advantages for the study of changes in neuronal firing associated with the development of a hostile response. The neurons mediating the behavioral responses to genital stimuli would be expected to exhibit certain properties. Since the behavior is triggered only by vaginal intromission, the system should have somatotopic specificity. Secondly, the system must be modulated by estrogen, since estrous responses to genital stimulation can be evoked from animals with intrahypothalamic implants of estrogen in amounts that are subthreshold for peripheral tissue effects (26, 27).

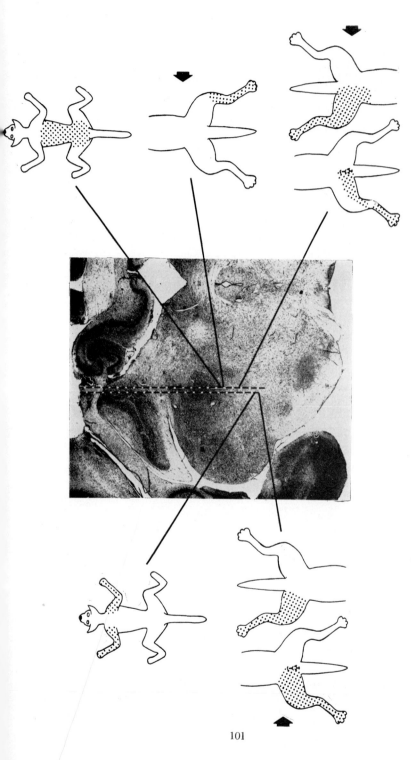

Fig. 5.6. Locations and receptive fields of neurons medial to magnocellular medial geniculate nucleus in the region of the medial lemniscus. Two micropipette tracks through the medial lemniscus of an estrous cat are indicated by the broken lines. Stippled areas on the body maps show the receptive fields in which mechanical stimulation-activated cells isolated along these tracks. Arrows indicate cells also driven by vaginal stimulation. From Rose and Sutin (33).

It must be kept in mind that in the cat, which ovulates reflexly, repeated vaginal stimulation leads to the release of luteinzing hormone and central nervous system events related to gonadotropin release must be separated from those concerned with behavioral manifestations.

Before considering our results in the cat, we want to mention briefly several pertinent studies in the rat. In this species the spontaneous firing rate of anterior hypothalamic neurons isolated from the rest of the nervous system in a "hypothalamic island" preparation is accelerated on the day of proestrus (28, 29). This increased firing can be mimicked to some extent by the administration of exogenous estrogen, but seems to be correlated mainly with the fall in blood levels of estrogen, for it occurs about 48 hours after the administration of the steroid. In intact rats, vaginal stimulation discharges many anterior hypothalamic and preoptic neurons, but is nonspecific since many of these cells are also fired by nociceptive or thermal stimuli (30–32). In the estrous rat, cervix stimulation reduces the firing rate of rostral hypothalamic neurons in contrast to the acceleration produced in the anestrous animal.

In both estrous and anestrous cats we found many cells which showed a general acceleration of firing during and after vaginal probing. However, the effect was nonspecific, for nociceptive or other sensory stimuli which produced electroencephalographic (EEG) arousal also increased the firing rate of hypothalamic cells. In a search for neurons which responded with a short latency burst of action potentials to vaginal stimulation, and to no other stimuli, we began exploring the genital projection upon the thalamus and at more proximal levels of the afferent pathway in the brain stem. Cells in the sacral projection zone of the ventrobasal thalamic nuclear complex had discrete tactile receptive fields which were contralateral, although some units were driven bilaterally from the tail or genitalia (Fig. 5.6). Receptive fields were usually confined to a portion of the tail or region of the skin adjacent to the base of the tail extending to the midline of the external genitalia and anus. Neurons fired with latencies of 10 to 25 msec. following tactile stimuli. Noxious stimuli consisting of pinching the skin outside of the tactile receptive field had no effect upon ventrobasal neurons. There were no discernible differences in the responses to tactile stimulation or receptive field size of units in estrous and anestrous animals. Since a number of the cells which had a tactile receptive field also responded to vaginal probing, we resorted to electrical stimulation of the vagina to avoid inadvertent tactile stimulation. Twenty-six percent of the cells tested responded to vaginal stimulation in the estrous cat, whereas only 7 percent of those examined in anestrous animals were affected by vaginal stimulation. There was no difference in the poststimulus firing pattern of cells driven by vaginal stimulation in the estrous and anestrous cats (33).

Moving further down the afferent path, we examined cells in the posterior thalamic nucleus and magnocellular portion of the medial geniculate nucleus. As expected, these cells showed no evidence of somatotopic organization of receptive fields, which differed greatly in size and shape from cell to cell. Cells in this region also exhibited polymodal response properties. Electrical stimulation of the vagina drove 19 percent of the cells tested, with no difference in the frequency of occurrence in estrous and anestrous animals. Since most of the neurons in both regions of the thalamus we examined responded to extravaginal stimuli, they cannot be considered specific genital sensory cells. As we continued to explore more caudally along the genital afferent path, a group of units was found in the lateral medulla which responded exclusively to vaginal probing (34). Figure 5.7 illustrates a lateral medullary neuron which responded to vaginal probing. Each probe initiated a burst of action potentials, and when the probe was removed the unit continued to exhibit an accelerated firing rate for several seconds. We studied 126 cells that responded to vaginal probing in cats anesthetized with urethane. These cells were localized to a region which included the medial portions of the lateral reticular nucleus and extended dorsomedially into the lateral medullary reticular formation and the vicinity of the nucleus ambiguus. We tried to mimic as much as possible the mating sequence of the cat.

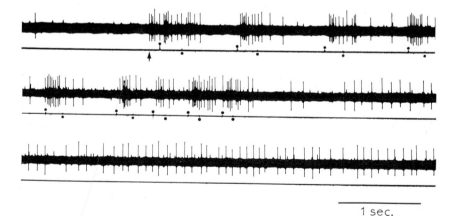

1 sec.

Fig. 5.7. Response of a unit to vaginal probing in an estrous decerebrate cat. Unit is located in the lateral tegmental field, dorsomedial to the lateral reticular nucleus. Arrow indicates introduction of probe. Upward and downward deflections of the stimulus marker represent inward and outward probe movements, respectively. Continuous traces. From Rose and Sutin (34).

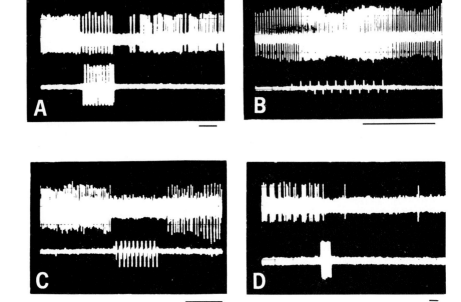

Fig. 5.8. Types of responses in lateral medullary neurons to vaginal probing. A different unit is shown on the top trace in each frame. The signal marker for vaginal probing is shown on the lower traces of each pair. (A) Probing elicited short bursts of spikes which were synchronized with thrusts, alternating with complete suppression of firing between thrusts. (B) Acceleration of firing throughout the period of vaginal stimulation. (C) and (D) Short and long duration suppression effects. Units A and D from estrous cats and B and C from anestrous cats. From Rose and Sutin (34).

Vaginal stimulation consisted of a series of thrusts over a period of 5 to 8 seconds. At least 15 minutes were allowed to elapse before a second epoch of vaginal stimulation was begun. All cats were ovariectomized several weeks before the acute experiment. The cats were brought into estrus by the administration of 200 μgm. of estradiol benzoate daily for several days until they were fully receptive and permitted intromission by a test male cat in a standard mating test (24). Discharge of lateral medullary neurons was measured both during vaginal probing and in the postprobe period. Eighty-six of the 126 cells studied responded only to vaginal probing and were unaffected by tactile, pressure or nociceptive stimulation in the coccygeal, sacral or lumbar dermatomes. The results described below are based upon that population of 86 cells which responded specifically to vaginal stimulation. Forty-one of the cells were obtained from estrous cats and 45 from anestrous animals. An example of the types of response

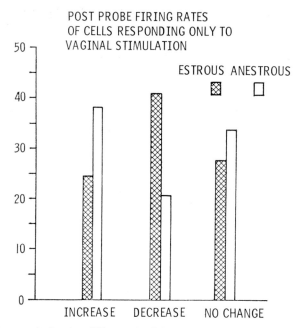

Fig. 5.9. Bar graph showing difference in firing rates of medullary neurons in estrous and anestrous cats.

patterns obtained is shown in Figure 5.8. Vaginal probing could lead to an acceleration of firing with each probe and continued increase in firing rate for a period of time following cessation of probing. Another response type consisted of an acceleration during probing with decreased firing rates after vaginal stimulation. In a smaller number of neurons, cessation of firing was seen during probing, with either an increase or decrease in the postprobe period. We found that the response *during* vaginal probing was not related to the hormonal condition of the animal. Sixty-nine percent of the cells in estrous and anestrous animals alike showed increased firing rates during vaginal probing, and 27 percent and 23 percent, respectively, demonstrated decreased firing. A difference in the response pattern between the two hormonal conditions does appear when the *postprobe* record is considered (Fig. 5.9). A response which outlasted the period of probing was seen in 72 percent of the units. In anestrous animals, 38 percent of the cells showed increased firing during vaginal stimulation, whereas 20 percent had a decreased discharge rate. In the estrous cats, only 25 percent showed an increase over the preprobe spontaneous firing rate after vaginal probing, whereas 42 percent had a reduced firing rate. The difference in the frequency of occurrence in these two postprobe response patterns is statistically significant ($P < 0.001$, χ^2, df $= 1$). The localization of cells responding only to vaginal probing is shown in Figure 5.10. In estrous cats, cells which showed an acceleration after vaginal probing were found within the boundary of the lateral reticular nucleus and in the adjacent reticular formation. In the anestrous cat, cells were largely confined to the region of the lateral reticular nucleus, particularly in its more caudal portions.

Because of the well known projections of the lateral reticular nucleus upon the cerebellum, we attempted to antidromically backfire lateral medullary neurons which responded to vaginal stimulation. Only 14 percent of the cells tested were antidromically discharged by cerebellar stimulation. Although anatomical studies have indicated that most cells of the lateral reticular nucleus project as mossy fibers to the cerebellum, our studies would indicate that at least a subpopulation has noncerebellar projections and is activated by afferent fibers from the genitalia.

Michael (27) has shown that ovariectomized cats can be brought to full sexual receptivity by intrahypothalamic implants of small quantities of estrogen without evidence of a systemic action of the steroid. This observation, together with evidence of a diencephalic uptake of labeled steroid, indicates that the steroid-sensitive cells which are concerned with the initiation of sexual receptivity in the cat are located in the basal diencephalon. The difference we found in the predominent response pattern in the lateral medulla in estrous and anestrous animals could be attributable to a modulation of excitability of medullary neurons by an estrogen-sensitive system in the hypothalamus. To test this possibility we examined the effect of 50-Hz. stimulation in the hypothalamus and midbrain upon lateral medullary cells that also responded to vaginal stimulation. Hypothalamic stimulation caused both increases and decreases in firing of medullary neurons. Although the action of stimulation of any hypothalamic site on an individual lateral medullary neuron was typically constant upon repeated tests, other nearby units might show a different response. The most marked effects of stimulation of the rostral brainstem were obtained when the electrodes were located in the central gray or adjacent reticular formation in the midbrain. Single pulse stimulation here also produced short latency responses in 16 units. An example is shown in Figure 5.11. In (A) the response of the cell to vaginal probing is shown. In (B) a short latency-driven action potential occurs during central gray stimulation. This is followed by a period of suppression of the spontaneous discharge (C). Fifty-Hertz stimulation of the central gray often completely suppressed the discharge of lateral medullary neurons.

In order to gather more information about the properties of descending projections from the hypothalamus to the midbrain, another series of

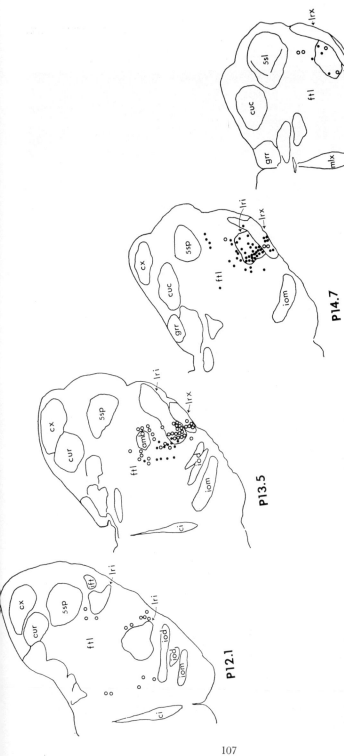

Fig. 5.10. Anatomical distribution of units responding to vaginal probing. ○, units recorded in estrous cats; ●, units from anestrous cats. amb, nucleus ambiguus; ci, inferior central nucleus; cuc, cuneate nucleus, caudal division; cur, cuneate nucleus, rostral division; cx, external cuneate nucleus; ftl, lateral tegmental field; grr, gracile nucleus, rostral division; ift, infratrigeminal nucleus; iod, dorsal accessory nucleus of the inferior olive; iom, medial accessory nucleus of the inferior olive; lri, lateral reticular nucleus, internal division; lrx, lateral reticular nuceus, external division; mlx, decussation of the medial lemniscus; 5sl, laminar spinal trigeminal nucleus; 5sp, alaminar spinal trigeminal nucleus, parvocellular division. From Rose and Sutin (34).

107

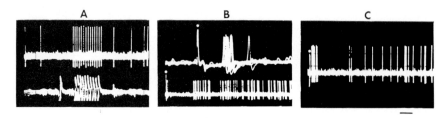

Fig. 5.11. Responses of a lateral reticular nucleus unit to vaginal or brain stimulation.
(A) Top trace is unit activity and the bottom trace indicates vaginal probes. (B) Short
latency driving of unit, followed by suppression of spontaneous discharge caused by
1-Hz stimulation of the midbrain just lateral to central grey. Upper superimposed
traces ($N = 10$) are displayed at higher gain and a faster sweep than the lower superimposed traces ($N = 20$). (C) Driven response followed by suppression of firing during
1-Hz. medial preoptic area stimulation ($N = 20$ superimposed sweeps). Time calibration:
A, 1 sec.; B, 1 msec. upper traces and 50 msec. lower traces; C, 20 msec.

experiments were undertaken on urethane-anesthetized male rats. As in
our studies of lateral hypothalamic neurons, cells in the midbrain and
pons were classified according to the response to single pulse stimulation
of the medial forebrain bundle. About half of the 237 cells tested responded to single hypothalamic stimuli, and 60 of these had short latency-
driven action potentials. Those cells which were not driven in a time-
locked fashion exhibited an increased poststimulus firing probability.
Only a few midbrain cells were inhibited by hypothalamic stimulation.
Figure 5.12, A and B, illustrates the response of a cell driven by hypothalamic stimulation. Cells of this type showed little spontaneous activity. In
C and D an example is shown of a cell which is not driven in the time-
locked fashion, but shows an increased probability of firing. E and F
illustrate a cell in which hypothalamic stimulation led to a brief period of
suppression followed by an increased probability of discharge.

The response of midbrain cells to 250-msec. trains of impulses delivered
at a frequency of 60 Hz. presented at intervals of 5 seconds or more was
also studied (Fig. 5.13). In order to control for possible generalized arousal
or vasopressor action of the stimulus, similar trains of pulses were applied
to the tail at intensities just sufficient to change the EEG from slow wave
to low voltage fast activity. Virtually all of the cells that were driven by
single lateral hypothalamic pulses showed an increased probability of
firing after a burst of stimuli. Tail stimulation generally had no effect on
this class of neurons. In contrast to this, 58 percent of the midbrain
neurons which showed a non-time-locked increase in firing rate following
single pulse lateral hypothalamic stimulation were also excited by tail
stimulation, suggesting that this group of cells may participate in nonspecific arousal responses.

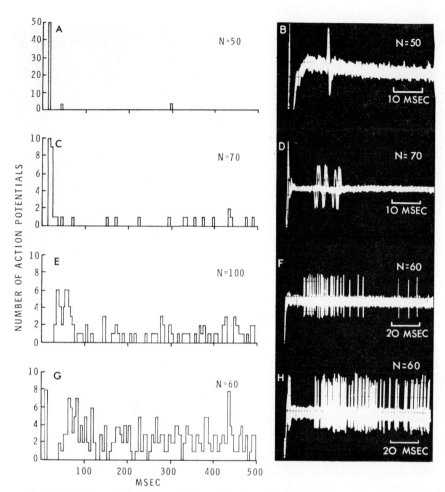

Fig. 5.12. Effects of single lateral hypothalamic stimuli on midbrain unit discharge. Poststimulus histograms for four different units are shown along with examples of superimposed recordings. N in each case indicates the number of stimulus presentations from which the record was made. A and B, driven unit; C and D, unit showing increased probability of firing, but which was not driven; E and F, cell showing a prolonged increase in probability of discharge; G and H, cell suppressed by stimulus with post-inhibitory increase in firing. (Unpublished observations of Thalmann and Sutin.)

Hypothalamic stimulation particularly affects groups of cells bordering the caudal midbrain central gray (Fig. 5.14). This is a region in which Malsbury, and co-workers (35) found units in the female rat which responded to tactile stimulation on the rear of the body, a region which would be contacted by the male during mating. The midbrain cells which we have found to be affected by hypothalamic stimulation are located in a

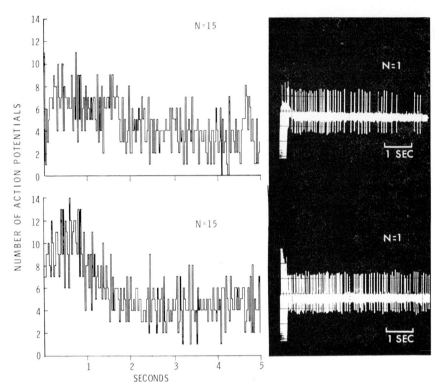

Fig. 5.13. Examples of a midbrain unit affected by repetitive stimulation of the hypothalamus (top) and by tail shocks (bottom). The poststimulus histograms on the left were
constructed from 15 presentations of stimulus trains. Right, an example of the response
during presentation of a single train of stimuli. The 50-Hz. stimulus artifacts occupy the
first 250 msec. of the sweep in the oscillographic recordings, whereas the poststimulus
histograms begin after the last pulse in the stimulus train. (Unpublished observations of
Thalmann and Sutin.)

region which preferentially accumulates labeled estradiol (36). Electrical
stimulation in this region in female rats produces tail and rump movements that resemble components of the receptive female's lordosis response (37).

DISCUSSION

Lorenz (38) has pointed out that sexual excitement results in an inhibition of aggression and preying long enough to permit mating in the
female of certain species such as the solitary carnivores. In the case of the
anestrous domestic cat, attempted intromission provokes aggressive behavior while in the estrous cat intromission results in a response, the copula-

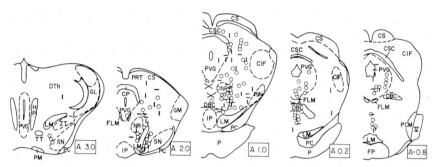

Fig. 5.14. Localization of response patterns of midbrain units to single pulse stimulation of the lateral hypothalamus. ○, driven unit; |, increased probability of firing, but not driven; —, suppression of spontaneous firing. CIF, inferior colliculus; CS, superior colliculus; CSC, commissure of the superior colliculus; DBC, decussation of the brachium conjunctivum; DTh, dorsal thalamus; FLM, medial longitudinal fasciculus; FP, fibers of the pyramid; GL, lateral geniculate; HP, habenulointerpeduncular tract; LM, medial lemniscus; PC, cerebral peduncle; P, pons; PM, mammillary peduncle; PRT, pretectal area; PVG, periventricular gray; SN, substantia nigra; TT, mammillotegmental tract; ZI, zona incerta; V, fifth nerve; A (in box with number), Horsley-Clare frontal coordinates.

tory cry and after-reaction (23, 39, 40), which is never seen in the anestrous animal. Denervation of the perigenital region does not prevent the copulatory cry and after-reaction, whereas denervation of the vagina eliminates these behavioral responses (41, 42). The specificity of vaginal stimulation which leads to the cry and after-reaction in the estrous female suggests that the study of brain stem neurons which fire *only* to vaginal stimulation will provide some insight into the neural coding which leads ultimately to receptive or agonistic behavior.

Studies of hypothalamic single cell responses to genital stimulation are not readily compared, for both cyclic (30, 43) and reflex (44–46) ovulators have been used. In addition, the hormonal and behavioral condition of the animal has varied. Some studies were done in conditions of constant light-induced persistent estrus (43), whereas others used postural criteria of estrus rather than mating tests. Still other differences relate to the anesthetic used and the nature of the data analysis. In view of the varied conditions, it is not possible to make valid general statements about the effects of genital stimulation upon hypothalamic neurons. We would point out, however, that there are relatively few reports of cells in the hypothalamus which are affected only by vaginal stimuli. For example, in an analysis of more than 300 cells Barraclough and Cross (30) found only three which were fired solely by genital stimulation, which included tactile stimulation of the vulva as well as vaginal probing. Lincoln and Cross

(43) reported a small number of probe-specific cells in the anterior hypo-thalamus and preoptic region of the rat.

Multiple unit activity which can be observed with 60-μ, low impedance microelectrodes inserted into the anterior and medial hypothalamus and midbrain tegmentum has been studied in estrous and anestrous cats (44, 45). Tactile and mechanical stimulation of the perineal area resulted in decreased firing rates in both estrous and anestrous animals. Vaginal stimulation led to increased firing in the estrogen-primed females while suppression of discharge occurred in anestrous cats (44). Later it was shown that the effect of stimulation involved the os cervix rather than the vaginal wall (45). Vaginal stimulation without involvement of the cervix often led to a suppression of hypothalamic discharge. In these studies in the cat, like those in the rat, other sensory stimuli also affected the multiunit activity recorded in the hypothalamus.

Our studies showing the extensive convergence of limbic and HVM inputs upon lateral hypothalamic cells may explain the paucity of neurons which respond only to genital stimulation. The specificity of lateral medullary neurons to vaginal probing provides an opportunity to study the firing patterns of this unique population under conditions in which genital stimulation leads either to an estrous cry and after-reaction or to attack and withdrawal behavior. The finding that differences exist in the postprobe firing pattern in estrous and anestrous animals in the afferent path at the level of the caudal medulla, while estrogen acts at more rostral brainstem levels, can be explained by assuming the existence of an estro-gen-sensitive system which descends from the hypothalamus.

The idea of hypothalamic modulation of lower brain stem neuronal networks in sexual behavior was first proposed by Bard (47). MacDonnell and Flynn (48) found that hypothalamic stimulation enlarges the perioral region in which tactile stimuli elicit reflexive head movement and jaw opening. These and other data (9) led to the concept of a hypothalamic sensory gate regulating cranial reflexes involved in stalking attack behavior.

Figure 5.15 presents a model to explain hormone-dependent differences in lateral medullary neuron responses to vaginal stimulation. Although the manner in which estrogen influences neurons is not known, we assume that the steroid modifies genome expression in cells scattered throughout the lateral hypothalamus or midbrain or both, resulting in the increased synthesis of transmitter. The estrogen-sensitive system would act as a tonic inhibitory control over signal transfer in lateral medullary neurons. A nonsteroid-sensitive descending system is also proposed, for hypothalamic or midbrain stimulation produces changes in lateral medullary cell firing

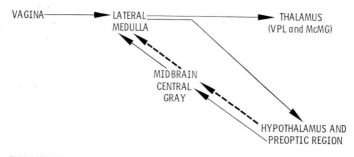

Fig. 5.15. Model proposed to explain the difference in firing patterns of lateral medullary neurons in estrous and anestrous cats.

in both anestrous and estrous animals. The evidence supporting this model can be summarized as follows.

1. Spontaneous unit activity in hypothalamic islands is greatest on the day of proestrus in rats (29).

2. Vagina and cervix stimulation in estrous rats leads to decreased firing of hypothalamic cells (30, 31).

3. Short latency-driven responses are recorded in the central gray and midbrain tegmentum after hypothalamic stimulation in rats (R. H. Thalmann and J. Sutin, unpublished observations). These cells do not respond to nociceptive or arousing stimuli.

4. There is anatomical evidence for direct medial forebrain bundle projections to the central gray and midbrain tegmentum (49, 50).

5. Estrogen implants into the hypothalamus of the cat lead to full sexual receptivity and acceptance of vaginal stimulation without evidence of a peripheral action of the steroid (51).

6. Cells that respond only to vaginal stimulation are found in the lateral medulla of cats. The poststimulation pattern differs in estrous and anestrous animals (34).

7. Central gray and hypothalamic stimulation can modulate the spontaneous discharge of lateral medullary cells which respond to vaginal sensory stimulation (34).

We visualize the system operating in the following manner. Stimulation of the vaginal wall leads to a burst of action potentials in the ascending path. In the anestrous animal, the descending tonic facilitatory path sums with the excitatory drive produced by the afferent burst of impulses to produce accelerated firing of lateral medullary cells which outlasts the duration of the vaginal probe. In estrous cats, the excitatory action of descending paths from the hypothalamus and midbrain is decreased because of the inhibitory effect produced by the steroid-sensitive system. The time course of the firing of lateral medullary cells is confined to the duration of the excitation produced by the afferent volley during a vaginal thrust.

The model presented here is a preliminary scheme. Further neurophysiological evidence is needed to confirm the existence of the estrogen-sensitive descending system. The nature of the response pattern along the spinal course of the genital afferent system also needs to be determined, and the pre- or postsynaptic site of action of the hypothalamo-midbrain-lateral medullary path must be defined.

We have found that lateral medullary lesions abolish or attenuate the copulatory cry and after-reaction in estrous cats (34), and Sprague and associates (52) noted that bilateral lateral midbrain lesions in estrous cats had a similar effect. Sprague and his co-workers also found that lateral midbrain lesions attenuated aggressive responses in cats that were vicious before the lesions were placed.

A more precise definition of the role of lateral medullary neurons in sexual receptivity and aggressive behavior elicited by genital stimulation is a goal for further experimental study.

SUMMARY

In order to study neural coding in a situation in which a sensory stimulus leads to aversive behavior, we have chosen the unique behavior triggered by vaginal probing in the estrous cat. We searched the hypothalamus and lower brain stem of urethane-anesthetized estrous and anestrous cats for cells which responded to vaginal probing but did not respond to tactile, pressure or nociceptive stimuli. Responsive neurons were classified according to changes in firing pattern both during vaginal probing and in the postprobe period.

We also studied the effects of limbic and sensory stimuli upon lateral hypothalamic neurons. Since stimulation of the ventromedial nucleus and perifornical region produces "affective-defense" reactions, we paid particular attention to these regions. Following limbic or ventromedial nucleus (HVM) stimulation, single cell recordings in the lateral hypothalamus showed two types of response. Seventy-six percent of the sample displayed fixed latency-driven action potentials, whereas the remainder showed a suppression of spontaneous activity for a period of 30 to several hundred milliseconds. The HVM was the most effective site of stimulation for influencing lateral hypothalamic cells. Almost exclusively excitatory effects were seen in perifornical neurons after HVM or limbic stimulation. There is extensive convergence of afferent projections upon lateral hypothalamic neurons, for 45 percent respond to stimulation of two or more sites. For this reason, it is not surprising that we were unable to find a population of neurons in the hypothalamus that responded only to vaginal probing. Many cells showed a general acceleration or decrease in firing rate during probing, but the same changes could be produced by arousing stimuli such as tissue compression or pinch. Although such cells may well be involved in the change from sexual receptivity to aversive behavior, it is not possible to experimentally assess their role.

In the lower brain stem we did find a group of cells that respond solely to vaginal probing among the stimuli tested. These neurons were located in the region of the medial portion of the lateral reticular nucleus and adjacent medullary reticular formation at the level of the obex. In estrous animals, a significantly greater proportion of cells showed a decreased firing rate in the postprobe period. These cells were found in the rostral portions of the lateral reticular nucleus and adjacent reticular formation extending to the region around the nucleus ambiguus. In the anestrous animals, the cells that responded to vaginal probing were most commonly characterized by increased firing during the postprobe period and tended to be located in the caudal half of the lateral reticular nucleus and adjacent reticular formation. The change to a predominance of decreased postprobe firing in the estrogen-treated animals suggests that the steroid affects a system which modulates brain stem cells. We found evidence for the existence of such a descending system by testing effects of hypothalamic stimulation upon the response evoked in medullary cells by genital stimulation.

REFERENCES

1. Maclean, PD, Delgado, JMR: Electrical and chemical stimulation of fronto-temporal portion of limbic system in the waking animal. Electroencephalogr Clin Neurophysiol 5: 91, 1953.
2. De Molina, FA, Hunsperger, RW: Central representation of affective reactions in forebrain and brain stem: electrical stimulation of amygdala, stria terminalis, and adjacent structures. J Physiol 145: 251, 1959.
3. Ursin, H, Kaada, BR: Functional localization within the amygdaloid complex in the cat. Electroencephalogr Clin Neurophysiol 12: 1, 1960.
4. Brown, JL, Hunsperger, RW: Neuroethology and the motivation of agonistic behaviour. Anim Behav 11: 439, 1963.
5. Hess, WR: Hypothalamus und Thalamus. Stuttgart, G. Thieme Verlag, 1956, p. 26.
6. Magnus, O, Lammers, HJ: The amygdaloid-nuclear complex. Folia psychiat neerl 59: 555, 1956.
7. De Molina, FA, Hunsperger, RW: Organization of the subcortical system governing defense and flight reactions in the cat. J Physiol 160: 200, 1962.

8. HILTON, SM, ZBROZYNA, AW: Amygdaloid region for defense reactions and its efferent pathway to the brain stem. J Physiol 165: 160, 1963.

9. FLYNN, JP: The neural basis of aggression in cats, in Neurophysiology and Emotion, edited by Glass, DC. New York, Rockefeller University Press, 1967, p. 40.

10. ROBERTS, WW, KIESS, HO: Motivational properties of hypothalamic aggression in cats. J Comp Physiol Psychol 58: 187, 1964.

11. EGGER, MD, FLYNN, JP: Effects of electrical stimulation of the amygdala on hypothalamically elicited attack behavior in cats. J Neurophysiol 26: 705, 1963.

12. MacDONNEL, MF, FLYNN, JP: Attack elicited by stimulation of the thalamus of cats. Science 144: 1249, 1964.

13. SIEGEL, A, CHABORA, J: Effects of electrical stimulation of the cingulate gyrus upon attack behavior elicited from the hypothalamus in the cat. Brain Res 32: 169, 1971.

14. SUTIN, J, EAGER, RP: Fiber degeneration following lesions in the hypothalamic ventromedial nucleus. Ann NY Acad Sci 157: 610, 1969.

15. CHI, CC: Afferent connections to the ventromedial nucleus of the hypothalamus in the rat. Brain Res 17: 439, 1970.

16. MILLHOUSE, OE: The organization of the ventromedial hypothalamic nucleus. Brain Res 55: 71, 1973.

17. NAUTA, WJH: Fiber degeneration following lesions of the amygdaloid complex in the monkey. J Anat 95: 515, 1961.

18. NAUTA, WJH: Neural associations of the amygdaloid complex in the monkey. Brain 85: 505, 1962.

19. HEIMER, L, NAUTA, WJH: The hypothalamic distribution of the stria terminalis in the rat. Brain Res 13: 284, 1969.

20. LEONARD, CM, SCOTT, JW: Origin and distribution of the amygdalofugal pathways in the rat: an experimental neuroanatomical study. J Comp Neurol 141: 313, 1971.

21. VAN ATTA, L, SUTIN, J: The response of single lateral hypothalamic neurons to ventromedial nucleus and limbic stimulation. Physiol Behav 6: 523, 1971.

22. VAN ATTA, L, SUTIN, J: Relationships among amygdaloid and other limbic structures influencing activity of lateral hypothalamic neurons, in The Neurobiology of the Amygdala, edited by Eleftheriou, BE, New York, Plenum Publishing Corp., 1972, p. 343.

23. BARD, P: The hypothalamus and sexual behavior. Res Publ Assoc Res Nerv Ment Dis 20: 551, 1940.

24. MICHAEL, RP: Observations upon the sexual behaviour of the domestic cat (Felis Cattus L.) under laboratory conditions. Behaviour 18: 1, 1961.

25. WHALEN, RE: Sexual behavior of cats. Behaviour 20: 321, 1963.

26. MICHAEL, RP: An investigation of the sensitivity of circumscribed neurological areas to hormonal stimulation by means of the application of oestrogens directly to the brain of the cat, in Regional Neurochemistry, edited by Kety, SS., Elkes, J. Oxford, Pergamon Press, 1961, p. 465.

27. MICHAEL, RP: Neurological mechanisms and the control of sexual behaviour. Sci Basis Med Ann Rev 316, 1965.

28. DYER, RG, PRITCHETT, CJ, CROSS, BA: Unit activity in the diencephalon of female rats during the oestrous cycle. J. Endocrinol 53: 151, 1972.

29. CROSS, BA, DYER, RG: Cyclic changes in neurons of the anterior hypothalamus during the rat estrous cycle and the effect of anesthesia, in Steroid Hormones and Brain Functions, edited by Sawyer, CH, Gorski, R.A. Los Angeles, University of California Press, 1972, p. 95.

30. BARRACLOUGH, CA, CROSS, BA: Unit activity in the hypothalamus of the cyclic female rat: effect of genital stimuli and progesterone. J Endocrinol 26: 339, 1963.
31. CROSS, BA: Electrical recording techniques in the study of hypothalamic control of gonadotrophin secretion. Excerpta Med Int Congr Ser 83: 513, 1965.
32. LINCOLN, DW: Unit activity in the hypothalamus, septum and preoptic area of the rat: characteristics of spontaneous activity and the effect of oestrogen. J. Endocrinol 37: 177, 1967.
33. ROSE, JD, SUTIN, J: Responses of single thalamic neurons to genital stimulation in female cats. Brain Res 33: 533, 1971.
34. ROSE, JD, SUTIN, J: Responses of single units in the medulla to genital stimulation in estrous and anestrous cats. Brain Res 50: 87, 1973.
35. MALSBURY, CW, KELLEY, DB, PFAFF, DW: Responses of single units in the dorsal midbrain to somatosensory stimulation in female rats, in Progress in Endocrinology, Proceedings of the Fourth International Congress of Endocrinology. Amsterdam, Excerpta Medica, 1972.
36. PFAFF, DW, KEINER, M: Estradiol-concentrating cells in the rat amygdala as part of a limbic-hypothalamic hormone-sensitive system, in The Neurobiology of the Amygdala, edited by Eleftheriou, BE. New York, Plenum Publishing Corp., 1972, p. 775.
37. PFAFF, D, LEWIS, C, DIAKOW, C, KEINER, M: Neurophysiological analysis of mating behavior responses as hormone-sensitive reflexes, in Progress in Physiological Psychology, Vol. V, edited by Stellar, E, Sprague, JM. New York, Academic Press, 1972.
38. LORENZ, K: On Aggression. New York, Bantam Books, Harcourt, Brace and World, Inc., 1969, p. 123.
39. YOUNG, WC: Observations and experiments on mating behavior in female mammals. Q Rev Biol 16: 135, 1941.
40. GREULICH, WW: Artificially induced ovulation in the cat (Felis Domestica). Anat Rec 58: 217, 1934.
41. BARD, P: The effects of denervation of the genitalia on the oestrual behavior of cats. Am J Physiol 113: 5, 1935.
42. ARONSON, LR: Sensory factors in mating behavior, in Symposium on Reproduction. Congress of Hungarian Society for Endocrinology and Metabolism, Budapest, Akadémiai Kiadó, 1967, p. 227.
43. LINCOLN, DW, CROSS, BA: Effect of oestrogen on the responsiveness of neurons in the hypothalamus, septum and preoptic area of rats with light-induced persistent oestrus. J Endocrinol 37: 191, 1967.
44. ALCARAZ, M, GUZMAN-FLORES, C, SALAS, M, BEYER, C: Effect of estrogen on the responsivity of hypothalamic and mesencephalic neurons in the female cat. Brain Res 15: 439, 1969.
45. BEYER, C, ALMANZA, J, DE LA TORRE, L, GUZMAN-FLORES, C: Effect of genital stimulation on the brain stem multiunit activity of anestrous and estrous cats. Brain Res 32: 143, 1971.
46. RATNER, A, KOENIG, JQ, FRAZIER, DT: Hypothalamic unit activity in the cat: effects of estrogen and vaginal stimulation. Proc Soc Exp Biol 137: 321, 1971.
47. BARD, P: Neural mechanisms in emotional and sexual behavior. Psychosom Med 4: 171, 1942.
48. MACDONNELL, MF, FLYNN, JP: Control of sensory fields by stimulation of hypothalamus. Science 152: 1406, 1966.
49. GUILLERY, RW: Degeneration in the hypothalamic connections of the albino rat. J Anat 91: 91, 1957.

50. Wolf, G, Sutin, J: Fiber degeneration after lateral hypothalamic lesions in the rat. J Comp Neurol 127: 137, 1966.
51. Harris, GW, Michael, RP: The activation of sexual behavior by hypothalamic implants of oestrogen. J Physiol 171: 275, 1964.
52. Sprague, JM, Chambers, WW, Stellar, E: Attentive, affective, and adaptive behavior in the cat. Science 133: 165, 1961.

DISCUSSION

Dr. Philip Bard (Baltimore, Maryland): Did you explore the medial surface of the cerebral cortex? There is good evidence that the external genitalia in the cat are represented there as far as tactile sensibility is concerned.

Dr. Jerome Sutin (Atlanta, Georgia): No, we did not.

Dr. Bard: It has also been reported that a tumor in that region in a woman produced rather marked nymphomania.

Dr. Dominick Purpura (Bronx, New York): I have been impressed by the concept of the hypothalamus as a continuous, extending pharmacological field. Whether the subject is preoptic area in relation to sexual dimorphism, or drinking and other kinds of behavior, or forebrain mechanisms controlling inhibition and sleep, we are dealing with systems where patterns emerge, not regional, localized centers. It is not surprising that there is difficulty picking up a discrete population of neurons in a hypothalamus responsive only to one kind of input from this extraordinarily complex forebrain diencephalic system. Still, I have difficulty with the concept of centers in the hypothalamus, and want to ask about the descending control. Are these on the input or output end of the system in the ventrolateral medulla? Are we dealing with upstream or downstream effects?

Dr. Sutin: I can only say that inasmuch as stimulation of the central gray fires cells in this region, there appears to be a descending system. Also, of course, the cat is a reflex ovulator, and there is information ascending from the genitalia relating to gonadotropin release as well as to the behavior I emphasized. The only other data we have are that lesions in the medulla block the estrous cry and greatly reduce the after-reaction without affecting other aspects of estrous behavior (J. Rose and J. Sutin, Brain Research, 56:350–354, 1973).

To answer your question, we do not have the type of data needed to determine whether the descending control system acts upon the input to lateral reticular neurons, that is, presynaptically or postsynaptically.

Dr. Paul D. MacLean (Bethesda, Maryland): With the monkey, we found that sensory stimulation is very ineffective in exciting any hypothalamic neurons, and we also found a very slow, spontaneous firing rate of the great majority of cells in the hypothalamus.

Dr. Sutin: I do not know why these cells do not respond more actively to sensory stimuli.

I should add that Dr. Maclean, in his work on penile erection in the monkey, and Dr. Pfaff, in his work on lordosis response in the rat, both find that they can obtain these effects from the lateral medullary region in which we found responses to genital stimulation.

Chapter 6

CENTRAL NEUROTRANSMITTERS IN AGGRESSION

Donald J. Reis

I. INTRODUCTION

That specific chemicals in the brain may be coded for specified behaviors has been an attractive concept to neuroscientists. Miller has used the term "the chemical coding of behavior" to describe this mode of neural organization (1). The implications of chemically mediated behavior are scientifically and socially far reaching; by extrapolation they lead to the possible realm in which behavior is manipulated by molecules.

Among the candidates for behavioral codons are several compounds of low molecular weight. These include the catecholamines, norepinephrine (NE) and dopamine (DA), the indole 5-hydroxytryptamine (5-HT, serotonin) and the amine acetylcholine (ACh). These agents are synthesized, stored and released in specific neural systems in the brain. They are believed to function in the central as in the peripheral neural system as neurotransmitters, *i.e.,* compounds which are released from nerve endings by nerve impulse activity at morphologically distinguishable synaptic junctions producing suitable changes in the excitability of the postsynaptic membrane (2, 3). In this paper I would like to examine the evidence that these agents may act in the brain to modify aggressive behavior. The possible role of NE in such behavior has been reviewed by me previously (4). However, I would now like to consider the role in aggression of not only this neurotransmitter but of DA, ACh and 5-HT, and to present evidence suggesting that these agents may have selective and independent actions on two neurologically distinct classes of aggression: affective and predatory aggression.

II. TWO NEUROLOGICALLY DISTINCT SYSTEMS MEDIATING AGGRESSIVE BEHAVIOR

Aggressive behavior may be defined as behavior which leads to damage or destruction of some goal entity (5). It is generally accepted that aggression is evolved as a complex behavioral response to environmental stimuli. In general, behavioral psychologists have tended to distinguish between different classes of aggression on the basis of the stimuli evoking the response. Thus, Moyer (5) has identified several classes of aggression of this basis including predatory, intermale, fear-induced, irritable, territorial, maternal and instrumental, and has suggested that the central neural mechanisms and neuroendocrine modulations of these aggressive states, in part, may differ.

In contrast, when aggressive behavior is classified by the type of *response* a simpler picture of the behavior emerges. There is substantial evidence that there are primarily two neurologically distinct patterns underlying the expression of aggressive or attack behavior. These may be termed *affective aggression* (affective attack (6)) and *predatory aggression* (biting attack (6)). They differ in their mode of expression, the provoking stimuli, the neuroanatomical substrate and, as will be developed later in this essay, their neurochemical modulation. Many of the differences between these two classes of aggression were recognized in pioneering studies of Flynn and his associates (see Reference 6) who first discovered that the two modes of aggression were differently organized in the brain (7). Some of the characteristics of these two types of aggression are outlined in Table 6.1.

A. Affective Aggression

Affective aggression has been the most intensively studied type of aggression. In the cat the prototype of this behavior has been called sham rage (8), the defense reaction (9) or affective attack behavior (10). It can be evoked in various species by brain lesions (*e.g.*, 8, 11), by electrical stimulation of brain (6, 7, 10, 16, 17), as a natural response to real or

TABLE 6.1

Some characteristics of affective and predatory aggression

Affective Aggression	Predatory Aggression
a. Intensive patterned autonomic activation, esp. sympathoadrenal	a. Little autonomic activation
b. Threatening and defensive postures	b. Stalking postures
c. Menacing vocalization	c. Little vocalization
d. Attack is with claws, frenzied, mutilating	d. Attacks by biting, lethally directed to back of neck
e. Initiated by somatic (esp. nocioceptive) as well as exteroceptive stimuli	e. Initiated by exteroceptive stimuli, usually visual
f. Generally lowered threshold for aggression (irritability), not always goal directed	f. No irritability
g. Intra- as well as interspecific	g. Interspecific
h. May be used only for display	h. Always aims at success
i. Not usually related to feeding	i. Related to feeding
j. Probably quite hormonally responsive	j. Probably less hormonally responsive

threatened attack (14, 18, 19) or to infliction of a painful stimulus (shock-induced aggression) (20, 21).

Affective aggression is the mode of aggressive display seen in aggressive states characterized as "irritable," intermale, territorial or maternal. It is probably a ubiquitous mode of aggressive behavior in vertebrates.

The behavior as represented in the cat has several characteristics (6, 8–14) (Table 6.1). a) It consists of an intense and patterned activation of the autonomic nervous system, particularly the sympathoadrenal axis, with a resultant increase in muscle blood flow, hypertension, increased cardiac output, decreased blood flow to viscera, pupillary dilation and piloerection (8, 22, 23). b) The animal assumes threatening and defensive postures including baring of the teeth and claws, arching of the back and retraction of the ears. c) There is threatening vocalization, particularly hissing and snarling (13). d) The object of aggression is primarily attacked with claws rather than teeth, the blows often inflicting widespread tissue damage (6). e) The initiating stimulus may be somatic (nocioceptive stimuli are particularly effective) or exteroceptive, especially visual. f) The threshold for aggression is often lower than normal, the animal being "irritable." g) The attack is likely to be intra- as well as interspecific. h) The affective display and threatening postures associated with this mode of aggression may be an end in itself serving to signal the intent of aggression. i) The mode of aggression is usually not related to feeding or predation. Indeed the intense vocalization of the affective display would be counterproductive for a predator, alarming prey before attack. j) It is the mode of aggressive expression which is probably hormonally responsive.

B. Predatory Aggression

Predatory aggression is that class of aggression which leads to destruction of a natural prey, usually for food. In the laboratory several paradigms have been used including the natural attack by rats against mice (muricidal killing (25)) or frogs (26). That predatory behavior could be evoked by brain stimulation was discovered by Wasman and Flynn in the cat (7) and has since been demonstrated in the rat (27, 28).

Predatory aggression is characterized by a) little autonomic arousal, b) the assumption, in predators, of characteristic stalking postures, c) minimal vocalization and d) an attack on the prey with precisely directed lethal blows to the back of the neck with little mutilation by claws. e) The behavior is usually triggered by exteroceptive, particularly visual, stimuli. f) It is not associated with increased irritability and, indeed, the animal is so actively concentrating on the prey that there is probably selective suppression of other sensory inputs (24). g) This mode of aggression is primarily intraspecific. h) Unlike affective aggression it is not elaborated only for display. Once initiated the predatory behavior aims at success. i) It is clearly related to feeding and j) it is probably not hormonally responsive.

C. Neural Systems Mediating Aggressive Behaviors

The two modes of aggression are probably subserved by different neural pathways. In support of this contention are the facts that electrical stimulation at discrete sites within the hypothalamus or lower brain stem may evoke only one of the two types of behavior in several different species and that lesions placed at sites from which only one of the types of aggression can be evoked by electrical stimulation results in degeneration along different pathways within the brain (30) (Fig. 6.1).

The neural pathway mediating affective aggression probably is widely distributed in the brain and spinal cord. The principal pathways as defined by electrical stimulation include a series of interlinked neuronal structures running from the amygdala caudally through its two major projections, the ventral amygdalofugal pathway and the stria terminalis, through the lateral hypothalamus and the periaqueductal gray matter into the caudal brain stem (13, 31). It is most likely that the representation of affective aggression is redundant. Portions of the behavior can be evoked by many levels of the neuraxis. It is a neuronal network which is, anatomically, closely related to the spinothalamic tract, a possible explanation for its close relationship to pain responses. The predatory responses are anatomically less well-characterized. From sites in the hypothalamus they seem to project into the ventral midbrain tegmentum (29, 31).

The neural networks from which attack behavior can be evoked by focal electrical stimulation are themselves under modulatory control by other brain regions. The modulatory regions are not themselves critical for the expression of the behaviors but can be demonstrated with excitation to inhibit or facilitate evoked natural aggression (32).

III. METHODS FOR STUDYING CENTRAL NEUROTRANSMITTERS AND BEHAVIOR

A. Criteria for Establishing the Essential Participation of a Central Neurotransmitter in Aggressive Behavior

To establish that an agent present in the brain acts as a neurotransmitter at specific synapses in the central nervous system, a set of generally accepted criteria need to be satisfied (2–4). These include the demonstration that the agent is synthesized, stored and released by specific neurons

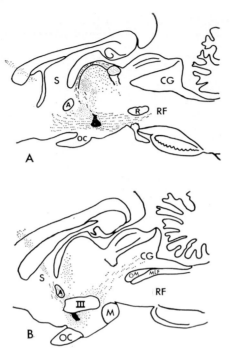

Fig. 6.1. Representative charts of neural degeneration plotted on sagittal sections of cat brain. A, after lesion of site from which electrical stimulation evoked rat killing without affective display (quiet biting); B, after lesion of site evoking affective attack. Note that the quiet killing site projects to the lower brain stem through the median forebrain bundle while the affective killing site projects to periaqueductal gray matter of midbrain. Abbreviations: A, anterior commissure; CG, central gray; M, mammillary body; MLF, medial longitudinal fasciculus; OC, optic chiasm; OM, oculomotor nucleus; RF, reticular formation; S, septum and III, 3rd ventricle. (From Reference 29.)

in the central nervous system, that it is locally inactivated, that it is released by stimulation of these neurons, that when applied to the postsynaptic neurons it mimics the action of the naturally released agent and that pharmacological agents which interact with the synaptically released transmitter should interact with the suspected transmitter in an identical manner. Implicit is the fact that no one single experimental methodology is sufficient to establish the role of a neurotransmitter function for a single compound. Biochemical, pharmacological, anatomical and neurophysiological methods must all be utilized.

Once having determined that a compound functions as a neurotransmitter at one synapse in the central nervous system, however, is not sufficient to establish its critical role as a transmitter mediating a specific

TABLE 6.2

Criteria for establishing the essential participation of a central neurotransmitter in a specific behavior

A. The neurotransmitter should be present in neurons within the central neural networks identified by other methods as necessary for expression of the specified behavior

B. The specific neural system harboring the transmitter should also contain precursors, intermediate metabolites and the enzymatic machinery required for its synthesis and rapid inactivation, either by degradation or reuptake of the transmitter

C. Increased local release of the transmitter should be demonstrated when the behavior occurs spontaneously and is evoked by focal electrical stimulation, brain lesions or both

D. Local application of transmitter at appropriate sites within the neuronal network should evoke the behavior

E. Chronic destruction of the specific neuronal systems harboring the neurotransmitter should abolish the specified behavior and result in disappearance of the neurotransmitter in regions to which the neurons project and which are essential to the behavior; replacement of the transmitter should reverse the effects of such destruction

F. Pharmacological agents which interact with the transmitter or its receptors to enhance or reduce its action should affect the behavior in a parallel manner

behavior. To accomplish this, different criteria need to be met (4). These take into account the facts that behavior in the brain is organized within extensive neuronal networks with regional localization of function and that different neurotransmitter systems in the brain are regionally distributed. The criteria which I believe necessary for establishment of the role of a specific transmitter in a specific behavior are indicated in Table 6.2.

To date no single putative neurotransmitter believed essential for the expression of aggression has satisfied all of the criteria required for establishing its critical role in either affective or predatory aggression.

B. Methods for Studying the Relationship of Neurotransmitters and Aggression

A number of research strategies have been employed in an attempt to determine the role of specific neurotransmitters in different classes of aggression (33). These techniques may be summarized:

1. The demonstration by biochemical methods of differences in the concentration or turnover of specific neurotransmitters in the brain between strains of a species differing in aggressivity, *i.e., natural* (spontaneous (33)) *aggression*. This includes strains of mice with a naturally

reduced threshold for affective aggression (34) or strains of rats with higher probabilities of killing a specified prey such as a mouse (25).

2. The demonstration of altered concentrations or turnover of these agents or their metabolites in the brains of animals made aggressive by a variety of manipulations including isolation, pain, electrical stimulation or selective lesions of the brain. Such aggressive states may be referred to as *evoked aggression* (induced aggression (33)).

3. The modification of natural or evoked aggression by drugs which facilitate or inhibit the availability of neurotransmitters at their receptors. Several classes of drugs have been used for this type of study.

a. The first class consists of drugs which inhibit the activity of enzymes required for the biosynthesis of the neurotransmitter. In this group are drugs such as α-methylparatyrosine, a specific inhibitor of tyrosine hydroxylase (35), the enzyme catalyzing the rate-limiting step in the biosynthesis of catecholamines (36), and parachloraphenylalanine (PCPA), an inhibitor of tryptophan hydroxylase (37), the enzyme catalyzing the rate-limiting step in the biosynthesis of 5-HT (38). The specificity of the enzyme blockade in altering behavior can be further tested by administration of the product of the enzymatic step which is blocked, thereby providing substrate for subsequent synthesis of the transmitter and reversal of the behavior. Thus, the administration of 3,4-dihydroxyphenylalanine (L-DOPA) will result in adequate synthesis of DA and NE after tyrosine hydroxylase is inhibited, and 5-hydroxytryptophan will allow 5-HT to be synthesized *in situ* after tryptophan hydroxylase is inhibited.

b. A second class of drugs consists of agents which facilitate the availability of the neurotransmitter at the receptor. These include (1) drugs which act to release the neurotransmitter directly from the nerve ending such as amphetamine (39) or tyramine, (2) drugs which block the inactivation of transmitters by reuptake into nerve endings such as the tricyclic antidepressants and finally (3) drugs which block enzymes metabolically degrading the transmitter such as the inhibitors of monoamine oxidase (MAO) or cholinesterase.

c. A third class of drugs consists of those which block intraneuronal storage. An example is reserpine.

d. A fourth class of drugs consists of agents which act to block the action of the neurotransmitter postsynaptically. Examples are chlorpromazine and haloperidol, which block central catecholamine receptors, and atropine, which blocks some central cholinergic receptors.

4. The intraventricular or intracerebral injection of the neurotransmitters or their agonists have been used to evoke behavior. Examples of the latter are apomorphine which acts to stimulate DA receptors (42) or carbachol, a powerful cholinomimetic.

5. Finally, attempts have been made by the use of chemicals which have a selective toxicity for specific neurotransmitter systems to selectively destroy neurotransmitter pathways. Examples of this are the use of 6-hydroxydopamine (6-OHDA) to destroy catecholamine pathways in the brain (41–46) or 6-hydroxydopa, which has a more selective action on noradrenergic neurons (45).

IV. THE ROLE OF SPECIFIC PUTATIVE NEUROTRANSMITTERS IN AGGRESSIVE BEHAVIOR

A. Noradrenergic Mechanisms

The neuronal systems in the brain which synthesize, store and release the neurotransmitter NE seem to play an important role in the elaboration of aggressive behavior. Indeed, there is more evidence implicating NE in this form of behavior than for any other neurotransmitter (4). The principal evidence supports the view that release of NE in the brain facilitates affective and inhibits the expression of predatory aggression.

1. Noradrenergic Systems in the Brain

The cell bodies of noradrenergic neurons reside in the mesencephalon, pons and medulla oblongata and send widely ramified axonal processes throughout the brain and spinal cord (Fig. 6.2). On the basis of lesion studies, Ungerstedt (46) has defined two principal pathways: a ventral NE

NORADRENALINE

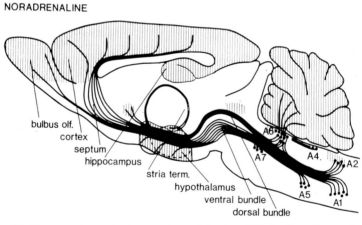

Fig. 6.2. The noradrenergic innervation of brain. Cell bodies of noradrenergic neurons are localized in lower brain stem (identified as A1 to A7) and widely innervate the remainder of the brain. The major nerve terminal areas are indicated by cross-hatching. (From Reference 46.)

system arising from cell groups in the medulla oblongata and pons and a dorsal NE system arising from cell bodies primarily localized in the nucleus locus ceruleus. The dorsal system ascends in the medial reticular formation and enters the median forebrain bundle. It primarily innervates cellular groups in the lower brainstem, mesencephalon and hypothalamus. It heavily innervates the bed nucleus of the stria terminalis, an area integrally involved in the expression of affective aggression (31).

The dorsal pathway arises from the relatively few cells comprising the nucleus of the locus ceruleus located paramedially along the floor of the 4th ventricle at the rostral end of the pons. The processes of these cells are widely ramified, their processes innervating cerebellum, neocortex, several portions of the limbic system including hippocampus and amygdala and also, in part, the hypothalamus. It is likely that collateral branches of the axons of individual neurons of this nucleus may send processes to widely divergent areas of the brain.

2. NE in Affective Aggression

There is considerable evidence that the neuronal release of NE facilitates or possibly initiates affective aggression. The evidence includes the demonstration of: a) increased concentrations or turnover of NE in the brain of animals in whom affective aggression has been induced; b) the initiation of several types of aggression by drugs which facilitate the action of NE within the brain; c) evidence that release of brain NE is closely linked to the affective display of sham rage behavior in the cat.

a. BRAIN NE IN INDUCED AGGRESSION. Rats in whom affective aggression is induced by isolation (see References 33, 47 and 48), the delivery of painful shocks (49, 51) or by forced restraint (52) seem to have increased concentrations or turnover of NE. One of the more interesting experiments in this regard has been recently reported by Lamprecht and his associates (51). In this study rats were repeatedly immobilized daily for 4 weeks. At the termination of the stress period, the rats showed an increase in the amount of shock-induced fighting as well as heightened activity of the peripheral sympathetic nervous system. Four weeks after cessation of daily periods of restraint sympathetic nerve activity, as evidenced by the presence of the enzyme dopamine-β-hydroxylase in the peripheral blood, had returned to normal. However, these animals still retained an increased propensity for fighting in association with a continued elevation in the hypothalamus of the activity of the enzyme tyrosine hydroxylase. The experiment suggests that the persistence of aggression was in some manner linked to the exalted capacity for synthesis of NE.

b. DRUG-INDUCED AGGRESSION. Aggressive behavior has been induced in several species by the systemic administration of drugs or pharmacologically active precursors of NE, all of which serve to increase the efficacy of central noradrenergic transmission. The nature of the aggression induced by noradrenergic-mimetic drugs seems to be attributable to increased irritability. Animals are thus more prone to fight in a group housing situation or when handled, and can thus be considered as expressing a form of affective aggression. Several examples may be cited. First, the precursor of NE, L-DOPA, which can increase the amount of available transmitter, increases fighting in groups of caged animals when administered by itself (53–55), after inhibition of MAO (56–58) or after blockade of 5-HT synthesis by the drug PCPA (59). Whether the effect of L-DOPA is related to the synthesis of DA or NE, or is secondary to the capacity of L-DOPA to release amines from nerve endings (60), has not yet been determined. Second, amphetamine, which excites central adrenergic receptors, increases spontaneous or isolation-induced fighting in rodents (48, 61–64) and facilitates aggressivity of rats during withdrawal from morphine (65). Third, tricyclic antidepressants or MAO inhibitors which increase NE availability centrally, either respectively by blocking the uptake inactivation or by inhibiting metabolic inactivation by deamination, also increase affective aggression (57, 66).

c. NORADRENERGIC MECHANISMS IN SHAM RAGE BEHAVIOR. The evidence for the participation of central noradrenergic pathways in the display of rage in the cat has been reviewed in detail elsewhere (4). The evidence may be summarized as follows.

Electrical stimulation of the amygdala or hypothalamus which produces sham rage behavior in the cat is associated with a fall in the concentration of NE but not DA or 5-HT in the brain (15, 16, 67). Electrical stimulation at adjacent sites failing to produce the behavior does not result in any change of the brain amines (Fig. 6.3). Thus electrical stimulation of the brain can selectively decrease brain NE concentrations but only when such stimulation can evoke the specific behavior.

A high decerebrating lesion which produces spontaneous recurrent attacks of rage (Fig. 6.4) also results, after several hours, in a fall in the concentration of NE but not 5-HT in the lower brain stem (11). A decerebrating lesion placed slightly caudal at the intercollicular level, and which fails to result in spontaneous rate (but leaves intact the display of rage to noxious stimulation (11, 68, 69)), does not result in any change in the amine concentration in the same areas of the lower brain stem (Fig. 6.5). This finding, taken together with the observation of selective decrease of brain NE when sham rage is evoked by electrical brain stimulation, is further evidence that the fall of NE concentration is specific for the behavior.

The fall of brain NE is the result of increased activity of noradrenergic

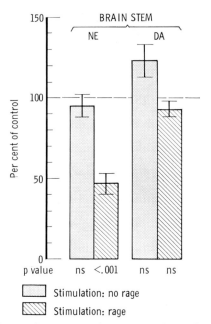

Fig. 6.3. Relative changes in concentration of norepinephrine (NE) and dopamine (DA) in brain stem and forebrain, respectively, after 3 hours of intermittent stimulation of amygdala in cat producing rage or no rage (Adapted from Reference 15.)

neurons and not the consequence of diminished amine synthesis. NE concentrations fall because the neurally mediated release of the transmitter is increased (70–72) and is in excess of the rate of neuronal resynthesis. It seems to occur in most, if not all, of the NE terminals throughout the brain stem (70, 71). The augmented neural activity of noradrenergic neurons is not the result of body movement or of changes in cardiovascular function associated with the induced behavior inasmuch as it occurs even after spinal cord transection abolishes all movement and reflex cardiovascular activity (11). The noradrenergic neuronal activity therefore probably represents a release of brain stem noradrenergic neurons from suprasegmental inhibition.

The release of NE in the brain is proportional to the intensity of the evoked behavior (73). Because drugs which facilitate the action of NE centrally enhance the behavior, whereas drugs which reduce the action of the amine attenuate it, we have proposed that the central neuronal release of NE may trigger parts or all of the behavior (4, 73). Furthermore, drug studies have suggested that it is only a small percentage of the NE in the brain, primarily that which is newly synthesized, which is required to trigger the attacks of rage (4, 56). The precise localization of regions in

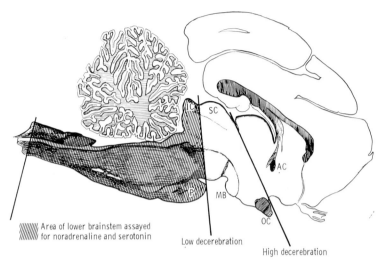

IC

SC

AC

P

MB

OC

//////// Area of lower brainstem assayed
//////// for noradrenaline and serotonin

Low decerebration

High decerebration

Fig. 6.4. Schematic representation of midsaggital section of cat brain showing plane of transection producing sham rage (high decerebration) or quiet behavior (low decerebration). The area of brain stem (cross-hatched) assayed for norepinephrine lies between line to left (at first cervical segment) and plane of low decerebration. Cerebellum and remainder of brain were not assayed. AC, anterior commissure; IC, inferior colliculus; MB, mammillary bodies; OC, optic chiasm and P, pons (From Reference 73.)

the brain harboring the critical noradrenergic terminals remains unknown.

When attack behavior evoked by electrical stimulation of the hypothalamus is prolonged by 3 days of intermittent stimulation, the activity of the enzymes tyrosine hydroxylase (the rate-limiting step in the formation of catecholamines) and phenylethanolamine-*N*-methyltransferase (PNMT) (the enzyme converting NE to epinephrine) is increased in the adrenal gland (74, 75). The increase in adrenal enzyme activity, probably because of an increase in enzyme molecules, is specific for the behavior and is neurogenically mediated. Stimulation at adjacent sites failing to produce the behavior fails to change the enzyme activity. There is also evidence that tyrosine hydroxylase activity is also increased by such stimulation in the brain (75). The importance of these observations is that they suggest that when attack behavior is prolonged it can produce more enduring changes in the biosynthetic machinery required for the production of the very neurotransmitter which is critical in the expression of the same behavior.

The mechanism by which NE produces its effect on the behavior is not entirely known. The transmitter may be acting to inhibit or excite neu-

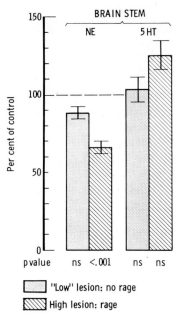

Fig. 6.5. Relative changes in concentrations of brain stem norepinephrine (NE) and serotonin (5HT) in the cat 3 hours after placement of low or high decerebration (Adapted from Reference 11.)

rons in specific areas of the brain. We have proposed that at least some parts of the behavior may result from inhibition by NE of neurons in brain stem regions which are themselves inhibitory to all or parts of the behavior. This conclusion is based on two lines of evidence. First, in the lower brain stem the density of NE terminals is maximal in regions which seem necessary for production of components of the behavior which are opposite in direction to those seen in sham rage. For example, the nucleus tractus solitarii receives a very rich innervation of NE terminals (46, 76). However, electrical stimulation in this nucleus evokes a fall of blood pressure, slowing of the heart rate and even the induction of sleep (77–81). This nucleus also receives an afferent input from carotid sinus baroreceptors (82, 83), stimulation of which facilitates the appearance of quiet behavior or sleep (84). Second, there is considerable evidence that NE, when applied iontophoretically to central neurons, tends to depress spontaneous activity (3, 85). Inasmuch as NE is released in rage in a region which produces behavior opposite to rage and at that site is presumably inhibitory to neuronal activity, it can only be concluded that the appearance of sham rage behavior or some of its components is the result of neural disinhibition. It is of interest that a similar mechanism of disinhibition has been proposed by Stein and Wise (86) as the principal mechanism through which NE acts to augment self-stimulatory behavior.

3. Brain NE in Predatory Aggression

Although there is ample evidence that the release of NE is facilitatory for affective aggression, central adrenergic mechanisms seem to inhibit predatory killing. The conclusion is primarily based on the observations that those drugs which presumably facilitate the action of NE centrally, such as amphetamines, L-DOPA or tricyclic antidepressants, are very effective in blocking muricidal killing in the rat (87–90). The suppression of predation occurs in spite of the fact that these drugs initiate affective aggression in the same species.

Attempts to explain in biochemical terms the opposing actions of the adrenergicomimetic agents in the two classes of aggression have not been altogether satisfactory. The "paradoxical" action of the tricyclic antidepressants in facilitating affective and inhibiting predatory aggression has been interpreted as related to their ability to suppress NE turnover *selectively* in muricidal rats (89). Others have suggested that drugs may, under some circumstances, act like a neuroleptic agent blocking noradrenergic transmission postsynaptically (91). I believe, however, that the contradictory findings can best be reconciled by assuming that it is the site at which NE neurons terminate rather than the NE neurons viewed as a uniform system which determines the role of the amine in specific behavior.

4. Some Contradictory Data

Although a large body of evidence supports the hypothesis that the release of NE from central noradrenergic neurons facilitates or even triggers affective aggression and suppresses predatory aggression, there are several experimental findings which are not easily reconciled with this view.

First are the complex changes in aggressive behavior reported in several recent studies (92–95) in which the drug 6-OHDA, which selectively destroys catecholaminergic neurons (41, 42, 44), or 6-OH-DOPA, a compound with more selective effects on noradrenergic neurons (45), were introduced into the brain. It would be predicted that if NE facilitates affective and inhibits predatory aggression, selective destruction of the NE neuron should result in opposing results, *i.e., inhibition* of affective and *facilitation* of predatory killing. The results, however, do not follow this simple prediction. Thoa and her associates have found that after the intraventricular injection of 6-OHDA or 6-OH-DOPA (45, 92, 93) there was a decrease in shock-induced fighting behavior in rats, a mode of affective aggression. The increase in fighting, however, appeared only gradually after a latency of several days, then continued to increase over several weeks. The delay in fighting did not correlate with the fall of brain NE which occurred much sooner (45), indicating that the reduction of the neurotransmitter was probably not itself the cause of the augmented aggression. It is conceivable that the delay in the increase of affective aggression was caused by the development of a denervation hypersensitivity of central noradrenergic receptors. Stimulation of these receptors could be by a small pool of remaining NE fibers or possibly by overflow from dopaminergic neurons in the critical area. If such is the mechanism of the augmented aggression in these animals, the findings would then be consistent with the NE hypothesis.

The effects of 6-OHDA on predatory aggression have recently been investigated by Jimerson and Reis (94). In these studies the effect of 6-OHDA bilaterally injected into the lateral hypothalamus of rats on the latencies for attack and killing of a natural prey, the frog, were observed. The drug resulted in a reduction in the probability that an individual rat would attack or kill a frog (Fig. 6.6), in the latencies for attack and kill, and in the intensity of the execution of the act of killing itself. The

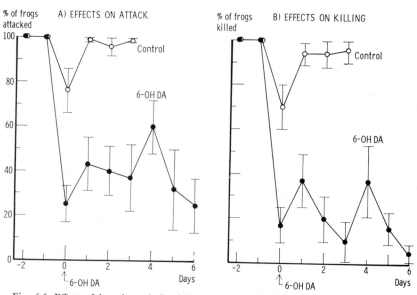

Fig. 6.6. Effect of intrahypothalamic injection of 6-OHDA on predatory behavior in rat. A, effects on attack; B, effects on killing. Each point represents percentage of frogs attacked or killed during five presentations for the group (*n* from 4 to 13) ± SEM for 2 days before and 6 days after intrahypothalamic injections of 32 μg. of 6-OHDA (From Reference 96.)

impaired behavior persisted but was characterized by daily fluctuations. On some days treated animals killed most frogs; on others, none. Although the latencies in treated animals for attack and kill were often increased, on other days these latencies were close to control. Motor activity and feeding and drinking behavior remained depressed throughout. The results of the study would suggest that destruction of catecholamine pathways passing through or terminating in the lateral hypothalamus would impair predatory aggression by interfering with the ability of the rat to initiate sustained killing (a motivational deficit), or in recognizing the frog as prey (a perceptual defect) or in both, and not in the ability to execute and perform the motor act of killing.

A second series of contradictory observations relate to the long standing observations that when NE is introduced intraventricularly it usually fails to produce aggression and indeed may even elicit sedation or sleep (95). Only rarely, when infused in very low (96) or extremely high (97) concentrations has any sort of behavior been elicited. These findings stand in contrast with the fact that intraventricularly administered ACh or carbachol will often produce affective aggression, thereby demonstrating that such behavior can be evoked through the intraventricular route.

The failure of NE, in most circumstances, to produce affective aggression when introduced intraventricularly may reflect the problem of achieving physiological levels of the amine at the appropriate site. For example, NE when microinjected into restricted areas of the upper brain stem has produced outbursts of affective attack in the cat (99).

However, another interpretation is that NE has multiple and possibly opposing actions in the brain. At some sites the amine produced behavioral inhibition, while in others it led to behavioral excitement and aggressive behavior. These contrasting actions possibly could be mediated by different types of adrenergic receptors, α and β. Thus, the diffuse application of NE to central neurons through the ventricles might result in a preponderance of behavioral inhibition masking any excitatory actions of the amine. Conversely, local application by microinjection of the amine might produce contradictory responses depending upon which receptors within the brain it was stimulating. Thus, it is probably the site at which the NE neuron terminates rather than the NE neuron of the uniform system which determines the role of the neurotransmitter in any specific behavior.

B. Dopamine in Aggression

1. Dopamine Systems in the Brain

The cell bodies of the neurons which synthesize, store and release the neurotransmitter DA reside within the substantia nigra and the interpe-

DOPAMINE

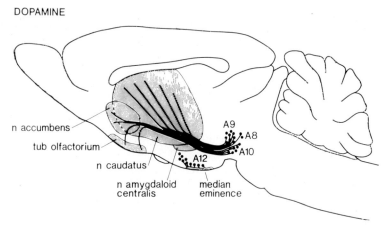

Fig. 6.7. The dopaminergic innervation of brain. Cell bodies of dopaminergic neurons are localized in mesencephalon (A8 to A10) and also in median eminence (A12). The major nerve terminal areas are indicated by cross-hatching. (From Reference 46.)

duncular nucleus (46, 76). The axons of these cells project into the striatum and basal forebrain, thereby exhibiting a far more restricted field of innervation than NE nerve cells (Fig. 6.7).

2. Dopamine in Affective Aggression

The possibility that central dopaminergic neurons, like noradrenergic neurons, facilitate the expression of affective aggression has been suggested by several recent investigations. First, it has been demonstrated that rats treated with apomorphine, a drug which is believed to act as a DA agonist (40), produces intraspecific fighting (99–101). The behavior, which is only seen in adult males (100), is facilitated by isolation (101) or by pain (100), and hence is clearly influenced by the environment. However, it is possible that apomorphine may also activate noradrenergic neurons (102). Second, Lycke and his co-workers (59) have demonstrated that mice infected with herpes simplex encephalitis have an increased synthesis of brain DA and a reduced synthesis of brain 5-HT. The infected animals are exceptionally aggressive and fight intensively among themselves. Since the aggressivity of these mice is reduced by inhibition of DA synthesis with α-methylparatyrosine, it seems likely that the behavior is related to the increased availability of DA, possibly facilitated by reduction of 5-HT. However, the possibility that changes in NE release may also influence the behavior has not been excluded conclusively.

The third line of evidence for the possible participation of DA in facilitating affective aggression is derived from the fact that many of the studies designed to demonstrate the role of NE in aggressive behavior do not exclude the possibility that DA is also involved. Thus, the finding that the production of sham rage by electrical stimulation of the brain results in a fall of brain NE but not DA does not rule out the possibility of augmented turnover of DA. Likewise, the excited and aggressive behaviors induced by the administration of L-DOPA or amphetamine to rats or cats conceivably could involve dopaminergic as well as noradrenergic mechanisms. Scheel-Kruger and Randrup (103), for example, have shown that the aggressivity produced in rats by the MAO inhibitor pargyline is facilitated by inhibiting the synthesis of NE by blockade of dopamine-β-hydroxylase. Everett and Borcherding (55) have demonstrated that the aggressivity in mice produced by L-DOPA is best correlated with levels of newly formed DA rather than NE. In addition, amphetamines, which evoke affective aggression, also increase the availability of DA as well as NE and their respective receptors (104). The amphetamine-induced aggression can be effectively blocked by neuroleptic agents believed more effective in blocking DA than NE (105).

Dopaminergic mechanisms, on the other hand, cannot account for all of the actions on affective aggression attributed to NE. For example, recurrent attacks of sham rage (which are facilitated by tricyclic antidepressants) can be evoked by decerebrating lesions (11) which destroy most of the DA terminals in basal ganglia and limbic forebrain (46).

3. Dopamine in Predatory Aggression

There have been no studies designed to examine the role of DA in predatory aggression. However, all drugs which would be expected to enhance the availability of DA at their receptors, such as amphetamine, L-DOPA and monoamine oxidase inhibitors, block predatory aggression (87, 88). Thus, if DA plays a role in modulating this class of aggressive behavior, it would be inhibitory.

C. Cholinergic Mechanisms

1. Cholinergic Systems

Those neurons synthesizing, storing and releasing the neurotransmitter acetylcholine (ACh) in the brain have a much wider distribution than those harboring the monoamine neurotransmitters. The absence of a specific histochemical method for identifying ACh has not permitted an extensive and specific mapping of the cholinergic neurons. However, by use of histochemical staining for cholinesterase Shute and Lewis have broadly outlined the probable cholinergic pathways (106, 107). These are much more extensively organized within the brain than are the monoaminergic projections and include intersegmental projections in reticular and limbic systems as well as locally restricted interneurons.

2. ACh and Affective Aggression

There is considerable pharmacological evidence that in addition to noradrenergic neurons, central cholinergic mechanisms participate in the neural organization of affective aggression. When introduced into the third or lateral ventricles of the cat, ACh or its congenor carbachol evoke a fully developed display of angry behavior (108, 109) and affective attack. In some studies (108–110) the behavior has been attributed to the development of seizure discharges in the hippocampus or amygdala. It has also been proposed that the behavior is triggered by the diffusion by the agent to critical sites located near the walls of the 3rd ventricle or the periaqueductal gray matter (108). However, the local injection of cholinergic agents into specific intercranial sites has produced affective display in the cat and rat (98, 111), without the appearance of seizure activity in simultaneously monitored EEGs (99).

3. ACh in Predatory Aggression

Whereas ACh can clearly elicit affective attack behavior, the most compelling evidence for the participation of central cholinergic networks in aggression is the demonstration of its role in the regulation of predatory killing, particularly in the elegant studies of Bandler. Using as a model predatory frog-killing behavior in the rat (26), Bandler demonstrated (112, 113) that a lethal attack on a frog could be facilitated by intracerebral injection of carbachol or ACh (in conjunction with a cholinesterase inhibitor) at specific sites in the lateral hypothalamus (Fig. 6.8), medial or midline thalamic nuclei and ventral midbrain tegmentum. The cholinergic effect seemed specifically related to evocation of predatory aggression by ACh because of the stereotyped nature of the killing response, the lack of increased irritability of the animals and the correspondence of sensitive sites to those areas in the rat or cat from which electrical stimulation could elicit or facilitate predatory aggression. Significantly, local injection of the cholinesterase inhibitor neostigmine at active hypothalamic sites also facilitated the behavior although systemic injection of atropine depressed it. These findings are important in that they suggest that it is the naturally occurring synaptic release of ACh which facilitates predatory killing. They also indicate that the effects of the topical application of cholinergic agents to the hypothalamus do not act indirectly by releasing other amines, particularly catecholamines (104).

More provocatively, Smith and his co-workers (114) have described the production of mouse-killing behavior in rats which were not constitutionally killers by intercerebral injection of carbachol into lateral hypothalamus. Neostigmine also produced killing in nonkillers, whereas atropine blocked predatory killing in "killer" rats. These experiments differed

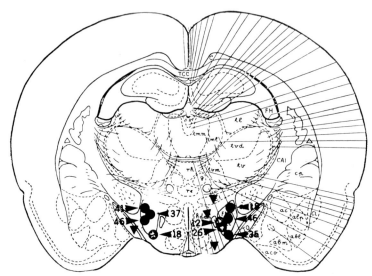

Fig. 6.8. Section of hypothalamus of rat indicating location of cannula tip from which cholinergic agents facilitated predatory aggression (dot) or no effect (triangle). The number beside each symbol refers to coded number of subject (From Reference 112.)

from Bandler's in that Bandler was unable, within the dose range that he used, to convert non-mouse-killing rats to mouse killers by cholinomimetic drugs.

The detailed anatomy of the cholinergic pathways subserving the predatory aggressive responses is as yet unknown. However, it is probable that they lie in part within the trajectories of the descending pathways which subserve predatory aggression as described by Chi and Flynn (29, 30), and overlap, in part, the central cholinergic systems described by Shute and Lewis (106, 107).

D. Serotonergic Mechanisms

The neural systems synthesizing, storing and releasing the neurotransmitter 5-HT are, within the brain, relatively restricted. The cell bodies of these neurons are localized to the raphe nuclei sending their axons rostrally and caudally to widely innervate the brain and spinal cord (46, 77).

The present evidence suggests that 5-HT is preponderantly inhibitory to several modes of aggressive behavior. Most of the data is pharmacological and based on experiments in which the synthesis of 5-HT is blocked by inhibiting the enzyme trytophan hydroxylase by PCPA. In this manner, it has been demonstrated that shock-induced spontaneous fighting or predatory killing in the rat (115–119), or aggressiveness and rat killing in the cat (120), are increased after treatment with PCPA. Sheard

(115) has shown that an increase in aggressivity in the rat is associated with a fall of brain 5-HT and of its principal metabolite, 5-hydroxyindole acetic acid, and may be returned to normal levels by treatment with a precursor, 5-hydroxytryptophan. These findings would indicate that the behavioral action of PCPA is attributable to its blockade of the synthesis of 5-HT. It has also been postulated that the antiaggressive action of lithium in rat and man (121, 122) is caused by an enhancement by the drug of the availability of 5-HT.

Drug-induced aggressivity is also facilitated by inhibition of 5-HT synthesis. For example, in mice, a dose of L-DOPA, which by itself fails to affect behavior, will, after PCPA pretreatment (59), evoke aggressivity. Likewise, aggressive pecking behavior in the chick can be evoked by amphetamines only after PCPA pretreatment (123).

There is little evidence that direct excitation of serotonergic neurons will inhibit predatory aggression. Kulkarni's observation that 5-HT will block muricidal behavior in the rat is consistent with the view that 5-HT release is inhibitory for predatory as well as affective aggression (124).

V. SUMMARY AND CONCLUSIONS

The expression of aggressive behavior in higher vertebrates is primarily mediated by two neurologically distinct systems. The first, ubiquitously distributed in vertebrates, subserves the expression of *affective* aggression. The second, possibly only developed in predators, subserves *predatory* aggression. The two classes of aggression differ in their autonomic, somatic and behavioral manifestations, the evoking stimuli and their sensitivity to hormones. Large portions of the neuronal network subserving each type of aggression also differ.

All available evidence suggests that several compounds including NE, DA, ACh and 5-HT, believed to act as neurotransmitters in the central nervous system, may have characteristic actions on each class of aggression (Fig. 6.9) implying, thereby, that specific neuronal systems which synthesize, store and release these agents are differently engaged. At present, the largest body of data suggests that the release of the catecholamine NE facilitates and in some cases may trigger the expression of affective aggression. Whether the amine acts to modulate all or merely portions of the behavior, as for example the intense alerting, is unknown. On the other hand, the same transmitter seems to inhibit predatory aggression. The mechanism whereby a single transmitter facilitates one and inhibits another closely allied behavior is unknown. Conceivably, it could relate to either the selective action of different neuronal groups releasing an identical transmitter or to differences in adrenergic receptor mechanisms in different regions of the brain.

ACTION OF SOME NEUROTRANSMITTERS
ON THE TWO CLASSES OF AGGRESSION

Neurotransmitter	Class of aggression	
	Affective	Predatory
Norepinephrine –	↑↑	↓
Dopamine -------	↑?	↓?
Acetylcholine ---	↑	↑↑
Serotonin-------	↓	↓

Fig. 6.9. Different actions of some central neurotransmitters on two classes of aggression.

Cholinergic mechanisms, on the other hand, seem primarily involved in the facilitation or triggering of the central neural networks mediating predatory aggression. ACh also seems to facilitate affective aggression. The roles of DA and 5-HT are uncertain. On the basis of the limited available data, DA seems to act like NE, facilitating affective and inhibiting predatory aggression. The action of 5-HT seems to be inhibitory for both classes of aggression.

The foregoing considerations lead to several conclusions. First, no single transmitter serves a unique codon for either class of aggression. Several and possibly many other neurotransmitters seem to interact in their expression. Second, the behavioral action of the various neural transmitters is not uniquely limited to aggression. Each of these agents has been considered to participate in other behaviors as well. For example, NE and ACh both have been implicated as neurotransmitters subserving the hypothalamic regulation of eating and drinking. Thus, each transmitter serves multiple behaviors while several behaviors are subserved by multiple transmitters.

Any consideration of the neurochemistry of aggression ultimately leads to reflections on the possible chemical control of violence and aggressive behavior in man. At present so little is known of neural substrates and the molecular basis of human behavior that extrapolations from animal investigations are at best dangerous and premature. There are, however, two considerations arising from animal studies which bear on the problem of the control of human aggression by drugs which act upon the central neurotransmitter systems. First, the plurality of neural transmitters mediating aggression suggests that blockade of the action of only one transmitter would be unlikely to control all types of aggressive behavior. Secondly, the multiplicity of behaviors subserved by any one transmitter raises the question of whether any drug would be able to have a selective action on aggression without affecting other types of behaviors.

Further elaboration of the problem must await more detailed studies of the neural pathways that subserve different types of aggressive behavior, the identification of the transmitters within each network and the critical applications of neurochemical, neurophysiological and pharmacological methods to identify the dynamic chemical changes which occur during the aggressive acts themselves.

REFERENCES

1. MILLER, NE: Chemical coding of behavior in the brain. Science 148: 328, 1965.
2. WERMAN, R: Criteria for identification of a central nervous system transmitter. Comp Biochem Physiol 18: 745, 1966.
3. PHILLIS, JW: The Pharmacology of Synapses. Oxford, Pergamon Press, 1970, p. 1.
4. REIS, DJ: The relationship between brain norepinephrine and aggressive behavior. Res Publ Assoc Res Nerv Ment Dis 50: 266, 1972.
5. MOYER, KE: Kinds of aggression and their physiological basis. Commun Behav Biol 2: 65, 1968.
6. FLYNN, JP, VANEGAS, H, FOOTE, W, EDWARDS, S: Neural mechanisms involved in a cat's attack on a rat, in Neural Control of Behavior, edited by Whalen, RE, Thompson, RF, Verzeano, M, Weinberger, NF. New York, Academic Press, 1970, p. 135.
7. WASMAN, M, FLYNN, JP: Directed attack elicited from hypothalamus. Arch Neurol 6: 220, 1962.
8. BARD, P: A diencephalic mechanism for the expression of rage with special reference to the sympathetic nervous system. Am J Physiol 84: 490, 1928.
9. ABRAHAMS, VC, HILTON, SM, ZBROZYNA, A: Active muscle vasodilatation produced by stimulation of the brainstem: Its significance in the defense reaction. J Physiol 154: 491, 1960.
10. HESS, WR: The Functional Organization of the Diencephalon. New York, Grune & Stratton, 1957.
11. REIS, DJ, MIURA, M, WEINBREN, M, GUNNE, L-M: Brain catecholamines: relation to defense reaction evoked by acute brainstem transection in cat. Science 156: 1768, 1967.
12. AKERT, K: Diencephalon, in Electrical Stimulation of the Brain, edited by Sheer, DE. Austin, University of Texas Press, 1961, p. 288.
13. FERNANDEZ DE MOLINA, A, HUNSPERGER, RW: Organization of the subcortical system governing defense and flight reactions in the cat. J Physiol (Lond) 160: 200, 1962.
14. DELGADO, JMR: Free behavior and brain stimulation. Int Rev Neurobiol 6: 349, 1964.
15. REIS, DJ, GUNNE, L-M: Brain catecholamines: relation to the defense reaction evoked by amygdaloid stimulation in the cat. Science 149: 450, 1965.
16. GUNNE, L-M, LEWANDER, T: Monoamines in brain and adrenal glands of cat after electrically induced defense reaction. Acta Physiol Scand 67: 405, 1966.

17. REIS, DJ, MOORHEAD II, DT, RIFKIN, M, JOH, T, GOLDSTEIN, M: Changes in enzymes synthesizing catecholamines resulting from hypothalamic stimulation producing attack behavior in cat. Trans Am Neurol Assoc 95: 104, 1970.

18. ADAMS, DB: The activity of single cells in the midbrain and hypothalamus of the cat during affective defense behavior. Arch Ital Biol 106: 243, 1968.

19. ADAMS, DB, BACCELLI, G, MANCIA, G, ZANCHETTI, A: Cardiovascular changes during naturally elicited fighting behaviour in the cat. Am J Physiol 216: 1226, 1969.

20. HUTCHINSON, RR, ULRICH, R, AZRIN, NH: Effects of age and related factors on the pain-aggression reaction. J Comp Physiol Psychol 59: 365, 1965.

21. ULRICH, R: Pain as a cause of aggression. Am Zool 6: 643, 1966.

22. FOLKOW, B, LISANDER, B, TUTTLE, RS, WANG, SC: Changes in cardiac output upon stimulation of the hypothalamic defence area and the medullary depressor area in the cat. Acta Physiol Scand 72: 220, 1968.

23. REIS, DJ, MOORHEAD, D, WOOTEN, GF: Differential regulation of blood flow to red and white muscle in sleep and defense behavior. Am J Physiol 217: 541, 1969.

24. HERNANDEZ-PEON, R, SCHERRER, H, JOUVET, M: Modification of electrical activity in cochlear nucleus during "attention" in unanesthetized cats. Science 123: 331, 1956.

25. KARLI, P, VERGNES, M, DIDIERGERGES, F: Rat-mouse interspecific aggressive behavior and its manipulation by brain ablation and brain stimulation, in Aggressive Behavior, edited by Garattini, S, Sigg, EB. Amsterdam, Excerpta Medica Foundation, 1969, p. 47.

26. BANDLER, RJ, MOYER, KE: Animals spontaneously attacked by rats. Commun Behav Biol 5: 177, 1970.

27. KING, MB, HOEBEL, BG: Killing elicited by brain stimulation in rat. Commun Behav Biol 2: 173, 1968.

28. PANKSEPP, J: Aggression elicited by electrical stimulation of the hypothalamus in albino rats. Physiol Behav 6: 321, 1971.

29. CHI, C, FLYNN, JP: Neural pathways associated with hypothalamically elicited attack behavior in cats. Science 171: 703, 1971.

30. CHI, C, FLYNN, JP: Neuroanatomic projections related to biting attack elicited from hypothalamus in cats. Brain Res 35: 49, 1971.

31. KAADA, B: Brain mechanisms related to aggressive behavior, in Brain Function. Vol. 5: Aggression and Defense: Neural Mechanisms and Social Patterns, edited by Clemente, CD, Lindsley, DB. Los Angeles, University of California Press, 1967, p. 95.

32. EGGER, MD, FLYNN, JD: Effects of electrical stimulation of the amygdala on hypothalamically elicited attack in cats. J Neurophysiol 206: 705, 1963.

33. VALZELLI, L: Drugs and aggressiveness. Adv Pharmacol 5: 79, 1967.

34. LAGERSPETZ, KMJ: Aggression and aggressiveness in laboratory mice, in Aggressive Behavior, edited by Garattini, S, Sigg, EB. Amsterdam, Excerpta Medica Foundation, 1969, p. 77.

35. SPECTOR, S, SJOERDSMA, A, UDENFRIEND, S: Blockade of endogenous norepinephrine synthesis by α-methyl-tyrosine, an inhibitor of tyrosine hydroxylase. J Pharmacol Exp Ther 147: 86, 1965.

36. NAGATSU, T, LEVITT, M, UDENFRIEND, S: Tyrosine hydroxylase. J Biol Chem 239: 2910, 1964.

37. KOE, BK, WEISSMAN, A: p-Chlorophenylalanine: a specific depletor of brain serotonin. J Pharmacol Exp Ther 154: 499, 1966.

38. GREEN, H, SAWYER, JL: Demonstration, characterization, and assay procedure of tryptophan hydroxylase in rat brain. Anal Biochem 15: 53, 1966.

39. CARR, LA, MOORE, KE: Effects of amphetamine on the contents of norepinephrine and its metabolites in the effluent of perfused cerebral ventricles of the cat. Biochem Pharmacol 19: 2361, 1970.

40. ERNST, AM: Mode of action of apomorphine and dexamphetamine on gnawing compulsion in rats. Psychopharmacologia 10: 316, 1967.

41. BLOOM, FE, ALGERIA, S, GROPETTI, A, REVUELTA, A, COSTA, E: Lesions of central norepinephrine terminals with 6-OH-dopamine: biochemistry and fine structure. Science 166: 1284, 1969.

42. URETSKY, NJ, IVERSEN, LL: Effects of 6-hydroxydopamine on catecholamine containing neurons in the rat brain. J Neurochem 17: 269, 1970.

43. SMITH, GP, STROHMAYER, AJ, REIS, DJ: Effect of lateral hypothalamic injections of 6-hydroxy-dopamine on food and water intake in rats. Nature New Biol 235: 27, 1972.

44. BREESE, GR, TRAYLOR, TD: Effects of 6-hydroxy-dopamine on brain norepinephrine and dopamine; evidence for selective degeneration of catecholamine neurons. J Pharmacol Exp Ther 174: 413, 1970.

45. THOA, NB, EICHELMAN, B, RICHARDSON, JS, JACOBOWITZ, D: 6-Hydroxydopa depletion of brain norepinephrine and the facilitation of aggressive behavior. Science 178: 75, 1972.

46. UNGERSTEDT, U: I. Stereotaxic mapping of the monoamine pathways in the rat brain. Acta Physiol Scand 367: 1, 1971.

47. WELCH, BL, WELCH, AS: Effects of grouping on the level of brain norepinephrine in white Swiss mice. Life Sci 4: 1011, 1965.

48. WELCH, BL, WELCH, AS: Aggression and the biogenic amine neurohumors, in Aggressive Behavior, edited by Garattini, S, Sigg, EB. Amsterdam, Excerpta Medica Foundation, 1969, p. 179.

49. KETY, SS, JAVOY, F, THIERRY, A-M, JULOU, I, GLOWINSKI, J: A sustained effect of electroconvulsive shock on the turnover of norepinephrine in the central nervous system of rat. Proc Nat Acad Sci 58: 1249, 1967.

50. MUSACCHIO, JM, JULOU, L, KETY, SS. GLOWINSKI, J: Increase in rat brain tyrosine hydroxylase activity produced by electronconvulsive shock. Proc Nat Acad Sci 63: 1117, 1969.

51. BLISS, EL, AILION, J, ZWANZIGER, J: Metabolism of norepinephrine, serotonin and dopamine in rat brain with stress. J Pharmacol Exp Ther 164: 122, 1968.

52. LAMPRECHT, F, EICHELMAN, BS, THOA, NB, WILLIAMS, RB, KOPIN, IJ: Rat fighting behavior: serum dopamine-β-hydroxylase and hypothalamic tyrosine hydroxylase. Science 177: 1214, 1972.

53. VANDER WENDE, C, SPOERLEIN, MT: Psychotic symptoms induced in mice by the intravenous administration of solutions 3,4-dihydroxyphenylalanine (DOPA). Arch Int Pharmacodyn Ther 137: 145, 1962.

54. RANDRUP, A, MUNKVAD, I: DOPA and other naturally occurring substances as causes of stereotypy and rage in rats. Acta Psychiat Scand 42: suppl. 191, 193, 1966.

55. EVERETT, GM, BORCHERDING, JW: L-Dopa: Effect on concentrations of dopamine, norepinephrine and serotonin in brains of mice. Science 168: 849, 1970.

56. REIS, DJ, MOORHEAD II, DT, MERLINO, N: DOPA-induced excitement in cat and its relationship to brain norepinephrine concentrations. Arch Neurol 22: 31, 1970.

57. EVERETT, GM, WIEGAND, RG: Non-hydrazide monoamine oxidase inhibitors and their effects on central amines and motor behavior. Biochem Pharmacol 8: 163, 1961.

58. Scheel-Kruger, J, Randrup, A: Stereotyped hyperactive behaviour produced by dopamine in the absence of noradrenaline. Life Sci 6: 1389, 1967.

59. Lycke, E, Modigh, K, Roos, BE: Aggression in mice associated with changes in the monoamine-metabolism of the brain. Experientia 25: 951, 1969.

60. Ng, KY, Chase, TN, Colburn, RW, Kopin, IJ: L-Dopa-induced release of cerebral monoamines. Science 170: 76, 1970.

61. Randrup, A, Munkvad, I: Stereotyped activities produced by amphetamine in several animal species and man. Psychopharmacologia 11: 300, 1967.

62. Lewander, T: Urinary excretion and tissue levels of catecholamines during chronic amphetamine intoxication. Psychopharmacologia 13: 394, 1968.

63. Lal, H, De Feo, JJ, Thut, P: Effect of amphetamine on pain-induced aggression. Commun Behav Biol 1: 333, 1968.

64. Lal, H, Nesson, B, Smith, N: Amphetamine-induced aggression in mice pretreated with dihydroxyphenylalanine (DOPA) and/or reserpine. Biol Psychiatry 2: 299, 1970.

65. Lal, H, O'Brien, J, Puri, SK: Morphine withdrawal aggression: sensitization by amphetamines. Psychopharmacologia 22: 217, 1971.

66. Schrold, J: Aggressive behaviour in chicks induced by tricyclic antidepressants. Psychopharmacologia 17: 225, 1970.

67. Gunne, L-M, Lewander, T: Monoamines in brain and adrenal glands of cat after electrically induced defense reaction. Acta Physiol Scand 67: 405, 1966.

68. Woodworth, RS, Sherrington, CS: A pseudoaffective reflex and its spinal path. J Physiol 31: 234, 1904.

69. Ellison, GD, Flynn, JP: Organized aggressive behavior in cats after surgical isolation of the hypothalamus. Arch Ital Biol 106: 1, 1968.

70. Fuxe, K, Gunne, L-M: Depletion of the amine stores in brain catecholamine terminals in amygdaloid stimulation. Acta Physiol Scand 62: 493, 1966.

71. Reis, DJ, Fuxe, K: Depletion of noradrenaline in brainstem neurons during sham rage behavior produced by acute brainstem transection in cat. Brain Res 7: 448, 1968.

72. Sweet, RD, Reis, DJ: Collection of (H³) norepinephrine in ventriculo-cisternal perfusate during hypothalamic stimulation in cat. Brain Res 33: 584, 1971.

73. Reis, DJ, Fuxe, K: Brain norepinephrine: evidence that neuronal release is essential for sham rage behavior following brainstem transection in cat. Proc Nat Acad Sci 64: 108, 1969.

74. Reis, DJ, Moorhead, II, DT, Rifkin, M, Joh, T, Goldstein, M: Changes in enzymes synthesizing catecholamines in attack behavior evoked by hypothalamic stimulation in cat. Nature 229: 562, 1971.

75. Reis, DJ, Moorhead II, DT, Rifkin, M, Joh, T, Goldstein, M: Changes in enzymes synthesizing catecholamines resulting from hypothalamic stimulation producing attack behavior in cat. Trans Am Neurol Assoc 95: 104, 1970.

76. Dahlström, A, Fuxe, K: Evidence for the existence of monoamine neurons in the central nervous system. II. Experimentally induced changes in the intraneuronal amine levels of bulbospinal neurone systems; IV. Distribution of monoamine nerve terminals in the central nervous system. Acta Physiol Scand 64: suppl. 247, 1, 1965.

77. Alexander, RS: Tonic and reflex functions of medullary sympathetic cardiovascular centers. J Neurophysiol 9: 205, 1946.

78. Brodal, A: The Reticular Formation of the Brainstem: Anatomical Aspects and Functional Correlations. Edinburgh, Oliver and Boyd, 1957.

79. MAGNES, J, MORRUZI, G, POMPEIANO, O: Synchronization of the EEG produced by low frequency electrical stimulation of the solitary tract. Arch Ital Biol 99: 33, 1961.

80. BIZZI E,, MALLIANI, A, APELBAUM, J, ZANCHETTI, A: Excitation and inhibition of sham rage behavior by lower brainstem stimulation. Arch Ital Biol 101: 614, 1963.

81. CRILL, WE, REIS, DJ: Distribution of carotid sinus and depressor nerves in cat brainstem. Am J Physiol 124: 269, 1968.

82. MIURA, M, REIS, DJ: The termination and secondary projections of carotid sinus nerve in cat brainstem. Am J Physiol 217: 142, 1969.

83. MIURA, M, REIS, DJ: The role of the solitary and paramedian reticular nuclei in mediating cardiovascular reflex responses from carotid baro- and chemoreceptors. J Physiol 222: 1, 1972.

84. BACCELLI, G, GUAZZI, M, LIBRETTI, A, ZANCHETTI, A: Prosso-ceptive and chemoceptive aortic reflexes in decorticate and decerebrate cats. Am J Physiol 208: 708, 1965.

85. BRADLEY, PB: The pharmacology of synapses in the central nervous system, in Recent Advances in Pharmacology, Ed. 4, edited by Robson, JM, Stacey, RS. Boston, Little, Brown & Co., 1968, p. 311.

86. STEIN, L, WISE, CD: Release of norepinephrine from hypothalamus and amygdala by rewarding medial forebrain bundle stimulation. J Comp Physiol Psychol 67: 189, 1969.

87. HOROVITZ, ZP, RAGOZZINO, PW, LEAF, RC: Selective block of rat mouse-killing by antidepressants. Life Sci 4: 1909, 1965.

88. KULKARNI, AS: Muricidal block produced by 5-hydroxytryptophan and various drugs. Life Sci 7: 125, 1968.

89. SALAMA, A, GOLDBERG, ME: Neurochemical effects of imiprimine and amphetamine in aggressive mouse-killing (muricidal rats). Biochem Pharmacol 19: 2023, 1970.

90. PANKSEPP, J: Effect of hypothalamic lesions on mouse-killing and shock-induced fighting in rats. Physiol Behav 6: 311, 1971.

91. YEN, HCY, KATZ, MH, KROP, S: Effects of various drugs on $3,4$-dihydroxyphenylalanine (DL-DOPA)-induced excitation (aggressive behaviour) in mice. Toxicol Appl Pharmacol 17: 597, 1970.

92. THOA, NB, EICHELMAN, B, NG, LKY: Shock-induced aggression: effects of 6-hydroxydopamine and other pharmacological agents. Brain Res 43: 467, 1972.

93. EICHELMAN, BS, THOA, NB, NG, LKY: Facilitated aggression in the rat following 6-hydroxydopamine administration. Physiol Behav 8: 1, 1972.

94. JIMERSON, D, REIS, DJ: Effects of intrahypothalamic 6-hydroxydopamine on predatory aggression in rat. Brain Res 61: 141, 1973.

95. MARLEY, E: Behavioral and electrophysical effects of catecholamines. Pharmacol Rev 18: 753, 1966.

96. SEGAL, DS, MANDELL, AJ: Behavioral activation of rats during intraventricular infusion of norepinephrine. Proc Nat Acad Sci 66: 289, 1970.

97. CORDEAU, JP, DE CHAMPLAIN, J, JACKS, N: Excitation and prolonged waking produced by catecholamines injected into the ventricular system of cats. Can J Physiol Pharmacol 49: 627, 1971.

98. HERNANDEZ-PEON, R, CHAVEZ-IBARRA, G, MORGANE, PJ, TIMO-IARIA, C: Limbic cholinergic pathways involved in sleep and emotional behavior. Exp. Neurol 8: 93, 1963.

99. SENAULT, B: Comportement d'aggressivité intraspécifique induit par l'apomorphine chez le rat. Psychopharmacologia 18: 271, 1970.

100. McKENZIE, GM: Apomorphine-induced aggression in the rat. Brain Res 34: 323, 1971.
101. SENAULT, B: Influence d'isolement sur le comportement d'aggressivité intraspécifique induit par l'apomorphine chez le rat. Psychopharmacologia 20: 389, 1971.
102. MAJ, J, GRABOWSKA, M, GAJDA, L: Effect of apomorphine on motility in rats. Eur J Pharmacol 17: 208, 1972.
103. SCHEEL-KRUGER, J, RANDRUP, A: Aggressive behavior produced by paragyline in rats pretreated with diethyldithiocarbamate. J Pharm Pharmacol 20: 948, 1968.
104. BESSON, MJ, CHERAMY, A, FELTZ, P, GLOWINSKI, J: Dopamine: Spontaneous and drug-induced release from the caudate nucleus in the cat. Brain Res 32: 407, 1971.
105. HASSELAGER, E, ROLINSKY, Z, RANDRUP, A: Specific antagonism by dopamine inhibitors of items of amphetamine-induced aggressive behavior. Psychopharmacologia 24: 485, 1972.
106. SHUTE, CCD, LEWIS, PR: The ascending cholinergic reticular system: neocortical, olfactory and subcortical projections. Brain 90: 497, 1967.
107. LEWIS, PR, SHUTE, CCD: The cholinergic limbic system: projections to hippocampal formation, medial cortex, nuclei of the ascending cholinergic reticular system and the subfornical organ and supraoptic crest. Brain 90: 521, 1967.
108. MacLEAN, PD: Chemical and electrical stimulation of hippocampus in unrestrained animals. II. Behavioral findings. AMA Arch Neurol 78: 128, 1957.
109. BAXTER, BL: Comparison of behavioral effects of electrical or chemical stimulation applied at the same brain loci. Exp Neurol 19: 412, 1967.
110. GROSSMAN, SP: Chemically induced epileptiform seizures in the cat. Science 142: 409, 1963.
111. MYERS, RD: Emotional and autonomic responses following hypothalamic chemical stimulation. Can J Psychol 18: 6, 1964.
112. BANDLER, RJ: Cholinergic synapses in the lateral hypothalamus for the control of predatory aggression in the rat. Brain Res 20: 409, 1970.
113. BANDLER, RJ: Direct chemical stimulation of the thalamus: effects on aggressive behavior in the rat. Brain Res 26: 81, 1971.
114. SMITH, DE, KING, MB, HOEBEL, BG: Lateral hypothalamic control of killing: evidence for a cholinoceptive mechanism. Science 167: 900, 1970.
115. SHEARD, MH: The effect of p-chlorophenylalanine on behaviour in rats: relation to 5-hydroxytryptamine and 5-hydroxyindoleacetic acid. Brain Res 15: 524, 1969.
116. TAGLIOMENTE, A, TAGLIOMENTE, P, GESSA, GL, BRODIE, BB: Compulsive sexual activity induced by p-chlorophenylalanine in normal and pinealectomized male rats. Science 166: 1433, 1969.
117. CONNER, RL, STOLK, JM, BARCHAS, JD, DEMENT, WC, LEVINE, S: The effect of parachlorophenylalanine (PCPA) on shock-induced fighting behavior in rats. Physiol Behav 5: 1221, 1970.
118. SHEARD, MH: Effect of lithium on foot shock aggression in rats. Nature 228: 284, 1970.
119. SHEARD, MH: Behavioural effects of p-chlorophenylalanine in rats: Inhibition by lithium. Commun Behav Biol 5: 71, 1970.
120. FERGUSON, J, HENRIKSON, S, COHEN, J, MITCHELL, G, BARCHAS, J, DEMENT, W: "Hypersexuality" and behavioral changes in cats caused by administration of p-chlorophenylalanine. Science 168: 499, 1970.
121. WEISCHER, ML: Uber die antiaggressive wirkung von lithium. Psychopharmacologia 15: 245, 1969.
122. SHEARD, MH: Effect of lithium on human aggression. Nature 230: 113, 1971.

123. Schrold, J, Squires, RF: Behavioral effects of a-amphetamine in young chicks treated with p-Cl-phenylalanine. Psychopharmacologia 20: 85, 1971.
124. Kulkarni, AS: Muricidal block produced by 5-hydroxytrytophan and various drugs. Life Sci 7: 125, 1968.

DISCUSSION

Dr. Paul D. MacLean (Bethesda, Maryland): That was a full and very interesting presentation. David Jacobowitz and I have been making a comparative study of aminergic pathways in mice, rats and monkeys; and I would like to know why you find most of the NE terminals in structures where you stimulate and get parasympathetic facts. You find the primary concentration of the NE terminals in the septum, in the medial preoptic area, the paraventricular nucleus and the superoptic nucleus. There are these fibers in the perifornical area, further forward in the hypothalamus. How do you explain this puzzling fact?

Dr. Donald Reis (New York, New York): We have addressed that problem in one of our papers. Sham rage in the cat, produced by acute decerebration, is characterized by a large variety of cardiovascular effects, including tachycardia and elevated blood pressure. In the lower brain stem, an important "parasympathetic" area with a large concentration of norepinephrine is the nucleus of the solitary tract (NTS). This is the site of termination of baroreceptors, activation of which inhibits the expression of sham rage. If you stimulate the NTS electrically, the outbursts of rage are inhibited and, in addition, such stimulation produces a fall of blood pressure and slowing of the heart rate. We have postulated that since norepinephrine release produces rage and that norepinephrine is released within the NTS, an area which when excited produces behaviors opposite to those in rage, the norepinephrine, at least in NTS, must act to inhibit systems themselves inhibitory for the behavior. Thus, we believe that the aggressive display of affective aggression represents, in a sense, neural or behavioral disinhibition rather than direct excitation of the behavior.

Dr. Seymour S. Kety (Boston, Massachusetts): I always enjoy Dr. Reis's work because he so nicely dissects complex problems and always makes the appropriate deduction from his studies. I am especially interested in his differentiation on the basis of new evidence between the affective types and the predatory types of aggression, and the implications that different neurotransmitters may be involved.

This raises another question, which stems from Dr. Raisman's presentation, the possibility that testosterone in some way may affect some of these neurotransmitters as a possible means of explaining the aggressivity of the male and the docility of the female. I know that in terms of the human race, it is an inflammatory subject. Still, it has been known for centuries that there is a difference between a bull and an ox; and the only difference, apparently, is in terms of circulating testosterone. It would be interesting if there were a mechanism by which testosterone could affect some of these neurotransmitters.

I find it interesting that dopamine and norepinephrine are both putative transmitters which apparently have different actions at synapses, although we do not understand exactly what those different actions are. It is even more interesting that dopamine is a precursor for norepinephrine and that the enzyme that makes the conversion, dopamine-β-hydroxylase, may be acting as a switch in terms of the relationship between dopamine reduction or the development of a dopamine pathway and the development of a noradrenergic pathway. This is not entirely a revolutionary concept, since Axelrod and Wurtman demonstrated a similar switch enzyme in the adrenal medulla, namely the enzyme PNMT which converts norepinephrine to epinephrine, and showed that corticosteroids played an important role in regulating the output from the adrenal medulla of epinephrine or norepinephrine.

Perhaps testosterone has some such effect on either the development of or the activity of dopamine-β-hydroxylase. If these two transmitters have different effects in terms of aggressivity, would there be the possibility that here may lie a possible interaction between the sex steroid and aggressive behavior?

DR. REIS: At present the possibility that dopamine-β-hydroxylase might be modulated by sex hormones has not been investigated. Personally, however, I suspect that sex hormones might in some manner work at the level of receptors rather than to modify the transmitter.

DR. MACLEAN: What were you going to say about the activation by apomorphine? I have been impressed by the way it seems to send monkeys, turkeys, possums and parrots on a kind of trip, making them hyperactive. They do not fight, but the possum will wake up in the middle of the day and run around, or the turkey will run through the flock. The parrot doesn't move around, but he goes on a kind of talking trip for 20 to 30 minutes.

DR. REIS: McKenzie and also Sennault have shown that apomorphine induces a curious kind of intraspecific fighting in rats dependent upon age and sex. Only older males are induced to fight by the drug. The fighting can also be facilitated by environmental stimuli such as pain. There is some evidence that apomorphine may also interact with noradrenergic systems.

DR. MURRAY GLUSMAN (New York, New York): I think you mentioned that serotonin inhibits attack and PCPA increases aggression. Could you say on what the information is based?

DR. REIS: When animals are given PCPA, which blocks the enzyme tryptophan hydroxylase, they become much more aggressive. You can reverse the aggressivity by the administration of 5-hydroxytryptophan, the product of tryptophan hydroxylase action, thereby short circuiting the block and producing serotonin. The evidence for an inhibitory action of serotonin, however, is primarily pharmacological and, at this moment, is reasonably soft.

Chapter 7

STEROID HORMONES AND AGGRESSIVE BEHAVIOR: APPROACHES TO THE STUDY OF HORMONE-SENSITIVE BRAIN MECHANISMS FOR BEHAVIOR[1]

OWEN R. FLOODY AND DONALD W. PFAFF

The search for brain mechanisms of hormone effects on aggression has several phases. The aggressive responses themselves must be described carefully to characterize stimulus-response sequences which will become the object of neurophysiological study. Hormones affecting agonistic behavior must be identified chemically. Their probable sites of action then can be discovered by techniques for tracing radioactive hormones and implanting hormones in nervous tissue. Finally, linking neurophysiological studies of aggressive responses with neuroendocrine studies of the relevant hormone effects should lead to hypotheses of how neural mechanisms of aggression are altered by hormones. Studies based on similar reasoning have successfully advanced our physiological understanding of the lordosis reflex, a primary mating response in the female rat (1, 2).

Evidence that androgenic hormones facilitate aggression has been provided by several studies with subhuman vertebrates, which are reviewed below. Yet, other studies have yielded conflicting or ambiguous results. We feel that valid generalizations about effects of androgens, and other hormones, on aggression will have to take into account the natural structure and context of the behavior considered, as well as the species and condition of the aggressive animal and its opponent. Emphasis in this review has been placed on studies of intraspecific fighting occurring "spontaneously" or as a consequence of isolation or the limited availability of specific commodities.

Our studies of steroid hormones and aggression have used the female hamster, a convenient laboratory animal which shows high levels of intraspecific aggression without artificial prodding. Description of a "flow chart" of aggressive responses in female-female encounters has proven useful in providing sensitive behavioral measures for behavioral studies, and eventually will facilitate neurophysiological analysis. In the female

[1] Supported by National Institutes of Health Grant HD-05751, a grant from The Rockefeller Foundation for the Study of Reproductive Biology, an NSF Predoctoral Fellowship to O.R.F., and a training grant from NIGMS.

hamster, combined treatment with 17, β-estradiol and progesterone inhibits fighting. Autoradiographic study shows that tritiated estradiol is concentrated by neurons in specific limbic and hypothalamic structures in the female hamster brain, thus providing some evidence for the neural localization of steriod effects on aggression in this animal.

STEROID HORMONES AND AGGRESSIVE BEHAVIOR IN SUBHUMAN VERTEBRATES

Androgens and Aggressive Behavior of Males

In a variety of species, the aggressiveness of a male is related closely to his reproductive condition (3). Such correlations have proved most conspicuous in developing individuals and among seasonal breeders. For example, in young male mice (*Mus musculus*), isolated except during brief daily encounters, the appearance of fighting at 34 to 36 days of age seems to coincide with the attainment of sexual maturity (4, 5).

In seasonally breeding species, the reproductive phase of the annual cycle may be associated with dramatic alterations in social organization (3). Increases in the frequency of male-male antagonism often may be instrumental in the establishment and defense of breeding territories. Gradual increases in the frequency of antagonistic interactions between individuals of the same sex accompany the breeding season in free-ranging ring-necked pheasants (*Phasianus colchicus*) (3, 6). Frequent aggressive episodes among males seem to represent instances of territorial defense and may be related to a seasonal increase in testes weight (see Reference 3 for additional examples in which variations in the frequency of intraspecific aggression may be correlated with breeding cycles, or changes in gonadal morphology).

Field studies of animal social behavior also have focused attention on correlations between the dominance rank or aggressiveness of individual males and their reproductive success. In Uganda kob (*Adenota kob thomasi* Neumann), the reproductive success of an adult male seems to depend upon his ability to successfully defend one of a limited number of territories frequented by sexually receptive females (7). Similarly, among free-ranging rhesus monkeys (*Macaca mulatta*), the sexual activity of individual males is related directly to their dominance ranks (8, 9).

The studies summarized above suggest that the tendency of a male to engage in aggressive interactions with male conspecifics may be related to some correlate of gonadal activity. A more direct approach to the investigation of correlations between gonadal activity and aggressivity has been used by Rose and his co-workers (10). Here, plasma testosterone concentrations of male rhesus monkeys have been measured directly and found to correlate positively with both dominance rank and frequency of aggressive behavior. At least in the case of dominance rank, however, the significant correlation with testosterone levels seems to be attributable largely to the relatively few animals occupying extremely high positions within the hierarchy. Thus, males in the highest quartile, with respect to dominance rank, had significantly higher concentrations of plasma testosterone than did less dominant animals. No significant differences in testosterone levels were observed among males in any of the lower three quartiles.

While strongly suggestive of a causal relationship between androgens and aggressive behavior, the above studies are limited to demonstrating correlations between some indices of male gonadal activity and dominance rank or frequency of participation in agonistic interactions. Such correlations might have arisen from the dependence of both sexual and aggressive activities on some third (internal or external) factor. Thus, while territorial and reproductive activities of the starling (*Sturnus vulgaris*) may bear a fixed temporal relationship to each other, the frequency of aggressive responses seems to depend upon levels of pituitary luteinizing hormone (LH) rather than upon gonadal androgens (11–13). More complete evidence establishing a direct dependence of aggression on gonadal androgens requires the demonstration that castration produces a decrease in the frequency of aggressive behaviors and that this change is reversed by androgen replacement therapy.

At least some strains of mice satisfy these criteria for the androgen dependence of aggressive behavior (e.g., see References 14–17). Beeman (14) staged extensive series of round robin encounters among inexperienced C57 black mice castrated at least 25 days before the beginning of testing. Twenty-five mice segregated among seven groups of 3 to 4 individuals exhibited no attacks or fights in a total of 198 encounters. Following the implantation of testosterone propionate (TP) pellets (estimated to be absorbed at an average rate of 0.15 mg. per day), a subset of the original group consisting of 14 males exhibited a total of 391 attacks and 234 fights in 108 encounters, levels of aggression comparable to those displayed by intact males. The complete removal of androgen pellets from a single group of three mice resulted in a profound decrease in the frequency of aggressive behaviors. Although this group had compiled 48 attacks and 18 fights in the 36 encounters during testosterone treatment, only three attacks appeared in the same number of encounters following the removal of the hormone pellets. Clearly, the castration of male mice typically is accompanied by a decrement in aggressive behavior. This decrease may be partially or totally reversed by treatment with TP. Similarly, hypophysectomy prevents the development of fighting behavior in male mice, and this decrement, also, may be at least partially alleviated by testosterone replacement therapy (16). Direct effects of androgens on neural mechanisms mediating aggression in the male mouse are presumed to be operating in each case.

Other species in which androgens have been implicated in the control of male-male aggressive behavior include the following: the gobiid fish, *Bathygobius soporator* (3, 18); the lizard, *Sceloporus grammicus microleptidotus* (19); domestic fowl, *Gallus domesticus* (20, 21); Japanese quail, *Coturnix coturnix japonica* (22); red grouse, *Lagopus lagopus scoticus* (23); ring doves, *Streptopelia risoria* (24, 25); valley quail, *Lophortyx californica vallicola* (26); the golden hamster, *Mesocricetus auratus* (27–29); the domestic laboratory rat, *Rattus norvegicus* (30); red deer, *Cervus elaphus* (31); roe deer, *Capreolus capreolus* (32) and a chimpanzee, *Pan troglodytes* (33). Inclusion in this list required the demonstration that castration reduces the incidence of aggression in adult males or that androgen treatment of intact or castrated adults occasions an increase in the incidence of fighting or advancement within a dominance hierachy or both. Factors limiting the hormonal dependence of aggression in some of these species are discussed below.

In several studies listed above, individuals subjected to androgen therapy were selected on the basis of low dominance rank or inability to defend a territory. Such individuals may have low levels of endogenous gonadal steroids (see Reference 10). Sexually immature males represent an analogous case. Androgen injections or implants have induced the early appearance of fighting behavior or dominance relations or both among immature males of a variety of species: the lizard, *Anolis carolinensis* (34); domestic fowl (35–37); herring gulls, *Larus argentatus* (38) and the laboratory mouse (39). In the last species, the neonatal castration of males results in a decrement in intermale aggressive behavior unless exogenous testosterone is administered within the few days imediately after birth (15, 40, 41).

Recent experiments have attempted to specify the chemical forms of androgen responsible for hormonally induced aggression. For example, the naturally occurring free alcohol form of testosterone effectively induces fighting behavior in castrated male mice confronted with relatively non-aggressive opponents (group-housed male castrates) (42). Androstenedione, the metabolically oxidized product of testosterone, was ineffective in the elicitation of intermale aggression under the same circumstances. However, castrated male mice confronted with intact, isolated (and presumably more aggressive) male opponents were responsive to the same androgen (43). Here, the implantation of 30-mg. pellets of androstenedione was associated with attack latencies which were significantly lower than those exhibited by cholesterol-implanted controls, and, in fact, were comparable to those associated with TP treatment. Androsterone, dehydroisoandrosterone and dihydrotestosterone are ineffective at inducing aggressive behavior in castrated male mice (42, 43). Orally administered methyltestosterone is similarly ineffective in doses of up to 0.8 mg. per day (44). Finally, administration of the antiandrogenic steroids cyproterone or cyproterone acetate to TP-treated castrated mice (45) or to intact gerbils (46) failed to induce a decrease in the incidence of aggressive behavior, although both antiandrogens exerted significant effects on androgen-sensitive peripheral tissues.

Pecking and bow-cooing directed at stimulus males have been elicited in castrated male ring doves by TP implants in the anterior hypothalamic-preoptic area of the brain (47). Similarly, some elements of aggressive behavior were exhibited by castrated male domestic fowl receiving TP implants in the lateral forebrain (48). TP implants in the preoptic area of capons elicit copulatory behavior, but not courtship or aggressive behaviors (49).

Studies summarized above include many relatively unambiguous demonstrations of the androgen dependence of aggressive behavior in a variety of species. In contrast to this array of consistent results, some other studies have failed to convincingly implicate androgens in the mediation of aggressive behavior. Male starlings and weaver birds (*Quelea quelea quelea* Ploceinae) provide particularly striking examples in that a specific hormone (LH) other than the gonadal androgens seems to underlie agonistic encounters not associated with competition for nest-building materials (11–13, 50). Further negative findings regarding the androgen dependence of aggression have been reported under some conditions for the males of a variety of other species: swordtail fish, *Xiphophorus helleri* (51); the lizard, *Anolis carolinensis* (3, 34, 52, 53); black-crowned night herons, *Nycticorax nycticorax hoactli* (54); pigeons, *Columba livia* (55, 56); ringdoves (57); dogs, *Canis familiaris* (58); the golden hamster (59); the laboratory mouse (15, 17, 40, 44, 60, 61); the laboratory rat (62, 63); roe deer (32) and rhesus monkeys, *Macaca mulatta* (64).

Factors Affecting Hormone Responsiveness

Differences among some of the results summarized above are most troublesome if aggression is considered as a monolithic behavior type, a viewpoint which certainly would be fallacious. Distinct categories of aggressive behavior have been defined according to the stimulus stituation provoking destructive attack (65). Different categories of aggressive behavior may be mediated by different physiological substrates. Thus, hormonal states which modulate aggressive responses in one stimulus context may have little effect when the stimulus situation is altered. For example, TP-treated male ring doves, housed in isolation or in male-female pairs, failed to differ from controls with respect to the incidence of aggressive behavior evoked by handheld conspecifics (57). In contrast, in group-caged unisexual flocks of doves, the administration of TP to low-ranking, submissive individuals resulted in an increased display of aggression and advancement within the social hierarchy (24).

These results emphasize the complexity and context dependence of agonistic behaviors. Factors which must be considered in the interpretation of inconsistent results regarding the hormonal dependence of aggressive behavior include the following: a) possible functions of aggressive behavior in relation to the natural social organization and ecology of the species; b) characteristics of the opponent; c) the species and strain of animal studied; d) the prior experiences and reinforcement history of the individual and e) the system of measurement employed to monitor variations in aggressiveness.

a. Intraspecific aggressiveness may facilitate the distribution of vital resources among the members of a community. Crook and Butterfield (50) have suggested that the degree to which a particular commodity is required for successful reproduction is related to the hormonal basis of competition for that commodity: "Hierarchies established in relation to competition for sexually relevant objectives are likely to be influenced by androgen whereas those in relation to quarrels without sexual significance will not be so affected" (50, p. 383). Accordingly, TP injections do not affect the relative dominance of male weaver birds in agonistic encounters stemming from individual distance infringements, but they do increase success in competitive encounters occasioned by the presence of nest-building materials (50).

b. Within the realm of intraspecific social behaviors, opponents differing in size, age, hormonal condition or all three may provoke distinct reactions on the part of an individual. Tested in treatment pairs in a neutral arena, female mice are quite nonaggressive unless treated neonatally with androgens (15, 66). Moreover, aggression among adult females is not readily modified by exogenous TP treatment in adulthood (15, 67–69). However, an ovariectomized female tested in her home cage against a prepuberal male exhibits significant levels of aggressive behavior, and the aggressiveness of such a female increases with adult TP but seems to be unresponsive to neonatal TP (15). Thus, in several important respects, changing the age/sex class of the opponent and other details of the testing situation reversed the results.

Regardless of hormonal condition, fighting may be observed in a normally nonaggressive animal if provoked sufficiently by a more aggressive opponent. Thus, castrated male rats encountering intact opponents in a neutral area exhibited low levels of several agonistic behaviors (30). Fighting within such pairs was extremely infrequent. Nevertheless, on the rare occasions that violent fighting did occur, castrates fought successfully and were not consistently submissive to their intact opponents. These results are reminiscent of the emphasis laid by Scott and Fredericson (70) upon the importance of pain as a primary releaser of aggressive behavior. As pointed out by the same authors, however, other stimuli, possibly including the sight of a fleeing animal, may bear a similar relation to aggressive behavior. Such a factor may have been instrumental in the unexpectedly high levels of aggression exhibited by ovariectomized female mice paired with prepuberal males (15).

c. Different species, and different strains within a single species, differ in their sensitivity to hormone treatment. For instance, although within treatment pairs of castrated male mice failed to fight in the absence of exogenous TP (14), prepuberally castrated male dogs competed as intensely among themselves for access to a receptive female as did a group of intact controls (58).

Among different strains of mice, the ability of neonatal TP treatment to induce aggression in females varies significantly and may be related to the aggressiveness exhibited by males of the same strain (71). The aggressive behavior of neonatally androgenized females was increased significantly only among females from inbred strains in which normal males exhibited high levels of aggression. Thus, the masculinization of females with respect to aggression apparently requires the activation of mechanisms which are shared with males, but which are normally inactive in females because of the absence of sex hormone during a critical developmental period.

d. Under certain circumstances, the prior experience and reinforcement history of an individual in agonistic interactions may be a more potent determinant of aggressiveness than hormonal state. Mice engaged in a competitive task motivated by aversive stimulation (foot shock) performed largely in accordance with the type of pretest training experienced (72). Individuals trained as "winners" exhibited longer and more intense bouts of fighting than individuals trained as "losers" or individuals receiving no prior training. While androgen status also affected competitive fighting, this seemed to represent an indirect effect exerted by virtue of a positive relationship between androgen treatment and body weight. Similarly, while spontaneous, or isolation-induced, fighting among inexperienced adult male mice requires endogenous or exogenous androgens (14), highly experienced male castrates confronted with a relatively nonaggressive opponent may continue to fight for at least 8 weeks after gonadectomy (60).

Social relationships among laboratory mice may be quite rigid. Having achieved dominance over a conspecific, a male mouse may maintain his high social rank despite severe debilitation induced by vitamin B_1

deficiency (70, 73). In more natural situations, the rigidity of social hierarchies in some species may be caused by the differing reinforcement
histories of individual group members. While the aggressiveness of free-
ranging male valley quail was increased by androgen administration, no
reversals in dominance rank resulted from hormone treatment of submissive individuals (26).

e. Finally, inconsistent results concerning the effects of hormones on
aggressive behavior may stem from idiosyncratic or ambiguous systems of
measurement. Behavioral measures sometimes are described incompletely
or in subjective terms. Moreover, classifications of behavioral responses
sometimes are ambiguous inherently, because some responses occur as
elements in other sequences (*e.g.,* sexual display) as well as in agonistic
ones (*e.g.,* see Reference 22). Even though the sensitivity and relevance
of behavioral elements as measures of aggressiveness may vary with their
placement in the agonistic sequence, measures sometimes are lumped
for the purposes of brevity and statistical analysis (74). The presentation of
a variety of distinct measures corresponding to different intensities of aggressive behavior seems to represent a more informative approach.

Effects of Progesterone and Estrogens on Aggression in Males

Progesterone (P) administration to intact male mice produces a significant decrease in the probability of fighting (17). Similarly, in castrated
male mice, the combinations of P and either TP or androstenedione are
associated with lower frequencies of aggressive behavior than those evoked
by either androgen alone (42, 43). Treatment of castrated male mice with P
alone results either in no significant effect on the incidence of aggression
(42, 43), or in a moderate, but possibly transient, induction of fighting (17).
Significant interactive effects of P upon behavioral events modulated by
androgens occur in the absence of interference with the maintenance of
androgen-dependent peripheral tissues (42, 43). This distinction, and the
ability of high doses of TP to reverse P-induced suppression of fighting
(42), suggests the occurrence of a direct competitive antagonism between P
and androgens at the level of the central nervous system (CNS). Consistent
with this notion is the observation of reduced uptake of tritiated testosterone by the rat brain as a consequence of P pretreatment (75).

Effects of P on bow-cooing in male ring doves (a behavior appearing in
both aggressive and sexual contexts) parallel many of those on male-male
fighting in mice. Systemic P administration suppresses bow-cooing in intact
males or TP-treated castrates (25). P alone does not induce bow-cooing in
castrated male doves. Moreover, the suppression of bow-cooing in intact

male doves during heterosexual pairings was associated with P implants in the anterior hypothalamus, preoptic nuclei and the lateral forebrain system (76). These neuroanatomical loci are similar to those at which TP implants elicited pecking and bow-cooing in castrated male doves during male-male encounters (47).

Effects of progestins on male aggression depend upon the species and conditions of testing. A particularly important consideration may be the age/sex class of the opponent. Progesterone treatment of castrated male hamsters results in enhanced success in encounters with intact nonreceptive females (28, see also 77).

Estrogens have been associated with suppressive effects upon aggressive behavior. In intact male individuals representing a variety of species, estrogens either have suppressed the incidence or vigor of aggressive behavior (immature domestic fowl (36); red grouse (23); mice (17, 78–80) and rats (81) or have had no significant effect (ring doves (57); an immature black-crowned night heron (54); valley quail (26); mice (82) and young rhesus monkeys (64)). Inhibitory effects of estrogens on the aggressivity of intact males could represent indirect effects involving some form of interference with the production, activity or both of testicular androgens. Neonatal injections of estradiol benzoate (EB) result in decreased body weights, decreased relative testes and seminal vesicle weights and a decrement in the amount of fructose in the seminal vesicles of intact male mice (79). The 72 per cent reduction in seminal vesicle fructose (a correlate of androgen titers) suggests that the decreased incidence of fighting among neonatally treated males stemmed from insufficient circulating levels of endogenous androgens, rather than from a direct effect of estradiol upon neural mechanisms involved in the mediation of aggressive behavior. Intact individuals may constitute inappropriate subjects for the investigation of exclusively CNS-mediated effects of exogenous estrogens on male aggressive behavior.

The administration of exogenous estrogens resulted in suppression of the aggressive behavior of castrated male herring gulls (38) and chimpanzees (33). The only clear instance of suppression described in the former study concerned a single male castrate receiving both estradiol dipropionate and TP. (As in the case of intact males, the decrement in aggressive behavior exhibited by this male may be attributable to indirect effects of estrogens upon the effectiveness of circulating androgens, rather than to a direct effect on brain mechanisms modulating aggressiveness.) Clark and Birch (33) describe a single, prepuberally castrated male chimpanzee which exhibited lower levels of success in food competition with an intact partner during periods of treatment with α-estradiol. However, the interpretation of changes in dominance status occurring during hormone treatment is complicated by variable results, and by concurrent changes in test location, known to have dramatic effects upon the social relations of the two males.

Recent studies of aggressive behavior in castrated male hamsters indicate that ovarian implants or exogenous estradiol benzoate (EB) facilitate intermale fighting (28, 29, 83). Untreated male castrates typically exhibit less aggression than, and are submissive to, their intact male opponents. Treatment with as little as 10 to 25 μg. per day of EB results in elevated frequencies of several agonistic behaviors and in increased relative dominance by the castrates. In this regard, EB replacement therapy seems to be at least as effective as is treatment with TP (29). Among Swiss-Webster albino mice, treatment of castrated males with EB facilitates the display of aggressive behavior in encounters with untreated male castrates (84). In contrast, despite similar opponents and test situations, castrated males of the CD-1 strain seem to be unaffected by EB replacement therapy even though TP did facilitate intermale fighting (42).

Administration of exogenous TP or EB to castrated male hamsters proves ineffective at inducing relative dominance over intact females (28). This is consistent with the dominance normally exhibited by intact females over intact males (74).

In summary, if estrogens affect the aggressive behavior of castrated males at all, they operate to increase the incidence of intermale fighting. Thus, in aggressive behavior, as in the case of at least some aspects of sexual behavior (84–86), estrogens may mimic behavioral effects of androgens. In each case, direct effects of estrogens upon central neural mechanisms mediating the behavior in question are presumed.

At least in some strains of mice, pituitary adrenocorticotrophic hormone (ACTH), adrenal steroids under the control of ACTH or both are capable of modulating aggressive behavior (16, 60, 87–89). Particularly in early encounters between inexperienced adult males, adrenalectomy or ACTH treatment results in a partial suppression of fighting behavior (16, 87, 89). Conversely, treatment with corticosterone, dexamethasone or hydrocortisone is associated with increased levels of isolation-induced aggression (16, 87, 89, 90). Deoxycorticosterone does not affect the latency or vigor of isolation-induced fighting in mice (90). Various combinations of adrenal and gonadal manipulations suggest that the adrenals and testes constitute independent systems modulating levels of intermale aggression in mice (89).

Hormones and Aggression in Females

The fighting behavior of many species is sexually dimorphic, females generally exhibiting lower frequencies of aggressive behaviors than males (3, 21). Direct comparisons of ovariectomized and intact females have yielded variable results. Six members of a flock of 12 hens decreased in social rank after ovariectomy (21); no ovariectomized hen occupied a hierarchical position above that of the least aggressive intact individual. Nevertheless, the preoperative ranks of the six operated birds with respect to each other survived gonadectomy, suggesting that not all manifestations of aggressivity were eliminated by ovariectomy. Female swordtails maintained their preoperative social ranks for 1 to 3 months after gonadectomy (51). Similarly, frequencies of aggressive responses exhibited by female rhesus monkeys in male-female encounters failed to vary significantly as a result of ovariectomy (91). In contrast, female lizards (*Anolis carolinensis*) exhibited elevated levels of aggression as a consequence of gonadectomy (52).

The aggressive behavior of adult female mice is relatively insensitive to treatment with TP or EB (15, 66, 67, 84, 92). Whereas fighting occurs in all male-male pairs in which both members have been gonadectomized at 30 days and treated with TP as adults, only 8 per cent of similarly treated female-female pairs exhibit fighting (66). The insensitivity of females to adult TP depends, in part, upon the age/sex characteristics of the opponent. Ovariectomized females tested in their home cages against prepuberal male opponents exhibit significant levels of aggression in the complete absence of hormone replacement, and are responsive to adult TP treatment (15).

Females of a variety of species have exhibited elevated levels of aggressive behavior during adult treatment with androgens: the lizard, *Sceloporus grammicus* (19); canaries, *Serinus canaria* (93); chickens (36, 94–97); herring gulls (38); immature black-crowned night herons (54); ring doves (24) and chimpanzees (98). An increased incidence of aggression among female swordtail fish subjected to prolonged androgen therapy seemed to be incidental to a more complete sex reversal (51). Only within a group of three ovariectomized chimpanzees did the facilitatory effect of TP seem to be duplicated by EB (98). In several other species, EB treatment of adult or immature individuals seems to have little or no effect on aggressivity: swordtails (51); canaries (93); chickens (36, 99) and night herons (54).

In contrast to results summarized above, the aggressive behavior of intact adult female valley quail is insensitive to treatment with either TP or EB (26). Similarly, no changes in dominance rank within groups of immature female rhesus monkeys occurred as a consequence of TP or EB therapy (64). However, at least some classes of aggressive responses exhibited by ovariectomized adult rhesus monkeys tested in male-female pairs may be subject to modification by EB (91). Although the overall level of aggression exhibited by untreated ovariectomized females persisted during EB treatment, aggressive responses which were not associated with mounting attempts by the male partner seemed to increase during hormone therapy.

Sexual dimorphisms in the spontaneous aggressivity of male and female mice, as well as in the responsiveness of gonadectomized individuals to adult TP, have been attributed to a sexually differentiated neural substrate ordinarily "organized" in the genetic male by (endogenous) neonatal androgens (66). The ability of neonatally administered TP to facilitate androgen-aroused fighting in adult gonadectomized female mice provides strong support for this interpretation (15, 66–68, 92, 100, 101). For example, fighting occurred in 95 per cent of the pairs of ovariectomized female mice treated neonatally with 0.5 mg. of TP and tested as adults under increasing doses of TP (66). In contrast, only 20 per cent of pairs treated with oil neonatally fought at any dosage of adult TP. Neonatal effects of TP upon later androgen-aroused fighting may be mimicked by neonatally administered EB (68) or testosterone, but not by androstenedione or the combination of testosterone and androstenedione (100).

The effectiveness with which exogenous androgen is able to "masculinize" the female CNS with respect to aggressive behavior depends upon the timing and extent of early hormone treatment (also on features of the test situation such as the age/sex class of the opponent (15) and on the measures accepted as criteria for the exhibition of aggression (67, 101)). The efficacy of a given dosage of TP seems to be related directly to its temporal proximity to birth (15, 67, 92, 101). Thus, 80 per cent of cages, each housing four females which had been treated with 0.4 mg. of TP within 2 hours after birth, contained at least one wounded individual (101). In contrast, females receiving the same dose of TP 48 ± 1 hour postbirth failed to engage in fighting severe enough to produce wounding. More sensitive indices of aggression demonstrate that single injections of TP (0.4 mg./gm. body weight) may significantly affect aggressive behavior in females treated as late as 12 days after birth (15, 67). In fact, females treated with 0.1 mg. of TP per day for 20 days beginning on the 30th day after birth exhibited significantly more androgen-induced fighting than females treated with oil according to the same schedule (92). While a "critical period" for androgenization may exist for any particular regime of neonatal TP treatment, the limits of this period are flexible. Different regimes of neonatal hormone treatment and different measures of aggression in adulthood may be associated with different critical periods.

Unlike female mice, nonestrous female hamsters (*Mesocricetus auratus* Waterhouse) are highly aggressive and tend to dominate males in heterosexual pairings (74, 102). In fact, the aggressive behavior that appears during interactions between nonreceptive females is very similar to that observed during male-male encounters (74, 102, 103). Various hormonal

manipulations have produced conflicting effects upon the aggressive behavior of female hamsters. Ovariectomy has been associated with a slightly
decreased incidence of female aggression in heterosexual (59, 77, 104) and
unisexual (105) pairings. Vandenbergh (29), however, has been unable to
distinguish between levels of aggression exhibited by ovariectomized and
intact females in unisexual pairings. Kislak and Beach (104) report a small
increase in female aggressiveness during heterosexual encounters consequent to the administration of large doses (0.225 mg. per day) of EB.
Lower doses of EB or TP have not significantly altered the aggressivity or
relative success of females encountering intact males (77). Similarly, EB
and TP therapy have proved ineffectual with regard to the aggressive behavior of ovariectomized females paired with intact females (29, 59, 105).

Progesterone (P) has been associated with increased levels of female
hamster aggression in male-female (77) and female-female (105) encounters. At least in the former situation, the change in female dominance
status consequent to the initiation of P therapy seems to be incidental to
a decrease in the intensity of male aggressive behavior. This suggests the
operation of a progesterone-dependent cue limiting male aggression, rather
than a direct effect of P upon female aggressivity. However, the increased
aggressiveness exhibited by P-treated ovariectomized females paired with
intact females suggests that P may exert both indirect and direct effects
upon female aggressivity. Kislak and Beach (104) have described the failure
of low doses of P to affect the aggressive behavior of two ovariectomized
female hamsters in heterosexual pairings.

The combination of EB and P has been associated with a profound decrement in female aggressivity in heterosexual pairings (59, 104). In female-female encounters, EB plus P also tended to suppress fighting (59).
Whereas 22 per cent of gonadectomized, untreated females initiated fights
during tests with estrous females, no female treated with 6 μg. of EB and
0.4 mg. of P fought under the same circumstances.

AGGRESSIVE BEHAVIOR IN FEMALE HAMSTERS

Behaviors Characteristic of a Typical Female-Female Encounter

An accurate description of the behavior sequences involved in fighting
is crucial in selecting sensitive indices of aggression. The agonistic behavior of male hamsters has been viewed as a somewhat stereotyped chain
of distinctive behavioral elements (103, 106). Figure 7.1 summarizes our
informal description of the sequence of social behaviors characteristic of
encounters between nonestrous adult female hamsters. This scheme is
based upon observations of many such encounters and on the informal
analysis of their records on movie film. This description probably is most

IMPRESSIONISTIC SCHEME OF FEMALE–FEMALE HAMSTER ENCOUNTERS

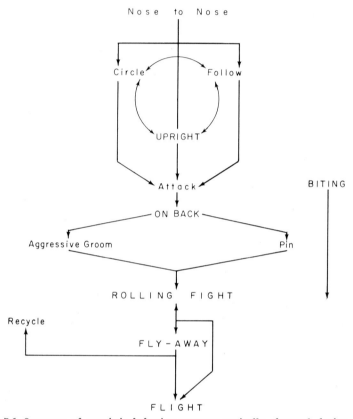

Fig. 7.1. Sequence of agonistic behavior patterns typically observed during a brief encounter between anestrous female hamsters. Capitalized terms denote behavior patterns selected as quantitative measures of aggressiveness. Thin lines connect patterns thought to represent similar levels of aggressiveness. Individual responses included in this scheme are defined in the text. This description of female-female encounters is based upon observations of many such encounters and on the informal analysis of their records on movie film.

representative of the initial encounters experienced by a pair of females. Interactions subsequent to the establishment of highly polarized dominance relationships may be characterized by omissions of some aggressive elements included in Figure 7.1.

The initial stage of an aggressive behavior sequence usually involves mutual investigation, with the noses of the antagonists in apposition and their vibrissae touching (*Nose to Nose* in Fig. 7.1). The timing for each

3-minute encounter was begun the instant that the nose of either individual approached any part of its opponent's body to a distance of 1 cm. or less. Following initial nose to nose contact, one or both females may continue social investigation, mild agonistic behaviors or both in an *Upright* posture (Fig. 7.1). Here, an individual has neither forepaw in contact with the substrate, and is within 1 body length of her opponent. These criteria are objective and may be scored easily from 2-frame per second movies used routinely to quantify the aggressiveneess of hormonally manipulated females. More detailed descriptions of our criteria will be published subsequently (Floody and Pfaff, in preparation).

Circle (Fig. 7.1) refers to a pattern of circular locomotion by both partners in which their bodies are antiparallel, the nose of each near the anogenital region of the other. *Follow* refers to a slow pursuit of one individual by the other, the nose of the following animal usually remaining in close proximity to, or in contact with, posterior regions of its opponent's body. Circling and following occupy positions in the hierarchy of female agonistic behaviors similar to that occupied by mutual sparring in an upright posture. Any of the three patterns may immediately succeed initial nose to nose investigation; they may alternate extensively among themselves, and any may serve as the immediate prelude to an *Attack*.

Attacks (Fig. 7.1) may be launched from either an upright or a sideways posture (in the latter, only the forepaw nearest the opponent is off the substrate, the upper body being rotated to the side accordingly). The sequence of behaviors involved in an attack have as common elements persistent movement by the attacking individual toward her opponent, and the creation of a situation in which an individual is lying on its back or side (*On Back* in Fig. 7.1) with its opponent typically in an upright posture, oriented at a right angle to and hovering over the supine individual. This relationship strongly recommends the on back position as an indicator of moderate levels of aggressive behavior.

A sequence of behaviors which commonly followed adoption of an on back position by one hamster involved intermittent bites of the supine individual by its upright opponent (*Aggressive Groom* in Fig. 7.1). During a bite, activity on the part of the supine hamster would cease, occasioning the release of the bite. In turn, termination of the bite would result in the resumption of movement by the supine individual, leading to another bite. Alternatively, an attacking female may be forced into an on back posture, but may then continue to attack from this position. The less aggressive opponent of such an individual, although in an upright posture, may be fully occupied attempting to hold the attacking female away from its abdomen with its extended forepaws (*Pin* in Fig. 7.1).

Biting is variable with respect to force and with respect to order of occurrence in the chain of hamster agonistic behaviors (Fig. 7.1). Substantial frequencies of biting usually occur first in association with attacks, but are even more closely associated with subsequent behaviors indicative of higher levels of aggressiveness.

Gradually increasing intensities of biting occurring in the course of aggressive grooming may provoke a *Rolling Fight*. This pattern of violent aggressive behavior is highly distinctive and has been described as "fighting" or "locked fighting" by Bunnell and his co-workers (106), Dieterlen (102), Kislak and Beach (104), Payne and Swanson (74) and Vandenbergh (29). Typically, the bodies of the two antagonists are perpendicular to and wrapped tightly around each other, their abdomens in close apposition. Severe and persistent biting, punctuated by frequent vocalization, may occur as the pair rolls wildly about.

Dieterlen (102) has described an aggressive maneuver in which a hamster engaged in a rolling fight disengages himself rapidly with an explosive extension of the hindlimbs. Such a *Fly-Away* (Fig. 7.1) provides an individual with a means of exiting rapidly from an unfavorable encounter. Moreover, the maintenance of a bite during this behavior could result in the severe wounding of an opponent (102). Fly-away represents a behavior typical only of extremely aggressive encounters.

During particularly violent encounters, fly-away sometimes was followed by an immediate resumption of rolling fighting, or by a "recycling" to some earlier phase of the agonistic sequence (Fig. 7.1). An alternative successor to fly-away (or rolling fight) was *Flight,* locomotion directed away from the opponent at a rate of at least 4 body lengths per second. If flight occurred, it defined the end of an encounter, and an opaque partition was immediately inserted between the two contestants. Otherwise, all encounters continued for 3 minutes from the initiation of nose to nose contact.

Measures of aggression scored from movies of encounters between pairs of female hamsters included the latency and total duration of the following: upright, on back, rolling fight and fly-away. The latency of flight and an estimate of the frequency of biting (the percentage of 20-frame (11-second) blocks in which at least one bite occurred) also were tabulated. Finally, the latency and duration of *Lordosis* provided some indication of the sexual receptivity of test females. Rigid and prolonged immobility, a slightly depressed abdomen, a vertical deflection of the tail and a slight elevation of the head were characteristic of this distinctive posture.

Relative latencies of behaviors selected as measures of aggressiveness provide a preliminary indication of the accuracy with which the scheme summarized in Figure 7.1 depicts the agonistic behavior of female hamsters. Each of five pairs of intact female hamsters was tested in six encoun-

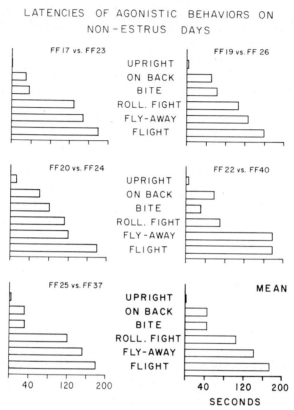

LATENCIES OF AGONISTIC BEHAVIORS ON
NON-ESTRUS DAYS

Fig. 7.2. Observed latencies of agonistic behaviors are compared with the order of occurrence predicted by the scheme of Figure 7.1. Vertical lists of our behavioral measures in the central part of this figure show the expected order of occurrence based on the scheme. Data included summarize all nonestrous encounters experienced by each of five pairs of intact adult female hamsters (*e.g.,* FF17 versus FF23) and the mean latencies averaged across all five pairs (lower right). Encounters lasted 3 minutes or less (maximum latency, 180 seconds).

ters on nonestrous days of the normal 4-day cycle. These were different encounters than those which generated the scheme. Behavior patterns described above have been listed in the central portion of Figure 7.2 in the order in which they appear in the scheme of Figure 7.1. The relative latencies of these behaviors (Fig. 7.2) provide convincing support for the scheme. Behaviors appearing early in the scheme, and considered to be indicative of relatively low levels of aggressiveness, have short latencies. Conversely, behaviors considered to represent intense aggression, and occupying later positions within the scheme, are characterized by relatively long latencies. The variability in the initial occurrence of biting also is incorporated into the "typical" sequence of Figure 7.1. Thus, to a first approximation, this description seems to reflect accurately the chain of behavioral elements characteristic of encounters between adult nonestrous hamsters. Indices of aggressiveness selected on the basis of this description seem well suited to describing variations in female aggressivity accompanying natural or experimentally induced fluctuations in hormonal state.

Variations in the Aggressive Behavior of Female Hamsters During the Normal Estrous Cycle

Each of five pairs of intact adult female hamsters experienced a series of eight 3-minute encounters in a clean neutral arena. The two members of each pair were cycling synchronously and were matched for body weight. For each pair, two tests were conducted on each of the 4 days of the normal estrous cycle. Different pairs began the sequence of eight regularly spaced tests at different stages of the estrous cycle. The aggressive response elements described above were scored from movies (2 frames per second) of each encounter. Any behavior which failed to appear during a particular encounter was assigned a latency equal to the duration of that encounter (180 seconds, or less if flight terminated the encounter).

Latencies of all agonistic behaviors considered indicate that levels of female-female aggression are lower on estrus day ("day 1") than on any of the other 3 days of the cycle (Fig. 7.3). Latencies of on back and rolling fight are significantly longer on estrus day ($P < 0.05$ for comparisons of day 1 with each of days 2, 3 and 4, sign test, see Reference 107). These results are remarkably consistent across all pairs of females (Figs. 7.4 and 7.5). Moreover, on back and rolling fight occur in fewer encounters on estrus day than on other days of the cycle (Table 1). The most pronounced cyclic variations in aggressiveness are shown by these moderate to high intensity agonistic behaviors. A more preliminary behavior, upright, tends to occur in a high percentage of encounters with low latencies. Conversely, the most intense responses, fly-away and flight, rarely occur (Table 1), and have average latencies close to 180 seconds throughout the estrous cycle (Fig. 7.3). Under our conditions of testing, latencies of biting are variable throughout the estrous cycle. Estrous female rodents sometimes are observed to gently bite the skin of inactive males, and this may account for the relatively high frequencies of biting by estrous female hamsters in these encounters. The development of severe biting, associated with high levels of aggressivity, may require particular responses on the part of the bitten individual to initial oral contact concerned with social investigation or sexual arousal as well as aggression. In contrast to agonistic behaviors, which occur less frequently and with longer latencies on estrus day, lordosis occurs with minimal latency on estrus day (Figs. 7.3 and

MEAN LATENCIES OF EACH BEHAVIOR

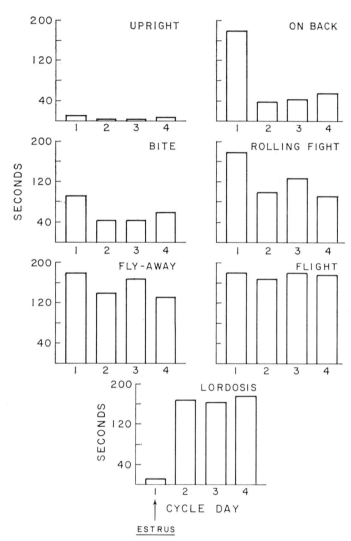

Fig. 7.3. Mean latencies of seven behavior patterns during the normal 4-day estrous cycle. Each bar summarizes the mean latency observed in 10 encounters (five female-female pairs) on a particular day of the cycle. Estrus day is designated day 1, and non-estrous days are days 2 to 4. The maximum latency attainable is 180 seconds. Latencies of On Back, Rolling Fight and Lordosis on day 1 differ significantly from those on days 2 to 4.

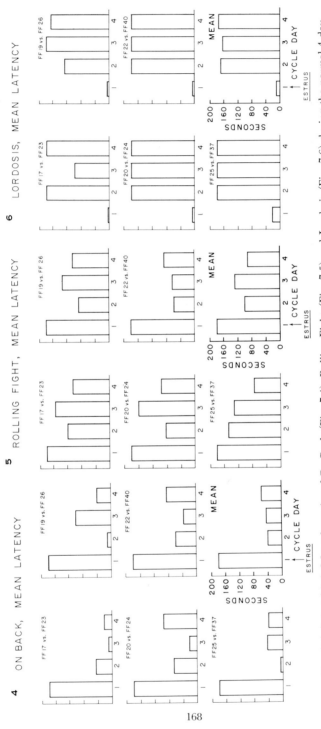

Figs. 7.4, 7.5, and 7.6. Mean latencies of On Back (Fig. 7.4), Rolling Fight (Fig. 7.5) and Lordosis (Fig. 7.6) during the normal 4-day estrous cycle. Each of five pairs of intact female hamsters (*e.g.,* FF17 versus FF23) experienced a series of eight 3-minute encounters (two on each of the 4-cycle days). Mean latencies compiled by each pair are summarized, as well as the mean across pairs (lower right). Estrus day is designated day 1, and nonestrous days are days 2 to 4. The maximum latency attainable is 180 seconds. Differences between day 1 and each of days 2 to 4 are statistically significant for each behavior pattern.

TABLE 7.1

Percentage of encounters during which behaviors occurred

Behavior Pattern	Cycle Day No.[1] (No. of Encounters)				Mean, Days 2–4 (30)
	Estrus 1 (10)	2 (10)	3 (10)	4 (10)	
	%				
Upright....................	100	100	100	100	100
On Back....................	0	100	100	90	97
Bite.......................	70	90	80	70	80
Rolling Fight..............	0	80	70	70	73
Fly-Away...................	0	40	20	40	33
Flight.....................	0	10	0	10	7

[1] Estrus day is designated day 1. Nonestrous days are days 2–4.

7.6). Thus, as is the case in heterosexual encounters (59, 74, 104), increased sexual receptivity on estrus day is associated with a profound decrease in the likelihood and severity of aggressive behavior.

The mean durations of moderate to high intensity agonistic behaviors lead to similar conclusions. Agonistic behaviors tend to be exhibited with shorter durations on estrus day (Fig. 7.7). These differences are statistically significant ($P < 0.05$, sign test) for the behaviors on back and rolling fight. For these behaviors, the cyclic variation is consistent across all pairs of females, even though the pairs differ markedly in basal (nonestrous) durations of aggressive responses (Figs. 7.8 and 7.9). In contrast, durations of lordosis are significantly longer ($P < 0.05$, sign test) on estrus days (Figs. 7.7 and 7.10).

Variations in aggressiveness during the estrous cycle of the intact female hamster may be related to our scheme (Fig. 7.1) describing sequences of aggressive behavior characteristic of this animal. Preliminary aggressive responses, such as the upright posture, occur with relatively short latencies in a high percentage of encounters throughout the estrous cycle. Responses corresponding to the most extreme forms of aggressiveness, such as fly-away and flight, must be preceded by a long chain of less intense aggressive responses, and occur with very long latencies or do not occur at all. Hormonal variations occurring during the estrous cycle have their most pronounced effects on moderate or high intensity aggressive responses such as the on back posture and rolling fight. The failure of the estrous female hamster to exhibit these aggressive responses quickly or often may reflect a failure of the estrous animal to attack (or to respond aggressively to an attack by) its opponent (see Fig. 7.1).

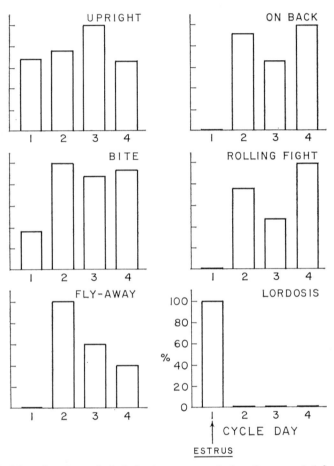

Fig. 7.7. Mean durations of six behavior patterns during the normal 4-day estrous cycle. Each bar summarizes the mean duration observed in 10 encounters (five female-female pairs) on a particular day of the cycle. The mean duration of each behavior is expressed as a percentage of the highest duration observed on any of the 4-cycle days. Estrus day is designated day 1, and nonestrous days are days 2 to 4. Mean durations of On Back, Rolling Fight and Lordosis on day 1 differ significantly from those on days 2 to 4.

The Hormonal Basis for Aggressiveness in the Female Hamster

In order to study the hormonal basis for variations in female aggressivity correlated with the estrous cycle, female hamsters were adrenalectomized and ovariectomized, thus removing all endogenous sources of sex

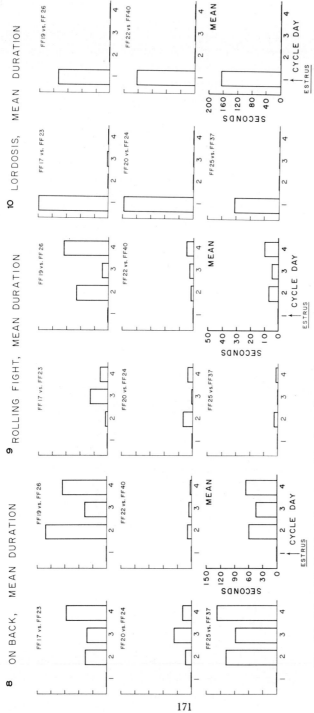

Figs. 7.8, 7.9, and 7.10. Mean durations of On Back (Fig. 7.8), Rolling Fight (Fig. 7.9) and Lordosis (Fig. 7.10) during the normal 4-day estrous cycle. Each of five pairs of intact female hamsters (*e.g.,* FF17 versus FF23) experienced a series of eight 3-minute encounters (two on each of the 4-cycle days). Mean durations compiled by each pair are summarized as well as the mean across pairs (lower right.) Estrus day is designated day 1, and nonestrous days are days 2 to 4. Differences between day 1 and each of days 2 to 4 are statistically significant for each behavior pattern.

steroids. Routine maintenance of these adrex-ovariex individuals included biweekly i.m. injections of 0.75 mg. of a long lasting mineralocorticoid preparation, deoxycorticosterone pivalate (Percorten pivalate, CIBA). Deoxycorticosterone (10 mg./kg.) has been reported by Kostowski and his co-workers (90) to have no significant effect upon isolation-induced aggression in mice.

Adrex-ovariex hamsters were tested under the following regimes of hormone treatment: TP (200 μg./day, 2 pairs), EB (10 μg./day, 2 pairs), P (500 μg./day, 2 pairs), or, EB plus P (10 μg./day of EB plus a single injection of 500 μg. of P approximately 4 hours before testing, 2 pairs) or oil vehicle alone (3 pairs). Tests were scheduled at 3- to 4-day intervals, and the 1st day of testing coincided with the 8th day of daily hormone treatment. Both members of a particular pair were subjected to identical treatments. Each pair of females was exposed to as many different hormone conditions as possible, with the order of conditions varied. Successive periods of treatment with different hormones were separated by at least 2 weeks. Encounters and data analyses were conducted as during the previously described experiment on naturally cycling females.

Adrex-ovariex female hamsters receiving only oil injections, fight at levels comparable to those exhibited by intact, nonestrous females, and considerably above levels of aggressivity characteristic of intact estrous females (Figs. 7.11 to 7.13). Replacement therapy with TP, P or EB individually did not exert consistent significant effects upon the aggressiveness of these females (Figs. 7.11 to 7.13), although further tests are being conducted to determine if EB alone can exert some facilitatory effect.

The combination of EB and P exerted a profound suppressive effect upon female aggressivity (Figs. 7.11 to 7.13). Levels of aggressive behaviors appearing under the influence of EB plus P resemble closely those exhibited by intact estrous females.

On the basis of these results, sex steroids seem to be reduced to a minor role in the stimulation of vigorous aggressive behavior during nonreceptive phases of the normal hamster estrous cycle. However, some combination of endogenous estrogen and progesterone could provide the endocrinological basis for the inhibition of aggressive behavior exhibited by the estrous female hamster.

SIGNALING SYSTEMS AND THE REGULATION OF FEMALE HAMSTER AGGRESSIVE BEHAVIOR

The ability to describe encounters between anestrous female hamsters in terms of a chain of somewhat stereotyped response elements (Fig. 7.1) suggests that the progress of a fight depends upon responses of each antagonist to signals from its opponent. Rapid communication regulating

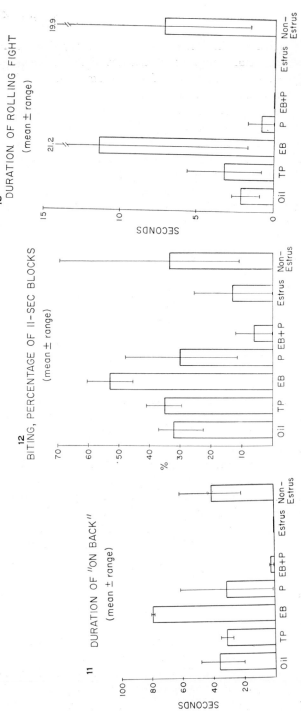

‡Figs. 7.11, 7.12, and 7.13. Effects of exogenous hormones on the mean durations of On Back (Fig. 7.11) and Rolling Fight (Fig. 7.13), and on the mean percentage of 11-second blocks during which Biting occurred (Fig. 7.12). Nine pairs of adrenalectomized-ovariectomized female hamsters experienced series of four 3-minute encounters under one or more of the following hormone regimes: testosterone propionate (TP, 200 μg./day), estradiol benzoate (EB, 10 μg./day) or progesterone (P, 500 μg./day). EB plus P tests (EB + P) were inserted into each EB series; daily EB treatment (10 μg./day) was supplemented by a single P injection (500 μg.) approximately 4 hours before testing. Mean durations of each behavior on Estrus (day 1) and Nonestrus (days 2 to 4) days of the normal estrous cycle are drawn from a previous experiment (see Figs. 7.7 to 7.10). In all three behaviors the combination of estradiol and progesterone reduced fighting to levels typical of normal estrus.

173

the progress of a fight might require visual and somatosensory signals. At a quite different stage in social interactions, distance signals indicating the overall state of aggressiveness (and receptivity) of a female might allow potential mates to concentrate sexual advances on estrus days, thus avoiding contact with aggressive anestrous females. In this regard, investigations have uncovered possible roles for olfactory and auditory signals.

Female hamsters exhibit a stereotyped form of scent marking associated with the deposition of an odorous vaginal secretion (108). The frequency of "vaginal marking" and the viscosity of the vaginal discharge may be correlated with the estrous cycle (108, 109). Male hamsters show a distinct attraction to the odors of estrous female vaginal secretions (108, 110). Under ideal conditions, this attraction is at least as pronounced as that shown by sexually experienced male rats for estrous female rat urine odor (111). Even sexually inexperienced intact male hamsters can show a significant preference for the estrus odor (110). Moreover, the degree of preference exhibited by male hamsters for the estrus odor is reduced after castration and can be reestablished with testosterone replacement therapy (110). Such an odor might not only attract male hamsters as mates, but also inform potential opponents of both sexes about the state of the female's estrous cycle, which in turn is linked to her aggressiveness.

Considering the female hamster as a source of olfactory signals is relevant in interpreting certain effects of hormones on aggression. When paired with intact male opponents, the relative success of gonadectomized male or female hamsters may be enhanced by progesterone treatment (28, 77). In each case, however, the increased success of the progesterone-treated partner seems to be an indirect effect involving a decrease in the level of aggressiveness exhibited by the intact male opponent. These results are consistent with the notion of a progesterone-dependent olfactory cue capable of inhibiting the aggressiveness of male hamsters. Ample precedents for such signaling mechanisms (relevant particularly to sexual differences in the display of aggressive behavior) are apparent in the work of Mackintosh and Grant (112) and Mugford and Nowell (113–116). The latter authors have linked relatively high levels of aggression displayed by isolated male mice toward androgenized females to the induction in these females of aggression-eliciting olfactory cues emanating from the preputial glands and other sources. In a variety of species, scent marking may be related to aggression among conspecifics (117).

Auditory signals also may be used to inform other hamsters of a female's estrous condition and thus of her state of aggressiveness. During informal observations, approximately 20 per cent of adult female hamsters in our colony have emitted distinctive vocalizations, ranging in their audible characteristics from sharp barks to forms resembling low hisses (ultrasonic components also seem to be present). Even within a "bout" (a brief series) of vocalizations by a single individual the full range of variability of these sounds may be exhibited. Rates of calling within a bout may be quite high, sometimes exceeding 15 vocalizations per minute. These distinctive vocalizations appear almost exclusively on estrus day, suggesting that this vocalization functions to attract males to a sexually receptive female, perhaps in part by signaling low levels of aggressiveness. Consistent with this speculation is the observation that rates of vocalization on estrus day may be increased by brief exposure to a male or to shavings from a male's home cage. For example, an estrous female hamster exposed to clean shavings in her home cage failed to vocalize during a 10-minute test. During the immediately succeeding 10 minutes, the female was exposed to shavings from the home cage of a male and 20 vocalizations were recorded. Finally, during a 10-minute test following a 30-second exposure to a male, the same female emitted 146 "estrus vocalizations."

In summary, several lines of evidence presented in this and other sections of the chapter indicate that signals between animals regulate the occurrence and progress of aggressive encounters. First, studies reviewed on p. 172–175 showed that characteristics of the opponent can influence aggressive responses of a test animal, implying a role for signaling between animals. It was pointed out that such influences can modulate effects of hormones on aggression in the test animals. Second, orderly stereotyped progress of fights between female hamsters suggests that responses of each individual are in some measure regulated by responses of the other, necessarily through a rapid signaling process. Finally, olfactory and auditory "distance" signals may indicate an overall level of aggressiveness, at least in the female hamster. Hormone effects on the emission and receipt of social signals may account for a significant part of the changes in aggressive behavior after hormone treatment (31).

ESTRADIOL CONCENTRATION BY CELLS IN THE FEMALE HAMSTER BRAIN

Of the steroid hormones important for regulating levels of aggression in the female hamster, 17β-estradiol and progesterone, estradiol has been easier to localize in neurons in specific regions of the brain. Previous work has demonstrated estradiol-concentrating neurons in a system of limbic and hypothalamic nuclei in the brain of the female rat (118–120).

In experiments with hamsters, five adult ovariectomized females weighing 90 to 110 gm. were injected intraperitoneally with 100 μc. of 17β-estradiol-2,4,6,7-H^3 (specific activity, 95 c. per mM., New England Nuclear) dissolved in ethanol. Two hours later, the hamsters were sacrificed by decapitation. Their brains were rapidly removed, blocked and frozen onto cryostat specimen holders. In the darkroom, frozen sections, unfixed and unembedded, were cut in the cryostat at a thickness of 6 microns, and were mounted directly onto slides precoated with Kodak NTB-3 nuclear emulsion. Darkroom procedures, modified from those used by Anderson and Greenwald (121), have been described (120). During the exposure period, autoradiograms were stored in light-tight plastic slide boxes equipped with desiccant and sealed with tape. These boxes were, in turn, stored in a lead box with additional desiccant and sealed against moisture, in a cold room at 4° C. After 8 months of exposure, slides were developed in Kodak D19 for 2 minutes at 16° C, rinsed for 45 seconds in Kodak Liquid Hardener stop bath and fixed in Kodak fixer for 18 minutes. Finally, the tissue was stained in cresyl violet acetate, dehydrated and cover slipped. Control experiments with brain tissue from uninjected animals and with autoradiograms exposed intentionally to light showed, respectively, that accumulations of reduced grains were caused by concentrations of radioactivity rather than by chemographic artifact, and that tissue chemicals did not damage the emulsion. Labeled cells, defined as having grain densities over their cell bodies greater than 5 times background levels, were detected and localized by systematic scanning and charting of complete transverse brain sections covering an anterior-posterior extent from the olfactory bulbs to the lower medulla.

Estrogen-concentrating cells were discovered in specific nuclei in the hypothalamus and limbic system. Labeled cells were found reliably in the medial preoptic area (Fig. 7.14b) and (in greater numbers) in the medial anterior hypothalamus (Fig. 7.14c). The arcuate nucleus of the hypothalamus contained well labeled cells throughout its extent (Fig. 7.14d). Estrogen-concentrating cells also were seen in the ventromedial and ventral premammillary nuclei.

In the limbic system, well labeled cells were found in the medial and cortical nuclei of the amygdala (Fig. 7.14d) and in the bed nucleus of the stria terminalis (Fig. 7.14b). Some estrogen-concentrating cells could be seen in the ventral half of the lateral septum (Fig. 7.14a). Labeled cells also were detected, in small numbers, in the ventral hippocampus and entorhinal cortex.

An apparent extension of this limbic-hypothalamic system of estrogen-concentrating cells was seen in the ventrolateral portion of the mesencephalic central gray (Fig. 7.14e).

With few exceptions, in this preliminary analysis, other regions of the female hamster brain had very few labeled cells, and even those few cells

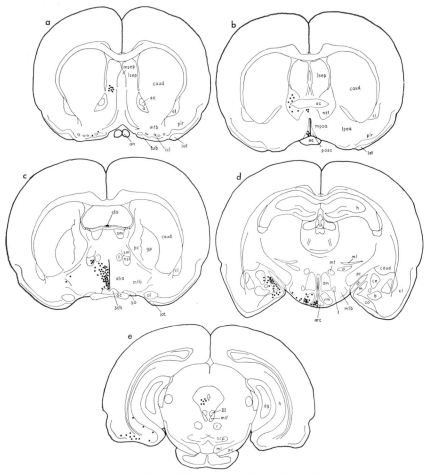

Fig. 7.14, a–e. Locations of estradiol-concentrating cells, indicated by ●, at five coronal levels of the female hamster brain. These preliminary maps are based on auto-radiograms from a female hamster representative of the sample of five. See text for description of the preparation of estradiol-H³ autoradiograms. Abbreviations: a, nucleus accumbens; ac, anterior commissure; aha, anterior hypothalamic area; arc, arcuate nucleus; b, basal amygdaloid complex; caud, caudate nucleus; ce, central nucleus of the amygdala; cl, claustrum; co, cortical nucleus of the amygdala; dg, dentate gyrus of the hippocampus; dm, dorsomedial nucleus of the hypothalamus; f, fornix; gp, globus pallidus; h, hippocampus; icl, Island of Calleja; lot, lateral olfactory tract; lpoa, lateral preoptic area; lsep, lateral septum; m, media nucleus of the amygdala; mfb, medial fore-brain bundle; ml, medial lemniscus; mlf, medial longitudinal fasciculus; mpoa, medial preoptic area; msep, medial septum; mt, mammillothalamic tract; nst, bed nucleus of the stria terminalis; oc, optic chiasm; ol, nucleus of the lateral olfactory tract; on, optic nerve; ot, optic tract; pc, cerebral peduncle; pir, prepiriform cortex; posc, preoptic area pars suprachiasmaticus; r, red nucleus; sch, suprachiasmatic nucleus; scp, superior cerebellar peduncle; sfo, subfornical organ; sm, stria medullaris; so, supraoptic nucleus; tub, olfactory tubercle; vm, ventromedial nucleus; zi, zona incerta and III, nucleus of the oculomotor nerve.

were not heavily labeled and were not found consistently in identified locations. One such exception is the very small amount of labeling seen in the nucleus of the solitary tract at the level of the obex.

The distribution of tritiated estradiol in the female hamster brain may be compared with the concentration of testosterone by neurons in the males of other species, since testosterone seems to facilitate aggression in many situations. In male rats, tritiated testosterone is concentrated by cells in certain limbic and hypothalamic regions, especially the medial preoptic area, lateral septum, olfactory tubercle and prepiriform cortex (122). In the male chaffinch, a songbird, testosterone-concentrating neurons have been discovered in the medial preoptic area, lateral septum, medial hypothalamus and in a specific midbrain region which may be involved in the control of hormone-dependent vocalizations (123, 124). In male domestic fowl, the preoptic region from which behavioral responses can be elicited by testosterone implantation contains significant numbers of testosterone-concentrating cells (Barfield and Pfaff, in preparation).

Sexual behaviors of female hamsters have been reported to be less sensitive to systemically administered estradiol than comparable behaviors of female rats (125). Notably, although the overall topography of estrogen-concentrating neurons is similar in the two species, this preliminary analysis suggests that fewer such neurons are present in the female hamster brain than in the female rat. Moreover, whereas the optimal placement of estradiol implants for the elicitation of mating behavior lies in the preoptic area in the female rat (126), it seems to be further caudal, in the medial anterior hypothalamus, in the female hamster (127). In turn, the ratio of anterior hypothalamic to medial preoptic labeling seems to be greater in the female hamster than in the female rat (120). Thus, comparisons of rat and hamster, on grounds of both overall estrogen sensitivity and the location of peak sensitivity within the preoptic-hypothalamic continuum, yield good correlations between estrogen binding and behavior.

In summary, estradiol is concentrated by cells in specific limbic and hypothalamic loci in the female hamster brain (Fig. 7.14). Steroid sex hormones (estradiol and progesterone in the female, testosterone or its metabolites in the male) might act on specific limbic and hypothalamic mechanisms to synchronize social behaviors, including aggression, with the reproductive state of an animal.

ACKNOWLEDGMENTS

Bibliographic assistance was obtained from The UCLA Brain Information Service. We thank Catherine Lewis and Gabriele Zummer for help with the experiments and in preparation of the manuscript.

REFERENCES

1. PFAFF, DW, LEWIS, C, DIAKOW, C, KEINER, M: Neurophysiological analysis of mating behavior responses as hormone-sensitive reflexes, in Progress in Physiological Psychology, Vol. 5, edited by Stellar, E, Sprague, JM. 1972, pp. 253–297.
2. PFAFF, DW, DIAKOW, C, ZIGMOND, RE, KOW, L-M: Neural and hormonal mechanisms underlying mating reflexes in the female rat, in The Neurosciences, Vol. 3, edited by Schmitt, FO, et al. Boston, MIT Press, 1973, pp. 621–646.
3. GUHL, A: Gonadal hormones and social behavior in infrahuman vertebrates, in Sex and Internal Secretions, Vol. 2, Ed. 3, edited by Young, WC. Baltimore, The Williams & Wilkins Co., 1961, p. 1240.
4. FREDERICSON, E: The effects of food deprivation upon competitive and spontaneous combat in C57 black mice. J Psychol 29: 89, 1950.
5. KIRKHAM, W: The life of the white mouse. Proc Soc Exp Biol Med 17: 196, 1920.
6. COLLIAS, N, TABER, R: A field study of some grouping and dominance relations in ring-necked pheasants. Condor 53: 265, 1951.
7. BUECHNER, H, MORRISON, J, LEUTHOLD, W: Reproduction in Uganda kob with special reference to behavior. Symp Zool Soc Lond 15: 69, 1966.
8. CONAWAY, C, KOFORD, C: Estrous cycles and mating behavior in a free-ranging band of rhesus monkeys. J Mammal 45: 577, 1965.
9. KAUFMANN, J: A three-year study of mating behavior in a free-ranging band of rhesus monkeys. Ecology 46: 500, 1965.
10. ROSE, R, HOLADAY, J, BERNSTEIN, I: Plasma testosterone, dominance rank and aggressive behaviour in male rhesus monkeys. Nature 231: 366, 1971.
11. DAVIS, D: Aggressive behavior in castrated starlings. Science 126: 253, 1957.
12. DAVIS, D: The physiological analysis of aggressive behavior, in Social Behavior and Organization Among Vertebrates, edited by Etkin, W. Chicago, University of Chicago Press, 1964, p. 53.
13. MATHEWSON, S: Gonadotropic control of aggressive behavior in starlings. Science 134: 1522, 1961.
14. BEEMAN, E: The effect of male hormone on aggressive behavior in mice. Physiol Zool 20: 373, 1947.
15. EDWARDS, D: Early androgen stimulation and aggressive behavior in male and female mice. Physiol Behav 4: 333, 1969.
16. SIGG, E: Relationship of aggressive behaviour to adrenal and gonadal function in male mice, in Aggressive Behavior, edited by Garattini, S, Sigg, EB. New York, John Wiley & Sons, Inc., 1969, p. 143.
17. SUCHOWSKY, G, PEGRASSI, L, BONSIGNORI, A: The effect of steroids on aggressive behaviour in isolated male mice, in Aggressive Behavior, edited by Garattini, S, Sigg, EB. New York, John Wiley & Sons, Inc., 1969, p. 164.
18. TAVOLGA, WN: Effects of gonadectomy and hypophysectomy on prespawning behavior in males of the gobiid fish, Bathygobius soporator. Physiol Zool 28: 218, 1955.
19. EVANS, L: Behavior of Sceloporus grammicus microlepidotus as modified by certain endocrines. Anat Rec 94: 405, 1946.
20. DOMM, L: Modifications in sex and secondary sexual characteristics in birds, in Sex and Internal Secretions, edited by Allen, E. Baltimore, The Williams & Wilkins Co., 1939, p. 227.
21. COLLIAS, N: Aggressive behavior among vertebrate animals. Physiol Zool 17: 83, 1944.

22. SELINGER, H, BERMANT, G: Hormonal control of aggressive behavior in Japanese quail (Coturnix coturnix japonica). Behaviour 28: 255, 1967.

23. WATSON, A: Territorial and reproductive behavior of red grouse. J Reprod Fertil (Suppl) 11: 3, 1970.

24. BENNETT, M: The social hierarchy in ring doves. II. The effect of treatment with testosterone propionate. Ecology 21: 148, 1940.

25. ERICKSON, C, BRUDER, R, KOMISARUK, B, LEHRMAN, D: Selective inhibition by progesterone of androgen-induced behavior in male ring doves (Streptopelia risoria). Endocrinology 81: 39, 1967.

26. EMLEN, J, LORENZ, F: Pairing responses of free-living valley quail to sex-hormone pellet implants. Auk 59: 369, 1942.

27. PAYNE, A, SWANSON, H: Neonatal androgenization and aggression in the male golden hamster. Proceedings of the Fourth International Congress of Endocrinology, Washington, D.C. Abstract 10, 1972.

28. PAYNE, A, SWANSON, H: The effect of sex hormones on the agonistic behavior of the male golden hamster (Mesocricetus auratus Waterhouse). Physiol Behav 8: 687, 1972.

29. VANDENBERGH, J: The effects of gonadal hormones on the aggressive behaviour of adult golden hamsters (Mesocricetus auratus). Anim Behav 19: 589, 1971.

30. BARFIELD, R, BUSCH, D, WALLEN, K: Gonadal influence on agonistic behavior in the male domestic rat. Horm Behav 3: 247, 1972.

31. LINCOLN, G, YOUNGSON, R, SHORT, R: The social and sexual behaviour of the red deer stag. J Reprod Fertil (Suppl) 11: 71, 1970.

32. BRAMLEY, P: Territoriality and reproductive behaviour of roe deer. J Reprod Fertil (Suppl) 11: 43, 1970.

33. CLARK, G, BIRCH, H: Hormonal modifications of social behavior. I. The effect of sex-hormone administration on the social status of a male-castrate chimpanzee. Psychosom Med 7: 321, 1945.

34. NOBLE, G, GREENBERG, B: Induction of female behavior in male Anolis carolinensis with testosterone propionate. Proc Soc Exp Biol Med 47: 32, 1941.

35. COLLIAS, N: Hormones and behavior with special reference to birds and the mechanisms of hormone action, in A Symposium on Steroid Hormones, edited by Gordon, E. Madison, University of Wisconsin Press, 1950, p. 277.

36. GUHL, A: The development of social organisation in the domestic chick. Anim Behav 6: 92, 1958.

37. NOBLE, G, ZITRIN, A: Induction of mating behavior in male and female chicks following injection of sex hormones. Endocrinology 30: 327, 1942.

38. BOSS, W: Hormonal determination of adult characters and sex behavior in herring gulls (Larus argentatus). J Exp Zool 94: 181, 1943.

39. LEVY, J, KING, J: The effects of testosterone propionate on fighting behaviour in young male C57Bl/10 mice. Anat Rev 117: 562, 1953.

40. BRONSON, F, DESJARDINS, C: Aggressive behavior and seminal vesicle function in mice: differential sensitivity to androgen given neonatally. Endocrinology 85: 971, 1969.

41. PETERS, P, BRONSON, F, WHITSETT, J: Neonatal castration and intermale aggression in mice. Physiol Behav 8: 265, 1972.

42. LUTTGE, W: Activation and inhibition of isolation induced inter-male fighting behavior in castrate male CD-1 mice treated with steroidal hormones. Horm Behav 3: 71, 1972.

43. ERPINO, M, CHAPPELLE, T: Interactions between androgens and progesterone in mediation of aggression in the mouse. Horm Behav 2: 265, 1971.

44. BEVAN, J, BEVAN, W, WILLIAMS, B: Spontaneous aggressiveness in young castrated C_3H male mice treated with three dose levels of testosterone. Physiol Zool 31: 284, 1958.

45. EDWARDS, D: Effects of cyproterone acetate on aggressive behaviour and the seminal vesicles of male mice. J Endocrinol 46: 477, 1970.

46. SAYLER, A: The effect of anti-androgens on aggressive behavior in the gerbil. Physiol Behav 5: 667, 1970.

47. BARFIELD, R: Activation of sexual and aggressive behavior by androgen implanted into the male ring dove brain. Endocrinology 89: 1470, 1971.

48. BARFIELD, R: Induction of aggressive and courtship behavior by intracerebral implants of androgen in capons. Am Zool 5: 203, 1965.

49. BARFIELD, R: Activation of copulatory behavior by androgen implanted into the preoptic area of the male fowl. Horm Behav 1: 37, 1969.

50. CROOK, J, BUTTERFIELD, P: Effects of testosterone propionate and luteinizing hormone on agonistic and nest building behaviour of Quelea quelea. Anim Behav 16: 370, 1968.

51. NOBLE, G, BORNE, R: The effect of sex hormones on the social hierarchy of Xiphophorus helleri. Anat Rec 78: 147, 1940.

52. EVANS, L: Behavior of castrated lizards. J Genet Psychol 48: 217, 1936.

53. GREENBERG, B, NOBLE, G: Social behavior of the American chameleon (Anolis carolinensis, Voight). Physiol Zool 17: 392, 1944.

54. NOBLE, G, WURM, M: The effect of testosterone propionate on the black-crowned night heron. Endocrinology 26: 837, 1940.

55. CARPENTER, C: Territoriality: A review of concepts and problems, in Behavior and Evolution, edited by Roe, A, Simpson, G. New Haven, Yale University Press, 1958, p. 224.

56. LUMIA, A: The relationships among testosterone, conditioned aggression, and dominance in male pigeons. Horm Behav 3: 277, 1972.

57. VOWLES, D, HARWOOD, D: The effect of exogenous hormones on aggressive and defensive behaviour in the ring dove (Streptopelia risoria). J Endocrinol 36: 35, 1966.

58. LE BOEUF, B: Copulatory and aggressive behavior in the prepuberally castrated dog. Horm Behav 1: 127, 1970.

59. TIEFER, L: Gonadal hormones and mating behavior in the adult golden hamster. Horm Behav 1: 189, 1970.

60. BURGE, K, EDWARDS, D: The adrenal gland and the pre- and post-castrational aggressive behavior of male mice. Physiol Behav 7: 885, 1971.

61. UHRICH, J: The social hierarchy in albino mice. J Comp Psychol 25: 373, 1938.

62. CONNER, R, LEVINE, S: Hormonal influences on aggressive behaviour, in Aggressive Behavior, edited by Garattini, S, Sigg, EB. New York, John Wiley & Sons, Inc., 1969, p. 150.

63. CONNER, R, LEVINE, S, WERTHEIM, G, CUMMER, J: Hormonal determinants of aggressive behavior. Ann NY Acad Sci 159: 760, 1969.

64. MIRSKY, A: The influence of sex hormones on social behavior of monkeys. J Comp Physiol Psychol 48: 327, 1955.

65. MOYER, K: Kinds of aggression and their physiological basis. Commun Behav Biol 2: 65, 1968.

66. EDWARDS, D: Mice: fighting by neonatally androgenized females. Science 161: 1027, 1968.

67. BRONSON, F, DESJARDINS, C: Neonatal androgen administration and adult aggressiveness in female mice. Gen Comp Endocrinol 15: 320, 1970.

68. Edwards, D, Herndon, J: Neonatal estrogen stimulation and aggressive behavior in female mice. Physiol Behav 5: 993, 1970.

69. Levy, J: The effects of testosterone propionate on fighting behavior in C57 Bl-10 young female mice. Proc W Va Acad Sci 26: 14, 1954.

70. Scott, J, Fredericson, E: The causes of fighting in mice and rats. Physiol Zool 24: 273, 1951.

71. Vale, J, Ray, D, Vale, C: The interaction of genotype and exogenous neonatal androgen: agonistic behavior in female mice. Behav Biol 7: 321, 1972.

72. Bevan, W, Daves, W, Levy, G: The relation of castration, androgen therapy and pre-test fighting experience to competitive aggression in male C57 BL/10 mice. Anim Behav 8: 6, 1960.

73. Beeman, EA, Allee, WC: Some effects of thiamine on the winning of social contacts in mice. Physiol Zool 18: 195, 1945.

74. Payne, A, Swanson, H: Agonistic behaviour between pairs of hamsters of the same and opposite sex in a neutral observation area. Behaviour 36: 259, 1970.

75. Stern, J, Eisenfeld, A: Distribution and metabolism of ^{3}H-testosterone in castrated male rats; effects of cyproterone, progesterone and unlabeled testosterone. Endocrinology 88: 1117, 1971.

76. Komisaruk, B: Effects of local brain implants of progesterone on reproductive behavior in ring doves. J Comp Physiol Psychol 64: 219, 1967.

77. Payne, A, Swanson, H: Hormonal control of aggressive dominance in the female hamster. Physiol Behav 6: 355, 1971.

78. Banerjee, U: Influence of some hormones and drugs on isolation-induced aggression in male mice. Commun Behav Biol 6: 163, 1971.

79. Bronson, F, Desjardins, C: Aggression in adult mice: modification by neonatal injections of gonadal hormones. Science 161: 705, 1968.

80. Terdiman, A, Levy, J: The effects of estrogen on fighting behavior in young male C57 Fl-10 mice. Proc W Va Acad Sci 26: 15, 1954.

81. Work, M, Rogers, H: Effect of estrogen level on food-seeking dominance among male rats. J Comp Physiol Psychol 79: 414, 1972.

82. Gustafson, J, Winokur, G: The effect of sexual satiation and female hormone upon aggressivity in an inbred mouse strain. J Neuropsychiat 1: 182, 1960.

83. Payne, A, Swanson, H: The effect of castration and ovarian implantation on aggressive behaviour of male hamsters. J Endocrinol 51: 217, 1971.

84. Edwards, D, Burge, K: Estrogenic arousal of aggressive behavior and masculine sexual behavior in male and female mice. Horm Behav 2: 239, 1971.

85. Davidson, J: Effects of estrogen on the sexual behavior of male rats. Endocrinology 84: 1365, 1969.

86. Pfaff, D: Nature of sex hormone effects on rat sex behavior: specificity of effects and individual patterns of response. J Comp Physiol Psychol 73: 349, 1970.

87. Brain, P, Nowell, N, Wouters, A: Some relationships between adrenal function and the effectiveness of a period of isolation in inducing intermale aggression in albino mice. Physiol Behav 6: 27, 1971.

88. Brain, P: Mammalian behavior and the adrenal cortex—a review. Behav Biol 7: 453, 1972.

89. Leshner, A: The adrenals and testes: two separate systems affecting aggressiveness. Hormones 3: Abstr 24, 272, 1972.

90. Kostowski, W, Rewerski, W, Piechocki, T: Effects of some steroids on aggressive behaviour in mice and rats. Neuroendocrinology 6: 311, 1970.

91. Michael, R, Zumpe, D: Aggression and gonadal hormones in captive rhesus monkeys (Macaca mulatta). Anim Behav 18: 1, 1970.

92. EDWARDS, D: Post-neonatal androgenization and adult aggressive behavior in female mice. Physiol Behav 5: 465, 1970.
93. SHOEMAKER, H: Effect of testosterone propionate on behavior of the female canary. Proc Soc Exp Biol Med 41: 299, 1939.
94. ALLEE, W, COLLIAS, N, LUTHERMAN, C: Modification of the social order in flocks of hens by the injection of testosterone propionate. Physiol Zool 12: 412, 1939.
95. DAVIS, D, DOMM, L: The influence of hormones on the sexual behavior of domestic fowl, in Essays in Biology. Berkeley, University of California Press, 1943, p. 171.
96. DOUGLIS, M: Social factors influencing the hierarchies of small flocks of the domestic hen: interactions between resident and part-time members of organized flocks. Physiol Zool 21: 147, 1948.
97. WILLIAMS, C, McGIBBON, W: An analysis of the peck-order of the female domestic fowl (Gallus domesticus). Poult Sci 35: 969, 1956.
98. BIRCH, H, CLARK, G: Hormonal modification of social behavior. II. The effects of sex-hormone administration on the social dominance status of the female-castrate chimpanzee. Psychosom Med 8: 320, 1946.
99. ALLEE, W, COLLIAS, N: The influence of estradiol on the social organization of flocks of hens. Endocrinology 27: 87, 1940.
100. EDWARDS, D: Neonatal administration of androstenedione, testosterone or testosterone propionate: effects on ovulation, sexual receptivity and aggressive behavior in female mice. Physiol Behav 6: 223, 1971.
101. WHITSETT, J, BRONSON, F, PETERS, P, HAMILTON, T: Neonatal organization of aggression in mice: correlation of critical period with uptake of hormone. Horm Behav 3: 11, 1972.
102. DIETERLEN, F: Das verhalten des syrischen goldhamster. Z Tierpsychol 16: 47, 1959.
103. LERWILL, C, MAKINGS, P: The agonistic behaviour of the golden hamster Mesocricetus auratus (Waterhouse). Anim Behav 19: 714, 1971.
104. KISLAK, J, BEACH, F: Inhibition of aggressiveness by ovarian hormones. Endocrinology 56: 684, 1955.
105. PAYNE, A, SWANSON, H: Hormonal modification of aggressive behaviour between female golden hamsters. J Endocrinol 51: xvii, 1971.
106. BUNNELL, B, SODETZ, F, SHALLOWAY, D: Amygdaloid lesions and social behavior in the golden hamster. Physiol Behav 5: 153, 1970.
107. SIEGEL, S: Nonparametric Statistics for the Behavioral Sciences. New York, McGraw-Hill Book Co., 1956.
108. JOHNSTON, R: Scent marking, olfactory communication and social behavior in the golden hamster, Mesocricetus auratus. Unpublished doctoral dissertation, The Rockefeller University, 1970.
109. ORSINI, M: The external vaginal phenomena characterizing the stages of the estrous cycle, pregnancy, pseudopregnancy, lactation, and the anestrous hamster, Mesocricetus auratus Waterhouse. Proc Anim Care Panel 11: 193, 1961.
110. GREGORY, E, ENGEL, K, PFAFF, DW: Behavioral responses of male hamsters to female hamster vaginal secretions. 1973, submitted for publication.
111. PFAFF, DW, PFAFFMANN, C: Behavioral and electrophysiological responses of male rats to female rat urine odors, in Olfaction and Taste, edited by Pfaffmann, C. New York, The Rockefeller University Press, 1969, p. 258.
112. MACKINTOSH, J, GRANT, E: The effect of olfactory stimuli on the agonistic behaviour of laboratory mice. Z Tierpsychol 23: 584, 1966.
113. MUGFORD, R, NOWELL, N: The aggression of male mice against androgenized females. Psychonom Sci 20: 191, 1970.

114. MUGFORD, R, NOWELL, N: The preputial glands as a source of aggression-promoting odors in mice. Physiol Behav 6: 247, 1971.

115. MUGFORD, R, NOWELL, N: The relationship between endocrine status of female opponents and aggressive behaviour of male mice. Anim Behav 19: 153, 1971.

116. MUGFORD, R, NOWELL, N: The dose-response to testosterone propionate of preputial glands, pheromones and aggression in mice. Horm Behav 3: 39, 1972.

117. RALLS, K: Mammalian scent marking. Science 171: 443, 1971.

118. PFAFF, DW: Uptake of estradiol-17β-H³ in the female rat brain. An autoradiographic study. Endocrinology 82: 1149, 1968.

119. PFAFF, DW, KEINER, M: Estradiol-concentrating cells in the rat amygdala as part of a limbic-hypothalamic hormone-sensitive system, in Proceedings: Neurobiology of the Amygdala, edited by Eleftheriou, BE. New York, Plenum Publishing Corp., 1972, p. 775.

120. PFAFF, DW, KEINER, M: Atlas of estradiol-concentrating cells in the central nervous system of the female rat. J Comp Neurol 151: 121, 1973.

121. ANDERSON, CH, GREENWALD, GS: Autoradiographic analysis of estradiol uptake in the brain and pituitary of the female rat. Endocrinology 85: 1160, 1969.

122. PFAFF, DW: Autoradiographic localization of radioactivity in rat brain after injection of tritiated sex hormones. Science 161: 1355, 1968.

123. ZIGMOND, RE, NOTTEBOHM, F, PFAFF, DW: Distribution of androgen-concentrating cells in the brain of the chaffinch. Excerpta Medica Int Cong Series 256, Abstract 340.

124. ZIGMOND, R, NOTTEBOHM, F, PFAFF, DW: Androgen-concentrating cells in the midbrain of a songbird. Science 179: 1005, 1973.

125. LISK, RD: Progesterone: Role in limitation of ovulation and sex behavior in mammals. Trans NY Acad Sci 31: 593, 1969.

126. LISK, RD: Diencephalic placement of estradiol and sexual receptivity in the female rat. Am J Physiol 203: 493, 1962.

127. CIACCIO, L, LISK, RD: Neuroendocrinology 1973, in press.

DISCUSSION

DR. DAVID HAMBURG (Stanford, California): I am interested in whether any aspects of aggressive behavior are related to fluctuations in gonadal steroids in the human. There has been some recent work both from our group and in England on this problem, particularly in relation to the so-called premenstrual tension syndrome. I refer not only to the irritability and depression felt during the few days prior to onset and the first 2 or 3 days of the menstrual period itself, but also to physical attacks. There does seem to be a disproportionate clustering of overtly aggressive acts during that time.

Both we and the English epidemiological group found that about one in five of young, highly educated, resourceful women reported that she was significantly impaired, unable to do important things that she wanted to do. In relation to hormonal correlate, there are some suggestions that the cycles that present the greatest risk are characterized by very rapid flow in progesterone and a tendency for estrogen to remain high. That is, a relatively high estrogen-progesterone ratio may predispose to these severe irritability problems in that period of cycle.

DR. PAUL D. MACLEAN (Bethesda, Maryland): Could Dr. Pfaff speak about the work with the unit recording?

DR. DONALD W. PFAFF (New York, New York): We do not have unit recording data directly relevant to the causality of aggression in the female hamster. However, with respect to androgen, we are certain that there are neurons in the preoptic area which are sensitive to androgens: single neurons, the firing of which can be altered by testosterone injected either directly into the preoptic area or systemically.

The current problem in all of this neuroendocrine work is to use neurophysiological methods to identify circuits from the sites of hormone-sensitive neurons to the regions where we know the sensory and motor aspects of the behavior are controlled. As far as I know, this problem has not yet been solved for any hormone-sensitive behavior.

Chapter 8

THE ROLE OF LIMBIC BRAIN DYSFUNCTION IN AGGRESSION

VERNON H. MARK AND WILLIAM H. SWEET

The word "role" in the title was used advisedly inasmuch as, in our present state of knowledge, it would be presumptuous to say that either environmental factors or brain factors cause aggression. All behavior is the result of environment-brain interaction.

Although the entire brain acts as a unit in responding to environmental stimuli and in initiating behavior, there is some differentiation and specialization within the nervous system. The limbic system is that part of the brain that is more intimately involved with the modulation and elaboration of the "fight or flight" responses that are so important for the preservation of vertebrate species when they are under attack. Papez (1) and other investigators have implicated the limbic brain in a large variety of emotional functions, and some investigators have called this the "emotional brain." In this context, we shall refer only to the limbic system, a term including not only the cingulum, hippocampus, septal nuclei and commissures of the older anatomists, but also some of the related portions of thalamus, hypothalamus, basal ganglia, midbrain and amygdala, as well as the orbital region of the frontal lobe.

There are two sources of evidence relating the limbic system of the brain to aggression, *viz.,* experimental and clinical. The focus of this presentation will be largely on the amygdala, although the evidence is equally impressive for other portions of the system, including the ventromedial hypothalamus.

The animal experiments can be divided into those related to brain stimulation and those related to brain destruction. Stimulation in or near the amygdala has been extensively studied and has produced defense or flight reactions in many species of unanesthetized mammals, reported in more than 40 publications (2). However, DeMolina and Hunsperger (3) and Ursin (4) emphasize that the area from which rage can be evoked is restricted to a small part of the amygdala. The converse response of placidity would be harder to establish in an animal, but Anand and Dua (5) have reported calmness progressing even to sleep. Egger and Flynn (6) report both types of behavior—facilitation of hypothalamically induced attack responses from lateral amygdala and suppression of such responses from more medial sites in the amygdala. Earlier, Alfonso-DeFlorida and Delgado (7) had obtained both positive and negative effects on aggressiveness upon prolonged stimulation of various points in the amygdaloid complex.

Destruction in and about the amygdala on both sides produces as its most common effect on attack or flight behavior, a marked reduction or taming. This is the conclusion of Ursin (8) upon a review of 20 articles. In a recent extensive study by A. Kling (personal communication) of a free-living monkey colony, bilaterally amygdalectomized monkeys were too placid for their own safety and were killed or otherwise rejected by the others when reintroduced to the colony. However, strikingly opposite findings have been reported by at least three groups. The cats of Bard and Mountcastle (9), some weeks after operation, exhibited sustained ferocity for months. The cats of Wood (10) were less consistent, but bilateral lesions of the central nucleus in 4 of 10 and of the basal nucleus in 5 of 10 animals were followed by increased aggressiveness. The bilaterally amygdalectomized monkey of Rosvold and his co-workers (11), having been number 3 in a colony of 8 monkeys, became aggressive postoperatively and drove the previous number 1 and number 2 beasts, respectively, down to the number 8 and number 7 positions in the colony, all others moving up two notches.

Clinical evidence relating to limbic system disease and assaultive behavior can be reviewed under three headings. The first of these is structural brain disease.

Limbic brain tumors have been associated with aggressive behavior. Specifically excluded from this section will be the small temporal lobe hamartomas which in one series were found in 22 per cent of the temporal lobe epileptics studied by Falconer and his associates (12). Other reports of tumors include one of Cushing (13), one of Alpers (14), one of Vonderahe (15), one of Dott, reported by Hill (16), four of Malamud (17), one of Reeves and Plum (18), three of Sweet and his co-workers (19) and one of Mullan (20). The lesions and sites were: 1 inferior posteromedial frontal abscess, 1 angioma of the temporal pole, 1 subfrontal meningioma, 4 invasive slow growing gliomas (3 temporal and 1 gyrus cinguli), 1 temporal glioblastoma, 3 hypothalamic tumors, 1 glioma of the optic chiasm and 1 colloid cyst of the 3rd ventricle. Although the mass was a postmortem finding in some, surgical attack on it was followed by cessation of the violence in five patients diagnosed antemortem.

Patients, especially young men, after craniocerebral injuries, often go through a phase of hyperactivity and belligerence. In many, the cerebral injury is too diffuse to permit correlation of one specific area of the brain with this symptom. However, McLaurin and Heimer (21) have reported as "restless and combative" 7 of 12 patients with contusions of the temporal lobe. In 9 of these 12 patients, the diagnosis was verified by open operation and in the other three, by clear-cut evidence in special radiographic studies.

Viral disease of the limbic system, such as herpes encephalitis, may be related to emotional changes and combativeness. Of course, rabies, whose name in French, German and Italian means rage, has as the most characteristic of its many lesion sites, inclusion bodies in Ammon's horn.

The second category of disease includes those patients with epilepsy who may have a structural or simply a functional derangement of the brain. By far the most common focal cerebral disorders associated with poor control of destructive impulses and rage are those which also give rise to limbic system epilepsy. Henry Maudsley, (22) almost a century ago, was able to study epileptic patients confined to an asylum who were untreated in terms of modern anticonvulsant and ataractic therapy. He described the auras of temporal lobe epilepsy (without anatomical correlations) and discussed at length the ictal and interictal violence and assaultive behavior of untreated epileptic patients.

The occurrence of abnormal aggressivity in epileptic patients has varied with the group of patients being studied. In some series, the clinical correlations of limbic epilepsy with aggression have generated comments by physicians on the frequent outbursts of anger, often appearing after minimal provocation in such patients. Thus, Gastaut and his co-workers (23) recorded paroxysmal rages in 50 per cent of their epileptics of the temporal lobe type. Falconer and his co-workers (24), in 50 patients whose temporal lobe epilepsy was associated with a predominantly unilateral spike focus, found as the commonest personality disturbance in 38 per cent a "pathological aggressiveness occurring in outbursts in an otherwise adjusted individual." Another 14 per cent had "an often milder but more persistent aggressiveness associated with a continued paranoid outlook." Rages, with typical French delicacy called "endogenous bouts of impulsiveness," became so severe in 38 epileptic patients of Roger and Dongier (25) that they had to be confined to mental hospitals. Everyone of the 38 had classical neurological symptoms of temporal lobe epilepsy, evidence of EEG foci in scalp leads from temporal or inferior frontal regions or both. In view of these facts one would anticipate that a feeling of anger might be reported in man as an aura ushering in a frank seizure of temporal lobe epilepsy, or that a directed assault may be a symptom occurring during such a seizure. However, in the published accounts in man, the majority of patients who describe any emotional component of their seizures classify it as fear. Other emotions such as anger, sadness, pleasure and joy, are all much less frequent. (Currie and his associates (26) studied

666 temporal lobe epileptics seen in a general hospital. Only 16 of their patients had rage attacks as part of the ictus.) In fact, Penfield and Jasper (27) stated that in their experience, "neither localized epileptic discharge nor electrical stimulation is capable of awakening the emotions of anger, joy, pleasure or sexual excitement." Gloor (28), speaking from the mass of experience of the Montreal Neurological Institute with patients having temporal seizures, mentions in particular that "rage with or without aggressive behavior, is an extremely rare ictal phenomenon." The data of Paillas (29) are in essential agreement. Of his 50 patients treated with surgery of the temporal lobe, 26 had affective symptoms as part of their seizure pattern. These consisted of fear or a generalized unpleasant feeling in 18; only 2 had "angry impulses" and 1 had a desire to bite himself. Fear, however, may precipitate attack behavior. This was true in 2 of the 4 patients to be described with inlying electrodes. Both of these patients had an aura containing an element of fear immediately preceding their destructive or assaultive acts. Abnormal aggressivity is clearly more frequent as an interictal rather than as a seizure phenomenon. Ounsted and his co-workers (30), for example, in a prospective study of 100 temporal lobe epileptics, found that 36 developed repeated episodes of "catastrophic rage" during the period of observation.

A third line of evidence is derived from the surgical removal of limbic structures. Surgical ablation of medial temporal lobe structures has most often been carried out in the form of a temporal lobectomy in patients with temporal lobe epilepsy. One recent representative of the many series of lobectomies is that of Walker and Blumer (31). In 50 temporal lobe epileptics, 17 of their patients had aggressiveness of such severe degree that it disrupted their entire environment, and 12 more had lesser degrees of aggressivity. After temporal lobectomy, only 5 had abnormal aggressivity.

Ablation of only part of the temporal lobe, namely in and around the amygdala, has been carried out bilaterally in mainly assaultive, hyperkinetic, self-mutilating individuals with mental retardation, psychosis or temporal lobe epilepsy. The early reports of Walker (32) on 4 psychotics described only a temporary increased placidity and no effect on the psychosis. Sawa and associates (33) did the operation on 5 schizophrenics, 5 epileptics and 1 assaultive, severely retarded individual. Rage reactions appeared early after operation; placidity appeared later and lasted longer. Narabayashi and Uno (34) reported on 98 mental defectives. The rages in the 13 adults in the series were dramatically improved in 4, recurred after improvement in 3 and were not improved in 6. Vaernet and Madsen (35), in 12 schizophrenics, achieved elimination or marked reduction of the aggressive episodes in 11. In 36 patients with psychomotor seizures, Vaernet did bilateral amygdalotomy in 7 and unilateral amygdalotomy plus contralateral anterior temporal lobe resection in 2 (personal communication to the authors). The behavioral disturbances were significantly improved in 4. Balasubramaniam and his co-workers (36) have the largest series—128 patients with bilateral amygdalotomies, of whom 53 were postepileptics. In only 9 was the destructive rage behavior eliminated. These patients did not need drugs and were able to mingle in society. Forty-five patients had some improvement with only occasional outbursts of rage behavior. The other patients were not affected by their surgery. Siegfried and Ben-Shmuel (37) have done the bilateral operation on 6 patients and found improvement of the aggressivity in 4. Hitchcock and his co-workers (38) report the same results from the same operation on 6 patients. Eric Turner (39) has done 63 bilateral temporal lobotomies 1 cm. from the tip in aggressive psychomotor epileptics. Psychomotor attacks were abolished in 65 per cent, and major rage attacks ceased in all of his patients.

There is some evidence to indicate that neighboring areas in the limbic system may have adversary roles. Animal experiments are suggestive of this for aggression, in both the hypothalamus and amygdala. Clinical observations of a discrete hypothalamic tumor associated with aggressive behavior (40) and iatrogenic hypothalamic lesions associated with placidity (41) correlate well with experimental observations. As far as the amygdala is concerned, there is some evidence of adversary systems in close topographic proximity.

In our clinical studies, (42, 43) patient E. had frequent rage attacks in which he would do great bodily harm to his wife and children, preceded by a rather typical temporal lobe epileptic aura. This aura, of face and chest pain, could be reproduced by *central* and *medial* amygdaloid stimulation. The patient would know that he was about to do something violent but would find it difficult to stop himself. However, his mood could be changed dramatically by stimulating in the lateral portion of the amygdaloid nucleus (Fig. 8.1). The patient would become calm and relaxed, and his subjective responses to lateral amygdala stimulation would reflect this.

Recently, Narabayashi has confirmed this observation by fractional destructive lesions in the amygdala of 47 abnormally aggressive epileptic patients (Fig. 8.2). He found 26 of 36 patients with medial or central amygdaloid lesions so relieved of their symptoms that they could return to work or school. However, only 1 of 11 patients with lateral amygdaloid lesions was so benefited.

It is our opinion that an individual with a diseased or malfunctioning limbic system decompensates, as far as abnormal or inappropriate aggres-

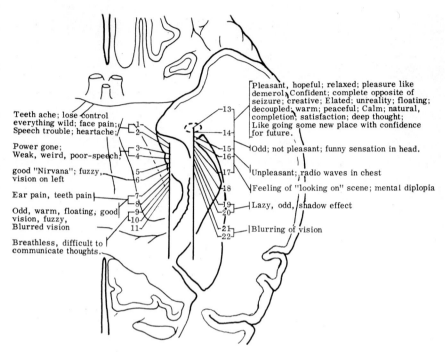

Fig. 8.1. Schematic drawing of electrode positions and responses to electrical stimuli in patient E., showing left temporal lobe with two strands of inlying electrodes. Strand with electrodes 1–11 is toward midline of head; strand 13–22 is 4 mm. lateral. Electrodes 1 and 13 are anterior, and 11 and 22 are posterior. Patient's subjective verbal responses were produced by passing a weak stimulating current through the electrode points into adjacent brain tissue. Stimulation frequency 60 c.p.s., biphasic square wave, pulse duration 1 msec., current 0.2 to 3.0 ma.

sive behavior is concerned, more readily than an individual with a normal brain, when both are subjected to environmental stress. The degree of decompensation and its relationship to environmental stimuli vary with the kind and severity of limbic system disease. The differing pattern of behavioral response can be shown, to some extent, by the effect of electrical stimulation within the amygdaloid nucleus in temporal lobe epileptic patients having inlying temporal lobe electrodes.

The first patient (U.) in our series had temporal lobe seizures accompanied by hallucinatory experiences of a very unpleasant and frightening nature, as well as seizures which were characterized by an overwhelming fear or rage. The patient was unsuccessfully treated by psychiatric and medical means for many years. The temporal lobe electrodes showed, in the first sequence with telemetered recording and stimulation, the effects of amygdaloid stimulation producing abnormal electrical discharges re-

Effect on Behavioral Abnormality	Lesion		
	medial		lateral
	15-17.5	17.5-20	
A''-A	Case 91 93 98	Case 61 101 71 110 74 112 75 113 76 117 82 121 86 122 92 124 94 125 97 126 99 127 100	Case 73
	Total (3 cases)	Total (23 cases)	Total (1 case)
B or B-C	Case 90 102 105	Case 85 109 115 118 123	Case 65 66 67 84 89 103 119
	Total (3 cases)	Total (5 cases)	Total (7 cases
C	Case 70 111		Case 95 104 107
	Total (2 cases)		Total (3 cases

Fig. 8.2. Roentgenogram measurements of amygdala lesion sites to midline of brain in 47 patients; 26 out of 36 patients with medial or central lesion sites were rehabilitated to job or school status, whereas only 1 of 11 patients with lesion sites in lateral amygdala achieved a similar result. Exact anatomical correlations, of course, cannot be made without postmortem pathological confirmation. (Supplied by Dr. Narabayashi of Tokyo. To be published in Proceedings of Third International Congress of Psychiatric Surgery, Cambridge, England, August 1972.)

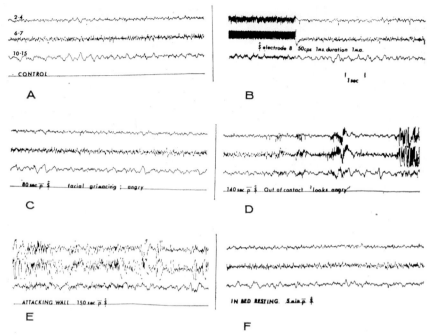

Fig. 8.3. Telemetered EEG tracings taken in patient U. during episode of attacking wall of room after stimulation. Remotely recorded brain waves from amygdala are seen in stimulus sequence: A, control recording (before stimulation); B, amygdala is remotely stimulated with weak current; C, electrical correlates of facial grimacing are not present; D, cascades of spikes are followed by frank amygdaloid seizures which precede attack behavior; E, patient's spring toward the wall occurs during amygdaloid seizure and, F, 5 minutes after attack behavior, brain wave record is similar to control recording.

corded in the amygdala, followed by attack behavior which was automatic and in which environmental factors played a relatively minor role (Fig. 8.3; see also Reference 44).

Another patient (A.), in spite of prolonged medical and psychiatric treatment, had as many as 150 temporal lobe epileptic attacks per day with bilateral foci. The patient's behavior, during and after the attacks, was quite variable. At times, it would be merely inappropriate, and occasionally assaultive. Electrical stimulation in the amygdala would, at times, produce staring and no other behavioral phenomenon, but with pronounced abnormal electrical discharges recorded from inlying electrodes in and around the amygdala. On one occasion, however, electrical stimulation produced a period of staring and absence followed by an episode of quite inappropriate and bizarre, stereotyped behavior ending

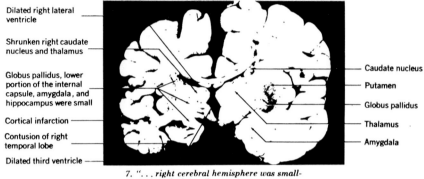

Dilated right lateral ventricle

Shrunken right caudate nucleus and thalamus

Globus pallidus, lower portion of the internal capsule, amygdala, and hippocampus were small

Cortical infarction

Contusion of right temporal lobe

Dilated third ventricle

Caudate nucleus

Putamen

Globus pallidus

Thalamus

Amygdala

7. *". . . right cerebral hemisphere was smaller than the left. . ."*

Fig. 8.4. Coronal section of brain of patient **D.**, showing atrophy subsequent to ischemic infarction of entorhinal cortex, basal ganglia, capsule, thalamus and hypothalamus. (Reprinted by permission from JAMA, 216: 1033, 1971.)

with a mild assault (in this case, pinching of the arm of one of the
attendants). At this time there was no electrical indication, at least from
electrodes in the amygdala, that a seizure was going on. Occasionally, the
assaultiveness in this patient was quite severe. However, there was no
memory for any of this behavior after the episode had been completed.

Patient **L.** had frequent episodes of interictal assaultiveness, and only
three reported episodes of aggression during the many seizures that he
had. However, he had an aura that was common to his attack behavior
and seizures. This aura was reproduced by electrical stimulation in the
amygdala. On a number of occasions, however, this failed to produce any
obvious behavioral change, only seizures, except on the one day in which
this patient was emotionally upset by his family. At that time, several
amygdaloid stimulations produced only one transient seizure. Four minutes
after the last stimulation, the patient had one of his most furious and
completely undirected episodes of attack behavior.

There are questions that must be asked of the limbic system-violence
hypothesis. One, do we know the exact mechanism of the environment-
brain interaction, or the exact kind of limbic system dysfunction or
discharge that will invariably produce violence or aggression? The answer
to that is no. Even though the evidence is suggestive, it is far from
complete. It is not surprising that this is true for emotional functions,
inasmuch as our understanding of neurological mechanisms in even less
complex situations, for example, spastic hemiplegia, is still incomplete.

A second question might be one that addresses the importance of the
role of limbic system disease in public violence. Here again, the role of

brain dysfunction in unknown. In fact, clinicians have difficulty in making the diagnosis of limbic brain disease even when it is present. The following case illustrates this point. Patient D. tried to kill a number of people and commit suicide while attempting to hijack an airplane. He did succeed in killing one pilot and wounding another. He received a concussion and was hospitalized, and a consultation was requested. This disclosed that he had had a penetrating brain wound 11 years before, with hemiparesis and dilated pupil. In spite of repeated neurological examinations, psychiatric interviews and psychometric tests, only the hemiparesis, mild difficulty with visual comprehension and memory and inferior quadrantic field defect were seen. No major sign of limbic system disease was found. Six hours of EEG examination showed very rare temporal slowing and two δ waves; it did not disclose the limbic abnormalities that were found in contrast roentgenograms of the brain. Six months later, this man committed suicide in jail. At postmorten examination, a large unilateral atrophic process including thalamus, hypothalamus, globus pallidus, lower portion of capsule, amygdala and hippocampus, characteristic of old ischemic infarction, was found (Fig. 8.4). The point in this case is not the relation of the pathological lesion to abnormal behavior, for this is quite unclear. It is, rather, the ineffectiveness of present neurological and psychiatric tests for the diagnosis of gross lesions of the limbic system when they are present (44).

SUMMARY

The steps needed to more clearly define the role of limbic disease in aggressive behavior include the development of simple, reliable clinical tests for the diagnosis of limbic system malfunction. At present, with the exception of limbic epilepsy, most patients with this disease defy diagnosis except by invasive procedures unsuitable for outpatient clinic or population studies. When this is accomplished, a statistical study needs to be carried out to answer the following questions.

1. Do a significant number of individuals with limbic disease have behavioral abnormalities such as inappropriate aggression?

2. Do a significant number of violent individuals have limbic disease?

As a corollary, it would be important to see what relation abnormal aggression has with disease of structures such as the parietal cortex. Parietal epilepsy as an isolated phenomenon is relatively infrequent, but patients with this disorder might serve as an excellent control.

Finally, even if limbic disease-related violence proves to be a small factor in the overall incidence of violence, it may still be worthwhile to investigate and treat those patients who are thus afflicted.

REFERENCES

1. PAPEZ, JW: A proposed mechanism of emotion. Arch Neurol Psychiatr 38: 725, 1937.
2. KAADA, BR: Brain mechanisms related to aggressive behavior, in Brain Function, Vol 5: Aggression and Defense: Neural Mechanisms and Social Patterns, edited by Clemente, CD, Lindsley, DB. Berkeley, Univ of California Press, 1967, p. 95.
3. DeMOLINA, AF, HUNSPERGER, BW: Central representation of affective reactions in forebrain and brainstem: electrical stimulation of amygdala, stria terminalis, and adjacent structures. J Physiol 145: 251, 1959.
4. URSIN, H: The temporal lobe substrate of fear and anger. Acta Psychiatr Neurol Scand 35: 378, 1960.
5. ANAND, BK, DUA, S: Stimulation of limbic system of brain in waking animals. Science 122: 1139, 1955.
6. EGGER, MD, FLYNN, JP: Further studies on the effects of amygdaloid stimulation and ablation on hypothalamically elicited attack behavior in cats. Progr Brain Res 27: 165, 1967.
7. ALFONSO-DeFLORIDA, F, DELGADO, JMR: Lasting behavioral and EEG changes in cats induced by prolonged stimulation of amygdala. Am J Physiol 193: 223, 1958.
8. URSIN, H: The effect of amygdaloid lesions on flight and defense behavior in cats. Exp Neurol 11: 61, 1965.
9. BARD, P, MOUNTCASTLE, VB: Some forebrain mechanisms involved in expression of rage with special reference to suppression of angry behavior. Res Publ Assoc Nerv Ment Dis 27: 362, 1948.
10. WOOD, CD: Behavioral changes following discrete lesions of temporal lobe structures. Neurology 8: 215, 1958.
11. ROSVOLD, HE, MIRSKY, AF, PRIBRAM, KH: Influence of amygdalectomy on social behavior in monkeys. J Comp Physiol Psychol 47: 173, 1954.
12. FALCONER, MA, HILL, D, MEYER, A, WILSON, JL: Clinical, radiological and EEG correlations with pathological changes in temporal lobe epilepsy and their significance in surgical treatment, in Temporal Lobe Epilepsy, edited by Baldwin, M, Bailey, P. Springfield, Ill., Charles C Thomas, Publisher, 1958, p. 396.
13. CUSHING, H: The Pituitary Body and Hypothalamus. Springfield, Ill. C.C Thomas, 1929.
14. ALPERS, BJ: Relation of the hypothalamus to disorders of personality: report of a case. Arch Neurol Psychiatr 38: 291, 1937.
15. VONDERAHE, AH: Forebrain and rage reactions. Trans Am Neurol Assoc 66: 129, 1940.
16. HILL, D: Cerebral dysrhythmia: its significance in aggressive behavior. Proc Roy Soc Med 37: 317, 1944.
17. MALAMUD, N: Psychiatric disorder with intracranial tumors of limbic system. Arch Neurol 17: 113, 1967.
18. REEVES, AG, PLUM, F: Hyperphagia, rage and dementia accompanying a ventromedial hypothalamic neoplasm. Arch Neurol 20: 616, 1969.
19. SWEET, WH, ERVIN, FR, MARK, VH: The relationship of violent behaviour to focal cerebral disease, in Aggressive Behavior, edited by Garattini, S, Sigg, EB. Amsterdam, Excerpta Medica Foundation, 1969, p. 336.
20. MULLAN, J: Violent behavior; a case report presented at the Central Neurosurgical Society. Chicago, March 1971.
21. McLAURIN, RL, HEIMER, F: The syndrome of temporal lobe contusion. J Neurosurg 23: 296, 1965.

22. MAUDSLEY, H: Responsibility in Mental Disease. New York, D. Appleton and Co., 1874.

23. GASTAUT, G, MORIN, G, LESÈVRE, N: Etude du comportement des épileptiques psychomoteurs dans l'intervalle de leurs crises; les troubles de l'activité globale et de la sociabilité. Ann Med Psychol 113: 1, 1955.

24. FALCONER, MA, HILL, D, MEYER, A, WILSON, JL: Clinical, radiological and EEG correlations with pathological changes in temporal lobe epilepsy and their significance in surgical treatment, in Temporal Lobe Epilepsy, edited by Baldwin, M, Bailey, P. Springfield, Ill., C.C Thomas, 1958, P. 396.

25. ROGER, A, DONGIER, M: Corrélations électrocliniques chez épileptiques internés. Rev Neurol 83: 593, 1950.

26. CURRIE, S, HEATHFIELD, KWG, HENSON, RA, SCOTT, DF: Clinical course and prognosis of temporal lobe epilepsy: a survey of 666 patients. Brain 94: 173, 1971.

27. PENFIELD, W, JASPER, H: Epilepsy and the Functional Anatomy of the Human Brain. Boston, Little, Brown, 1954.

28. GLOOR, P: Discussion of B. R. Kaada; Brain mechanisms related to aggressive behavior, in Brain Function, Vol. 5: Aggression and Defense: Neural Mechanisms and Social Patterns, edited by Clemente, CD, Lindsley, DB. Berkeley, Univ of Calif Press, 1967, p. 118.

29. PAILLAS, JE: Aspects cliniques de l'épilepsie temporale, in Temporal Lobe Epilepsy, edited by Baldwin, M, Bailey, P. Springfield, Ill., C.C Thomas, 1958, p. 411.

30. OUNSTED, C, LINDSAY, J, NORMAN, R: Biological Factors in Temporal Lobe Epilepsy. England, The Lavenham Press Ltd., 1966.

31. WALKER, AE, BLUMER, D: Temporal lobe epilepsy and violent behavior. Lecture at The Johns Hopkins Hospital, Baltimore, March 1970.

32. WALKER, AE: Discussion of Scoville et al. Res Publ Assoc Res Nerv Ment Dis 31: 370, 1953.

33. SAWA, M, VEKI, Y, ARITA, M, HARADA, T: Preliminary report on amygdaloidectomy in psychotic patients, with interpretation of oral-emotional manifestation in schizophrenics. Folia Psychiatr Neurol Jap 7: 309, 1954.

34. NARABAYASHI, H, UNO, M: Long range results of stereotaxic amygdalotomy for behavioral disorders. Confin Neurol 27: 168, 1966.

35. VAERNET, K, MADSEN, A: Stereotaxic amygdalotomy and basofrontal tractotomy in psychotics with aggressive behaviour. J Neurol Neurosurg Psychiatr 33: 858, 1970.

36. BALASUBRAMANIAM, P, RAMANUJAM, PB, RAMAMURTHI, B, KANAKA, TS: Stereotaxic surgery for behavior disorders, in Psychosurgery, edited by Hitchcock, E, Laitinen, L, Vaernet, K. Springfield, Ill., Charles C Thomas, Publisher, 1972, p. 156.

37. SIEGFRIED, J, BEN-SHMUEL, A: Neurosurgical treatment of aggressivity: stereotaxic amygdalotomy versus leukotomy, in Psychosurgery, edited by Hitchcock, E, Laitinen, L, Vaernet, K. Springfield, Ill., Charles C Thomas, Publisher, 1972, p. 214.

38. HITCHCOCK, E, ASHCROFT, GW, CAIRNS, VM, MURRAY, LG: Preoperative and postoperative assessment and management of psychosurgical patients, in Psychosurgery, edited by Hitchcock, E, Laitinen, L, Vaernet, K. Springfield, Ill., Charles C Thomas, Publisher, 1972, p. 164.

39. TURNER, E: A new approach to unilateral and bilateral lobotomies for psychomotor epilepsy. J Neurol Neurosurg Psychiatr 26: 285, 1963.

40. REEVES, AG, PLUM, F: Hyperphagia, rage, and dementia accompanying a ventromedial hypothalamic neoplasm. Arch Neurol 20: 616, 1969.

41. SANO, K, YOSHIAKI, M, SEKINO, H, OGASHIWA, M, ISHIJIMA, B: Results of stimulation and destruction of the posterior hypothalamus in man. J Neurosurg 33: 689, 1970.

42. STEVENS, JR, MARK, VH, ERVIN, FR, PACHECO, P, SUEMATSU, K: Deep temporal stimulation in man: long-latency, long-lasting psychological changes. Arch Neurol 21: 157, 1969.
43. MARK, VH, ERVIN, FR, SWEET, WH, DELGADO, JMR: Remote telemeter stimulation and recording from implanted temporal lobe electrodes. Confin Neurol 31: 86, 1969.
44. MARK, VH, SOUTHGATE, MT (eds.): Violence and brain disease: clinical pathological conference. JAMA 216: 1025, 1971.

ADDENDUM

Since the presentation of this work, two important papers and one editorial have supplied additional information on this topic:

ADDITIONAL REFERENCES

1. WALKER, AE: Man and his temporal lobes (John Hughlings Jackson Lecture). Surg Neurol 1: 69, 1973.
2. FALCONER, MA: Reversibility by temporal-lobe resection of the behavioral abnormalities of temporal-lobe epilepsy. N Engl J Med 289: 451, 1973.
3. GESCHWIND, N: Effects of temporal-lobe surgery on behavior (editorial). N Engl J Med 289: 480, 1973.

DISCUSSION

Note. Before Dr. Mark read his paper, the representative of a protest group made the following statement.

We have come here today to express our outrage, contempt and utter revulsion for institutional psychiatry and its repressive and inhuman exploitation carried out under the guise of legitimate medicine. We specifically point to psychosurgery and the brain butchers who would hack and cut away all vestiges of social dissent to satisfy the appetite of a society that is obsessed with utter and absolute conformity.

Dr. Peter Breggan has estimated that 600 persons are lobotomized each year. Given the political climate in this country and psychiatrists' appetites for human experimentation, the number could easily reach 6000 or perhaps 60,000 victims a year.

Psychosurgery is but one method of behavior and social control that is being employed, but it is the most sure since it is irreversible.

Dr. Mark joined forces with Dr. Ervin and Dr. Sweet after the Detroit ghetto uprising of 1967 in sending a letter to one of the psychiatric journals in which they stated that those ghetto dwellers who participated in the Detroit rebellion and committed acts of violence have low violence thresholds and were suffering from diseased brains. They recommended psychosurgery. Their proposed treatment carries the explicit warning that ghetto inhabitants who rebel against racism and social and economic oppression shall be dealt with by having their brains cut open. A lobotomy is a partial murder.

We of the coalition unequivocally demand an end to psychosurgery in this country. We hold it illegal and a high crime against humanity.

DR. VERNON H. MARK (Boston, Massachusetts): I would like to acknowledge the assistance of Dr. William Sweet and Dr. Ira Sherwin with this presentation without suggesting their responsibility for any of my statements.

Note: Dr. Mark then presented his paper.

SHERVERT H. FRAZIER (Chairman) (Boston, Massachusetts): Is social control a legitimate function for the practice of medicine? Doesn't social control presume to function in the interest of society and thus contradict the Hippocratic oath? "Do no harm. My patient's health comes first."

DR. MARK: I essentially agree. The patients who are candidates for medical and psychiatric treatment, and only as a last resort surgical treatment, are patients who are sick. To deny them the opportunity for medical care is infringing on their human rights.

DR. FRAZIER: The next question: "In your book, *Violence and the Brain,* you defined acceptable violence as the controlled, minimal, necessary action to prevent personal physical injury or wanton destruction of property. The shooting of the four Kent State students was justified by the state troopers as necessary to prevent injury to themselves. During the Detroit uprising, the mobilization of the militia was justified by the threat to property. The mobilization resulted in the Algiers Motel murders, as well as scores of other killings of Detroit residents. How would you defend your definition of acceptable violence in these cases?"

DR. MARK: The definition of violence used in that book was taken from the humanist, Jones, at Harvard University. In the book it is specifically stated that killings or other violent acts done by troopers or police are just as unacceptable as any other kind of violence (1).

DR. FRAZIER: The next question is: "You have performed amygdalotomies on patients with temporal lobe epilepsy and rage reactions. The operations, while not eliminating the epilepsy, have eliminated the rage reactions. The procedure seems to be effective against rage reactions. Under what circumstances would you consider using the operation on an individual with rage reactions but no demonstrable brain disease?"

DR. MARK: First of all, we did a 3-year follow-up on some of the patients reported in the book. One patient, who had been described as not having had her epilepsy affected, did get a beneficial effect on the epilepsy. Her seizure went from 20 a day to 20 a year. As for using the operation on an individual with rage reactions but no demonstrable brain disease, I would not consider that an acceptable procedure.

DR. FRAZIER: The next question is: "In a 1967 letter to the Journal of the American Medical Association, coauthored by yourself and Drs. Sweet and Ervin, you asked, Is there something peculiar about the violent slum dweller that differentiates him from his peaceful neighbor? You go on to note that we need to intensify clinical studies of the individuals committing the violence. The goal of such studies would be to pinpoint, diagnose and treat people with low violence thresholds before they contribute to further tragedies. The President's Commission on Civil Disorders concluded that most, if not all, of the deaths occurring during the urban rebellions were attributable to National Guardsmen and police officials. Would you recommend therapeutic ablations on the officers of the National Guard, on the governors who called out the Guard, or on the oppressed black and Latin inner city residents?"

DR. MARK: Our book indicates that it is worthwhile and necessary to look at the people who carry guns, whether supposedly in the public interest or not. We have had patients who were public officials, who carried guns and who had this kind of response. We hospitalized these patients, and they were treated. There is no difference here in our outlook.

DR. FRAZIER: The next question is: "Would you recommend mental status examinations of the prisoners at Attica who rebelled in support of such demands as adequate medical care, or of Nelson Rockefeller who ordered in the police who caused the deaths? Do you consider potentially violent the students at the Southern University of New Orleans who demonstrated against racist cutbacks in the University budget? What about the governor who ordered in the police who committed the only violence that took place? When you review recent history, Dr. Mark, whom would you diagnose as violent—those who rebel against the intolerable conditions in our society, or those who impose intolerable conditions on others?"

DR. MARK: I think the incident at Southern University indicates that perhaps we need to look at the public officials who carry guns to see whether they are normal or abnormal. At present, our ability to test patients is very limited, but there are some psychological tests which may be useful in this kind of investigation.

DR. DOMINICK PURPURA (Bronx, New York): First, I would like to speak to the young people who are here today. It is regrettable that you have taken it upon yourselves to make this mission against psychosurgery. You are injecting yourselves upon the problem which we are all concerned about. This organization is devoted to the exploration of problems of nervous and mental diseases. It has a history of concern for the problems you are concerned about. Our responsibility is to get at the facts, whereas some of you have, rather distressingly, taken a very anti-intellectual attitude. This is the kind of problem we face in this society and in this organization.

REFERENCE

1. MARK, VH, ERVIN, FR: Violence and the Brain, New York, Harper & Row, 1970, p. 151.

Chapter 9

AGGRESSION IN CHILDREN

LAURETTA BENDER

Child psychiatrists and psychologists studying child behavior, both normal and abnormal, have had to deal with Freud's teachings (1) that aggression in children is hostile, a promordial reaction to ever present frustration, an instinctive drive equated with the death instincts leading to death wishes as a normal developmental feature.

Although these theories have not been accepted by all psychoanalysts (2) the child analysts following Anna Freud and Melanie Klein have made these concepts basic to their studies of child development and to their educational and psychotherapeutic practices.

Anna Freud (3), while studying the English children evacuated from London in the Hampstead Nurseries, wrote: "It is one of the recognized aims of education to deal with the aggressiveness in child nature in the first four or five years." She stated: "The dangers of the war lie in the fact that the destruction raging in the outer world may beget the very real aggressiveness which rages on the inside of the child." She claimed that the child must be safeguarded from the primitive forces of the war "not because horror and atrocities were so strange to them but because of the need to estrange the young child from the primitive and atrocious wishes of their infantile nature." However, the psychoanalytic literature does not record child atrocities as a result of stimulation from war experiences or as a result of primary aggressive drives.

In her more recent writings (1965) Anna Freud (4) still says "Greed, demandingness, possessiveness, extreme jealousy and competitiveness, impulses to kill rivals and frustrating figures, i.e., all the elements of the infant's instinctual life become nuclei for later dissociability if permitted to remain unmodified and the social growth implies adoption of a compliant defensive attitude toward them. As a result of defenses on the part of the ego some of them are eliminated from the conscious self altogether (by repression) others are turned into their opposite which are more acceptable (by reaction formation) or deflected into noninstinctual aims (by sublimation) others are ... displaced onto images of others (by projection)."

Although she here speaks of these processes as "normal elements in the infants instinctual life," elsewhere she speaks as though the processes denote pathology. She says "But such early delinquency-like behavior need not develop into a delinquent or criminal but an obsessional character or neurosis." She goes on to say, "Many children who begin with phobia or anxiety hysteria grow later into true obsessionals ... (and) are predestined to develop in later life not obsessional neuroses but schizoid and schizophrenic states instead."

In my own experience with disturbed children in New York City and State, where I have worked since 1934, I have never been able to confirm these theories. Wherever aggression, hostile or destructive, has been shown in the behavior of children, it has been the result of some form of real developmental pathology in the context of an unsympathetic or actively disturbing social and environmental situation which has disorganized the normal constructive patterned drives and behavior of the developing child.

I have postulated the normal drives in child development in the following way (2).

1. An inherent drive for normality determined by biological maturation, patterned with a direction towards a goal, and which can never be completely blocked or diverted by any pathology within the child or in his outer world.

2. An inborn capacity to relate and identify with other humans such as the mother, and thus experience love, social relations, communication and language.

3. An inborn capacity for fantasy, symbol formation and projection in all his experiences, and to communicate these experiences, thus reconstructing and mastering the outer world with creativity.

Therefore, destructiveness and hostile aggression in a child is a symptom complex caused by developmental pathology which disorganizes the normal constructive patterned drives, so that inadequate gratification leads to frustration.

My experience with aggressiveness in children is best demonstrated by presenting the case material on children I have known, who have actually been involved in the death of another human being. If the psychoanalytic theories were correct, instances of children causing a death should not be uncommon. But in 35 years of psychiatric practice in New York City and New York State, I have been able to collect 34 cases of children under the age of 16 years, who have apparently been responsible for a death. These 34 cases were collected from the New York City Bellevue Psychiatric Hospital, the children's courts of New York City, the New York State mental hospital system and correctional institutions. Included were children that I personally was able to study psychiatrically and where all hospital, court and follow-up records were available to me. All cases were followed up at least 5 to 25 years after the homicidal incident.

By 1945 eight children had been observed at Bellevue who were held responsible for a death (5, 6). The conclusions were overwhelming—the death was always accidental and unexpected by the child. Neither had the child any concept of the irreversibility of death. The death occurred because the victim happened to be in the path of the activity initiated by the child and was unintentionally fatal. The child then responded with a severe depressive grief or mourning reaction. His life pattern changed critically from that point. He tried by every means in fantasy and by acting out to deny the act and its consequences, the death of the victim and its irreversibility. He might even attempt to repeat the whole experience in order to prove that it could not have happened. These children needed long periods of careful psychiatric care to ameliorate their emotional disturbance and protect them from repeating the experience.

These eight children had all experienced early social deprivation but also had endogenous pathology such as schizophrenia, encephalitis, epilepsy and primary learning disabilities. Subsequent follow-up into adulthood showed that their latent pathology was more severe than recognized at the time of observation following the incident. Three were chronically hospitalized as psychotic schizophrenics. Two epileptics were impossible to rehabilitate. Two others repeatedly failed in community adjustment. Only one child, a girl, subsequently made an adequate social adjustment at 25 years when her mother was in a mental hospital and father and brothers were known to social agencies as inadequate.

In 1959 (7) and again in 1969 (8) more extensive studies were reported on 25 additional boys and girls to the age of 16 years who had caused a death, and since then a 26th case has been added. The conclusions this time are that a constellation of factors is always present when a boy or girl caused a death. There needs to be a disturbed, poorly controlled, impulsive child, a victim who acted as an irritant, an available lethal weapon and always a lack of protective supervision by some third person who could have stopped the fatal consequences.

Of the total 34 death-causing children studied psychiatrically, some combination of the following factors were found.

1) Organic brain disease with an impulsive disorder, an abnormal electroencephalogram, and/or epilepsy in 15 of the 34 cases; 2) schizophrenia with preoccupations with death and killing in the pseudoneurotic phase of younger children or with antisocial paranoid preoccupation in the pseudopsychopathic phase of the adolescent children in 13 of the 34 cases; 3) compulsive fire setting in 13 cases; 4) defeating school retardation with reading disabilities in 13 cases and 5) extremely unfavorable home

conditions and life experiences. As indicative of the last factor, 6 children had one or both parents and a sibling who were mentally ill in a hospital and 2 children had observed their father being killed, 1 by the mother.

Data on the religious and ethnic background showed that there were 23 white and 11 black children. There were 19 Catholics, of whom 6 were Italian, 4 Irish and 3 Puerto Rican. Twelve were Protestant, of whom 10 were black and 2 white. There was 1 Jew, 1 Mormon and 1 German Lutheran.

The I.Q. range was from 18 to 127, with a mean I.Q. of 87; there were four with an I.Q. under 70.

The mode of death in younger children was by fire (6 children), drowning (5 children), pushing off of heights (3 children) and choking (1 child). Deaths by fire and drowning were all purely incidental. The child's subsequent severe depression and grief ridden reaction required psychiatric care. Nevertheless, of these 15 young children, 10 years and under, 7 were schizophrenic and 3 were grossly defective with developmental brain damage. The five involved in a drowning were all fire setters. They had all been known to threaten to kill before the drowning. None were free from family, social and personal disorders of grossly damaging degree. Multiple deaths (two and three) were caused by drowning and fire.

The 19 older boys, ages 11 years through 15 years, caused deaths by stabbing with sharp weapons (7 boys), by repeated blows with a heavy object (6 boys) and by shooting (6 boys). Four younger boys, ages 6, 8 and 9, are included in these categories. This group showed the most pathology with clinically recognizable schizophrenia, epilepsy and/or significant brain damage diagnosed in all cases.

Our more recent studies have shown that definite pathology could always be recognized in these homicidally aggressive children or young adolescents inasmuch as we have acquired more clinical experience with diagnostic procedures. Furthermore, the pathology was confirmed and seemed more obvious when follow-up reports were obtained. This was true of adolescent schizophrenics with pseudoneurotic and pseudopsychopathic defenses, who often seemed to be symptom-free and not psychotic at the time (9). There is a strong tendency in our culture, and even among professionals, not to recognize psychoses or endogenous pathology in young people, to deny or not ask for previous histories and to seek only for sociological or psychogenic factors. Subsequent course, however, has confirmed the presence of pathology in all these youngsters.

An adequate and, preferably, repeated use of electroencephalograms has revealed impulse disorders and latent epilepsy even before it was clinically demonstrable in a surprising number of adequately studied homicidal adolescents. Twelve children, 10 years and older, had electroencephalograms; eight were pathological and only one questionable.

There was a total of 41 victims, of whom 30 were children and 11 were adults. Of the 30 children, 13 were siblings, 2 were cousins and 15 unrelated. Of the related children 10 died by fire started by 5 children, 2 younger siblings were pushed out of windows, 1 infant was choked by a defective blind brother, 1 child was drowned and 1 struck by an ax. Only one of the siblings who caused these deaths was older than 10 years.

Of the 15 unrelated children, 4 were drowned, 4 stabbed, 3 hit with heavy objects, 2 shot, 1 pushed off a roof and 1 girl had bricks dropped on her from a roof by two boys. The age of the children who caused these deaths ranged from 9 to 15 years.

Of the eleven adults who died, 6 were relatives, 1 14-year-old boy shot his mother and older sister, 1 13-year-old shot his stepmother, 1 8-year-old stabbed his mother and father and 1 14-year-old stabbed his aunt.

Five unrelated adults were killed by five boys, 12 to 15 years of age, by fire, shooting, stabbing and bludgeoning, the last was for robbery.

Thanks to Dr. Don Winn of Queens Childrens Hospitals (formerly the Children Service of Creedmoor State Hospital), I have data on six young adolescents 13½ to 16 years of age examined in that hospital between September 1969 and March 1972, and who had each caused a death. They had all been referred from Brooklyn. Three had been observed and diagnosed and released from the hospital before they had caused the death and three after.

There were five boys and one girl. Five were black and one Puerto Rican. The 13½-year-old girl started a fire that killed three people. Four boys stabbed their victims; one boy held his mother while his friend stabbed her. One boy raped his woman victim first.

All six of these adolescents were diagnosed as schizophrenic. Four were considered to be latent with psychopathic features or what I have called pseudopsychopathic schizophrenia (9); the girl and one boy also had definite signs of organic brain disease and suspected epilepsy. Three had psychotic parents and two had experienced a homicide in the family. Of course there is no follow-up on these recent cases but they fall into the same pattern as the other cases in this study.

The psychodynamics of the prepuberty child after he had caused a death is that he does not believe that he is able to kill or that death is irreparable (10) and he attempts, by fantasy and acting out, to prove that it is not possible. An adolescent makes an effort to deny both guilt and feelings of guilt for his part in the act that caused the death and to claim amnesia or other repressive defenses. Both are usually misunderstood and dangerous. Eight of the boys who had caused a death, afterwards were still threatening to kill whenever they were frustrated. Several expressed fear of their own ability to kill. Sixteen of the 34 boys and girls, because of their early disturbed behavior, had psychiatric evaluation before the incident that led to the death. In many of these, recommendations had been made which had not been followed. Five boys and one girl had been reported as very dangerous. Of course, it cannot be denied that many children are reported as dangerous who have not proven to be so later.

Dr. Renatus Hartog, who examined Lee Harvey Oswald as a delinquent boy, is reported (11) to have said after the assassination of President Kennedy that he had found the boy "potentially dangerous." He also estimated that 15 per cent of the youngsters in the Youth House, a retention home for delinquents of New York City, who were referred to him for psychiatric evaluation, were "potential killers." Dr. Hartog does not report, however, that any of them actually did kill.

We are faced with the problem of determining why there is not more violence committed by the potentially dangerous recognizable by psychiatrists (12). This reinforces the concept that a constellation of factors is required: endogenous pathology, unfavorable social environment, an irritating victim, a lethal agent and a lack of protection.

In such a psychiatric evaluation of known child and young adolescent killers there is no place for the psychoanalytic concepts of universal inborn aggressiveness or death instincts or death wishes, as formulated by Freud and many of his followers.

REFERENCES

1. FREUD, S: Beyond the Pleasure Principle. London, International Psychoanalytic Press, 1922.
2. BENDER, L: Genesis of hostility in children. Am J Psychiatr 105: 241, 1948.
3. FREUD, A, BURLINGHAM, DG: War and Children. New York, Medical War Books, 1922.
4. FREUD, A: Normality and Pathology in Childhood: Assessments of Development. New York, International Universities Press, Inc., 1965.
5. BENDER, L, CURRAN, F: Children and adolescents who kill. J Crim Psychopathol 1: 297, 1940.
6. KEELER, WR: Children's reaction to death in the family, in A Dynamic Psychopathology of Childhood, edited by Bender, L. Springfield, Ill., Charles C Thomas, Publisher, 1954, p. 172.
7. BENDER, L: Children and adolescents who have killed. Am J Psychiatr 116: 510, 1959.
8. BENDER, L: Hostile aggression in children, in Aggressive Behavior, edited by Garattini, S, Sigg, EB. Amsterdam, Excerpta Medica Foundation, 1969, p. 322.
9. BENDER, L: The concept of pseudopsychopathic schizophrenia in adolescence. Am J Orthopsychiatr 29: 491, 1959.
10. SCHILDER, P, WECHSLER, D: Attitude of children towards death. J Genet Psychol 46: 406, 1934.
11. SIBLEY, J: Youth problems studied in the light of the Oswald case. The New York Times, Jan. 5, 1967. p. 75.

12. RAPPEPORT, JR: Clinical Evaluation of the Dangerousness of the Mentally Ill. Springfield, Ill., Charles C Thomas, Publisher, 1967.

DISCUSSION

DR. SALEEM SHAH (Rockville, Maryland): I agree about the incidence of psychiatric pathology among youngsters involved in homicide and delinquency. I am troubled, however, about some of the base rate problems that are often ignored in these discussions. Dr. Bender mentioned something like 35 cases in the entire state of New York. If one looks for all the youngsters who have experienced severe developmental stress or emotional deprivation, who have some vague, questionable indices of organic brain damage and who may also be diagnosed as schizophrenic or depressive, you might find several hundred thousands. I suspect that the developmental and other characteristics of Lee Harvey Oswald could be multiplied by a few thousand. My concern is that if we base our distinctions on small, highly selected samples, hoping to make some preventive effort, we will run into the problem of massive false positive predictions, the same problem that we face in regard to civil commitments.

I wonder about the policy implications. We have commitment laws for individuals who show violence and who are mentally ill. Yet I would suspect that more people have been killed by drunken drivers than by all the schizophrenics who have lived in the past century. When we consider the policy implications, we should keep in mind the very low base rates of the phenomena Dr. Bender is discussing.

DR. LAURETTE BENDER (New York, New York): I certainly agree. It is not an inborn instinct that leads children to kill. There does have to be a constellation of factors, one of which has to be endogenous pathology, but the other factors must be present too. We have to do more about our social-cultural situation so that less children come from handicapped homes. We have to do more to provide that such children should be well supervised and not left to their own devices so much. We have to do more in every field of psychiatry and social endeavor.

I agree that 34 is a small number, but it is because I have not really tried to collect these cases over the years.

DR. MELMAN (Philadelphia, Pennsylvania): What types of epilepsy were found in your patients?

DR. BENDER: Almost every type. Very often the epilepsy did not assert itself until after the act had been committed and the child had been institutionalized. Then the epilepsy would come forward and have to be treated. There was no specific incidence of limbic epilepsy but this was, after all, 20 to 40 years ago when such diagnoses were not made. Neither was there a diagnosis of temporal lobe epilepsy.

MISS MATHEA FALCO (Washington, D.C.): Were the victims of these children relatives or playmates?

DR. BENDER: Many of them, especially with the drownings, were playmates. In the fires, they were more usually strangers, although in one case a defective boy started a fire that killed his two defective brothers while he himself got out.

In another fire, three siblings were killed because the mother could rescue only two of her five children. There was an incident in which a boy had his mother stabbed by another boy. There were two situations in which a sister was burned by an older sister, apparently accidentally. There was almost every combination. I would say the minority of the cases were siblings and even fewer were parents. Otherwise they were playmates.

Chapter 10

DRUG USE AMONG YOUTHFUL ASSAULTIVE AND SEXUAL OFFENDERS[1]

JARED R. TINKLENBERG AND KENNETH M. WOODROW

INTRODUCTION

In recent years, there has been rising concern about the assaultive crime rate in the United States, especially crime committed by youthful offenders (1). During this same period, there has been a burgeoning of drug abuse by young people. Exotic new chemicals such as dimethyltryptamine (DMT) and 2,5-dimethoxy-4-methylamphetamine (STP) have been added to the illicit pharmacopoeia, and high dose intravenous injections of several substances have become popular in some parts of the country. Because of changes in drug use and rates of aggressive crime, we thought it timely to assess patterns of drug use by youthful offenders. We were especially interested in four interrelated questions:

Which drugs were reported to enhance assaultive tendencies, and which were reported to reduce assaultiveness?

Which drugs were actually associated with assaultive and sexually offensive behavior?

Were there differences in drug preferences among assaultive delinquents, sexual offenders and nonassaultive individuals?

Were there different patterns of drug use among physically assaultive delinquents, sexual offenders and nonassaultive offenders?

SUBJECTS

All of the subjects interviewed in this study were male adolescent offenders incarcerated during January 1971 to October 1972 at Karl Holton School, a moderate security facility of the California Youth Authority in Northern California. Since most delinquents in California are not incarcerated but are handled by probation or facilities within their communities, these subjects represent some of the most serious youthful offenders in the state. Only 2 to 3 per cent of those youths convicted of felonious crime are not eligible for confinement in moderate security facilities, usually because of psychiatric disturbance or security risk.

---

[1] This work was supported by National Institute of Mental Health Grant A-0498 and by the van Ameringen Foundation.

Three groups of subjects were studied. The *physically assaultive* group of 50 subjects and the *sexual offender* group of 22 people were obtained from a population roster of 327 youths convicted of at least one crime against persons involving sexual or assaultive behavior, *i.e.*, murder, manslaughter, assault and battery, robbery, rape or other sexual misconduct. From this population random selections were made at monthly intervals of about 20 per cent of the individuals who had been incarcerated for at least 6 months and who were scheduled for appearance before the parole board. Sampling over time was done for administrative reasons and to avoid possible biases inherent in either consecutive or cross-sectional sampling. The *nonassaultive* group of 80 subjects was selected from a second population of 782 youths who had never been charged or convicted of any assaultive or sexual offenses but who had committed other crimes. The sampling procedure was identical with that involving the assaultive and sexual groups except a 10 per cent sample was obtained each month.

The 50 assaultive study subjects admitted committing the following offenses, all of which resulted in death or actual tissue damage to the victim: 3 murders, 7 cases of manslaughter, 6 episodes of rape with battery and 34 offenses of assault and battery. Inclusion in the assaultive group depended on admitted behavior, which was corroborated by official records of assaults that resulted in definite injury to the victim, usually necessitating medical attention or hospitalization. If the offense entailed threats of violence or attempted violence, but no injury ensued, such as during a robbery or a gunshot that missed, the subjects were excluded from this study. There were 16 such cases of attempted or threatened assault which were excluded, out of a total of 116 cases incarcerated at Karl Holton during the study period.

The 22 youths in the sexual group were those for whom there was corroboration in official records and interview data of sexually aggressive activity directed against the definite wishes of the victim. Their admitted crimes included 11 offenses of pedophilia and 16 episodes of forcible rape in which there was coercion usually by threat of violence but no battery. An additional four subjects were excluded from further analysis because they denied the use of force and claimed the victim was willing. By chance our sample included no individuals charged with voyeurism or exhibitionism, perhaps because relatively few of these people are treated in the security facilities of the Youth Authority.

The 80 individuals in the nonassaultive group were convicted of the following most serious offenses: narcotic and drug law violations, 30; burglary, 25; escape and runaway, 11; auto theft, 9; camp failure, 8; petty theft, 5 and miscellaneous other offenses. Multiple offenses account for the larger number of episodes than subjects. It should be emphasized that our research strategy was to examine various dimensions of drug use after obtaining a random sample from two populations who differed in terms of officially recognized aggressive behavior; one population consisted of youthful offenders who were clearly physically or sexually assaultive and the second population of individuals who had demonstrated no assaultive behavior which resulted in official charges, but who had been extensively delinquent. Although the sampling criteria resulted in a large proportion of individuals charged with drug law offenses to be included in the nonassaultive group, the bias is mitigated by the fact that some of the assaultive group were also initially charged with possession or use of drugs only to have the charge dropped when the more serious conviction was obtained. One potential advantage of studying California youth stems from the fact that a wide array of psychoactive substances has been used in California for a longer time period than most parts of the world; relationships between drug use and assaultive or sexual behavior might first be discernible in these people.

SOURCES

Data were obtained from 1) semistructured, private interviews conducted by either an experienced psychiatrist or a professional clinical interviewer and 2) concurrent analysis of official documents such as police records and laboratory reports. This form of corroboration, which permits immediate cross-validation and resolution of discrepancies, was used to maximize validity. Interview reports had to closely coincide with official records; if these sources did not agree, the data were not used. As described above, 4 subjects, all charged with sexual offenses, out of 156 were in this category, leaving a sample size of 152. To enhance reliability, the same interviewing format and scoring techniques were used for all of the subjects and the two investigators met at biweekly intervals to resolve ambiguities of processing the data.

Respondents were told the purpose of the study, and knew that information was purely voluntary and completely anonymous. The youths knew that the investigators were from Stanford University and could not influence in any way treatment conditions or length of incarceration. Only one subject refused to be interviewed. To further reduce possible distortion and denial, all interviews were conducted at least 6 months after arrest and after 90 per cent of the subjects had already made their parole board appearance for progress determination, or after all reports had been submitted to the board. Denial is often maximal immediately after arrest when verbal reports of drug use during criminal activities are sometimes markedly erroneous, especially with certain drugs such as barbiturates and amphetamines (2). Denial generally diminishes during the first 4 to 6 months of incarceration, perhaps because inmates learn from each other that their crucial concern, the time of their release, is not determined by specific details of their committment offense such as drug involvement, but on the general nature of their crime, their performance within the institution and the prevailing policies of the parole board. The subjects seemed candid about their behavior and usually either confirmed the official records, or described the official records as under-reporting their drug use and the involvement of drugs in the committ-ment offense.

Throughout the study, we had excellent cooperation from the Califor-nia Youth Authority, which was able to provide important ancillary information concerning the precise details of the offense. The personnel of the Youth Authority made it clear to the respondents that their participation or nonparticipation was not being recorded and would in no way influence their incarceration.

CHARACTERISTICS OF THE SUBJECTS

All three groups had a mean age at interview of 18.5 years with a range of 15 to 22 years. The racial composition of the assaultive group was 40 per cent Caucasian, 36 per cent Black and 24 per cent other (Mexican-American and American Indian); the sexual offender group consisted of 68 per cent Caucasian, 14 per cent Black and 19 per cent other; and the nonassaultive group included 80 per cent Caucasian, 15 per cent Black and 6 per cent other. The higher ratio of non-Caucasian to Caucasian in the assaultive group may reflect racial differences in arrest and convictions as well as rates of deviancy. Data were analyzed for racial variables, but only a few minor differences existed among the races in terms of drug use patterns. The three study groups were similar in coming almost entirely from lower socioeconomic backgrounds (Classes 4 and 5 on the Hollings-head-Redlich 2-factor index), having spent most of their adolescence in California, generally having opportunies to use a wide range of drugs and having been previously committed for approximately the same amount of time to a correctional facility.

RESULTS

The first three tables depict patterns of drug use by the study groups. Table 10.1 indicates the number of subjects who reported using at least once a drug in 1 of the 12 categories. "Volatiles" refers to glues, aerosols, lighter fuel, kerosene, gasoline, and so forth. "Other Barbiturates" in-cludes short and intermediate acting barbiturates, especially pentobarbi-tal (Nembutal) and secobarbital-amobarbital (Tuinal), and rarely, the longer acting barbiturates, usually phenobarbital. Under the heading

TABLE 10.1

Subjects having at least one episode with each drug

Drugs	Offenders					
	Assaultive (n = 50)		Sexual (n = 22)		Nonassaultive (n = 80)	
	n	%	n	%	n	%
Alcohol	49	98	22	100	79	99
Marihuana[1]	45	90	16	73	76	95
Secobarbital[1]	36	72	12	55	70	88
Amphetamines[2]	33	66	8	36	68	85
Volatiles	30	60	10	45	52	65
Psychedelics[2]	26	52	7	32	69	86
Hashish[2]	25	50	4	18	61	76
Other barbiturates[2]	19	38	5	23	51	64
Cocaine[2]	13	26	5	23	48	60
Heroin[2]	9	18	3	14	42	53
Other opioids[2]	6	12	2	9	26	33
Miscellaneous[2]	8	16	2	9	31	39

[1] $P < 0.01$, by 3-way χ^2 analysis, comparison of study groups.

[2] $P < 0.001$, by 3-way χ^2 analysis, comparison of study groups.

"Other Opioids" are morphine, opium, hydromorphone (Dilaudid) and occasionally meperidine (Demerol). It should be emphasized that these data reflect reported drug use, therefore inadvertent or deliberate distortions are possible. In addition, with illicit drug taking people often do not get the putative drug and adulteration is common.

The highest percentage of all three study groups used alcohol at least once; marihuana was in second rank for all three groups and secobarbital was third. Perhaps the most intriguing finding in this table is that, with the exception of alcohol, compared with the other two groups higher percentages of nonassaultive subjects reported using at least one drug in each of the 12 categories. This result does not simply reflect nonassaultive group-sampling criteria, which included offenders convicted of drug law offenses, because separate analysis of subjects convicted of drug law violations indicated their overall drug use was slightly less than that for the other nonassaultive subjects. Sexual offenders represented the other extreme; with the exception of alcohol, the lowest percentage of sexual offenders used one drug from each category as compared with the assaultives and with nonassaultives. The assaultive group was intermediate. This distribution was significant by χ^2 analysis, with the exception of alcohol and volatiles.

Table 10.2 depicts *multiple* drug use by displaying how many subjects

TABLE 10.2

Multiple drug use

Drug Category[1]	Offenders					
	Assaultive (*n* = 50)		Sexual (*n* = 22)		Nonassaultive (*n* = 80)	
	n	%	*n*	%	*n*	%
No Drugs...............	—	—	—	—	1	1
1 category.............	5	10	5	23	—	—
2 categories..........	3	6	2	9	2	3
3 categories..........	3	6	7	32	3	4
4 categories..........	5	10	—	—	3	4
5 categories or more..	34	68	8	36	71	89
Total.................	50	100	22	100	80	100

[1] $P < 0.001$, by Kruskal-Wallis test ($\chi^2_2 = 17.02$). Average ranks: nonassaultive, 87.9; assaultive, 71.9 and sexual, 45.7.

TABLE 10.3

Median of past drug use for those who used the drug

Drug[1]	Offenders		
	Assaultive (*n* = 50)	Sexual (*n* = 22)	Nonassaultive (*n* = 80)
Marihuana[2].................	139	24	600
Alcohol[3]...................	118	88	201
Amphetamines..............	38	—	60
Secobarbital...............	23	14	60
Psychedelics[4]...............	23	—	130
Hashish[4]..................	15	—	73
Other barbs...............	14	—	31
Cocaine...................	7	—	24
Heroin[4]..................	7	—	47
Volatiles..................	6	4	11
Other opiates.............	—[1]	—	5
Misc.....................	—	—	6

[1] Medians computed only for drugs used by nine or more subjects.

[2] $P < 0.001$, by Kruskal-Wallis test ($\chi^2_2 = 30.63$). Average ranks: nonassaultive, 8.54; assaultive, 5.22 and sexual, 3.83.

[3] $P < 0.05$, by Kruskal-Wallis test ($\chi^2_2 = 7.15$). Average ranks: nonassaultive, 8.42; assaultive, 6.79 and sexual, 6.10.

[4] $P < 0.05$ between assaultives and nonassaultives, by Mann-Whitney U test.

reported using drugs from only 1 of the 12 drug categories, how many reported using drugs from 2 of the 12 drug categories, and so forth. Nonassaultives were the most extensive multiple drug users, the sexual offenders used the smallest variety of drugs and again, the assaultive group was intermediate. There was a significant difference among the groups by the Kruskal-Wallis test.

The third table indicates the median number of episodes that the users of each drug within each group had with the drug. An episode was defined as a period of being continuously "high," under the influence of a drug, without "coming down to your usual non-drug self." These data were obtained by first asking the subject for the total number of episodes per drug in his life. If the number was over 50, computation was made by first ascertaining when the drug was initially used, an event which most of our young subjects could recall with considerable clarity. Then, a determination was made of the average usage per week with corrections for periods of incarceration, drug unavailability, and so forth. Although we strove to maximize accuracy, great precision should not be attributed to these figures. The relative ranking of these drug use frequencies, however, is probably accurate as the rankings were also obtained by a separate query in which subjects were asked, for example, "Did you use alcohol more often than marihuana, or marihuana more often than alcohol?" This line of questioning was continued using pairs of drugs. As will subsequently become important, secobarbital was reported fourth in frequency of use among the assaultives, after marihuana, alcohol and amphetamines. We computed the median only for those drugs which nine or more people reported using. The nonassaultive group again had the most extensive experience with all 12 drug categories compared with the other two groups.

Figure 10.1 addresses a different question: How did these delinquent subjects, most of whom had wide drug experience, expect that various drugs would alter their propensities for assaultive behavior? Specifically, they were asked: "Of all the drugs you've mentioned using, was there one drug you'd most likely get into a fight on or hit someone when you were mad or angry?" and "Of all the drugs you've used was there one drug that helped you 'cool it' when you got angry or mad, so you didn't get into a fight?" Inasmuch as people who had had experience with only one drug were excluded from analysis, the numbers in the middle column under *Users* represent the number of subjects from each study group who had used the particular drug and at least one other drug. The striking finding is the high percentage of subjects in all three groups who selected secobarbital as the drug most likely to *enhance* assaultiveness. Almost 80 per cent of the 36 secobarbital users of the assaultive group, representing some of Northern California's most aggressive juvenile delinquents, chose secobarbital. When asked to explain their choice, these comments emerged:

"You're struggling to stay awake. Like a drunk but you don't get sick. You get mad much easier ... You don't give a damn. You're a big man on reds. You go

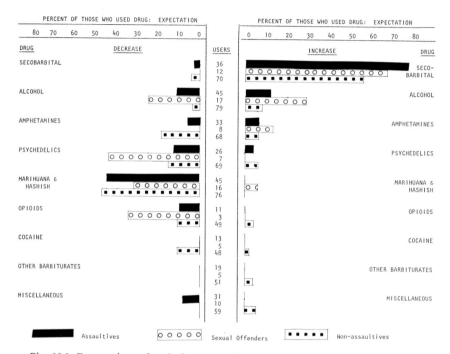

Fig. 10.1. Expectations of each drug regarding the increase or decrease of assaultiveness.

out and look for a gun. Usually take three or four reds. Let's go to a party. Let's do something."

Those youths in our nonassaultive group who had no legal indications of assaultive behavior in their past made substantially the same comments:

"You don't feel any pain, you're more headstrong than on alcohol. You're about to pass out but you don't ... It gets me, just builds up in me. I don't usually like to fight but on reds I just love to fight ... For one reason, you're stumbling and you might stumble into someone and they might say 'Watch it' and you might start mouthing off. You think you own the world. And you think you're really bad when you're loaded."

Conversely, as also shown in Figure 10.1, marihuana, hashish, psychedelics and the opioids were in general felt to *decrease* assaultiveness. The effects of marihuana were described as follows:

"It just made me relax. I didn't forget the trouble, but I saw it from a different point of view and saw it wasn't worth fighting over. . . . You'd be so busy trippin' you wouldn't pay any attention."

Data on the other drug categories, including alcohol and ampheta-mines, were less conclusive, perhaps reflecting individual variation or the fact that subjects were forced to choose a single drug.

Figures 10.2, 10.3 and 10.4 show the relationship of drug preference and expected decrease in assaultiveness. Subjects, who had had experience with at least two drugs, were asked, "Of all the drugs you've tried, which one did you prefer?" Figure 10.2, the nonassaultive group comparison, and Figure 10.3, the sexual offender group, both show concordance between the lines depicting expectations of decreased assaultiveness and drug prefer-ence. In other words, both nonassaultive and sexual offender groups expressed a preference for the drugs expected to reduce assaultiveness. Marihuana and its concentrated form, hashish, were the drugs for which the nonassaultive group both expressed the strongest preference and thought most markedly reduced assaultiveness; the psychedelics were the drugs most preferred and thought most likely to decrease assaultiveness by the sexual offenders group. Inexplicable on the basis of the available data is the marked discrepancy between the two study groups of expectation and preference for alcohol.

Figure 10.4 shows responses of the assaultive group on these two parame-ters—drug preference and expectations of decreased assaultiveness. In

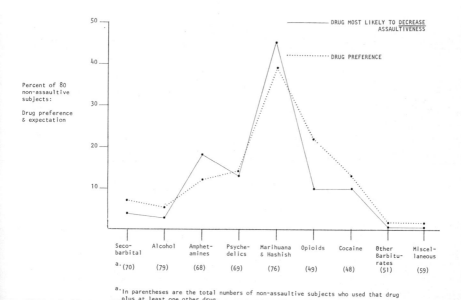

Fig. 10.2. Relationship between drug preferences and drug expected to decrease as-saultiveness: nonassaultive group.

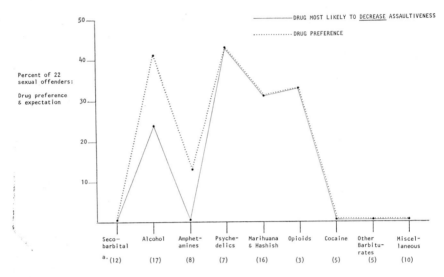

Fig. 10.3. Relationship between drug preferences and drug expected to decrease assaultiveness: sexual offenders group.

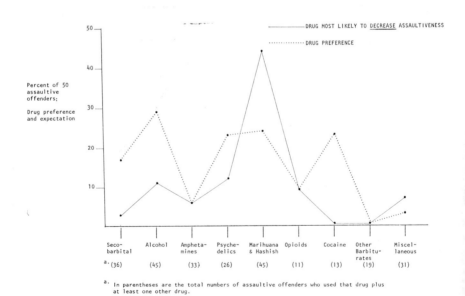

Fig. 10.4. Relationship between drug preferences and drug expected to decrease assaultiveness: assaultive group.

contrast to the nonassaultive and sexual groups, there is no close correspondence of drug preference with expectations of decreased assaultiveness.

A comparison of Figure 10.2, 10.3 and 10.4 shows that while the assaultive delinquents reported no definite correlation between drug preferences and expectations of decreased assaultiveness, the nonassaultive and sexual offenders preferred drugs expected to reduce aggression. This finding is consistent with the conclusions of Allen and West that the heavy users of lysergic acid diethylamide (LSD) and marihuana preferred these drugs because the effects facilitated their personal "flight from violence" (3).

Thus, the nonassaultive and sexual delinquents generally preferred drugs expected to reduce aggression, whereas assaultive subjects showed no definite correlation between drug preferences and expectations of decreased assaultiveness.

Figure 10.5, which portrays data from the assaultive group on preferences and expectations of *increased* assaultiveness, indicates no concordance between preference and expectations of increased assaultiveness; assaultive subjects did not prefer drugs that were expected to enhance aggression.

Drug involvement with corroborated offenses is shown on Table 10.4.

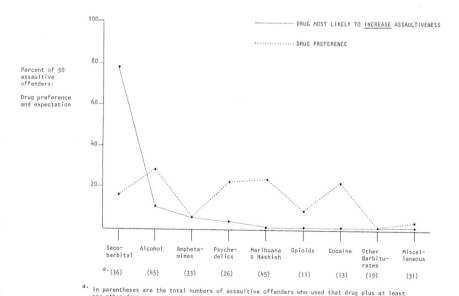

Fig. 10.5. Relationship between drug preferences and drug expected to increase assaultiveness: assaultive group.

TABLE 10.4

Drugs involved with corroborated offenses

Offenders and Drug	n	%	Deaths
Assaultive Offenders (n = 50)			
Alcohol	17	30	3
Secobarbital	8	14	2
Alcohol, secobarbital and marihuana	3	5	1
Alcohol and secobarbital	2	4	1
Marihuana	2	4	—
Amphetamines	1	2	1
Alcohol, amphetamines and marihuana	1	2	—
Volatiles	1	2	—
Miscellaneous	1	2	—
Total drugs	36	64	8
No drugs	20	36	2
Total	56	100	10
Sexual Offenders (n = 22)			
Alcohol	9	32	
LSD	1	4	
Total drugs	10	36	
No drugs	18	64	
Total	28	100	

The subjects averred they were under the influence of the drug at the time of the crime; in most instances reports from accomplices, witnesses, analytic laboratories, and so forth provided ancillary support for these statements. Despite the plethora of exotic chemicals available and used by these California youths, alcohol was the drug most frequently involved in serious assaultive offenses. Out of a total of 36 offenses involving drugs, alcohol was implicated alone or in combination with other drugs in 23 offenses, 5 of which resulted in death. This close link between the use of alcohol and violence in adolescents is similar to associations in adult offenders (4–6). Secobarbital, alone or in combination, was in second rank with a total of 13 serious assaultive offenses, including four deaths. This finding should be juxtaposed with the previously emphasized data that secobarbital ranked fourth, after marihuana and amphetamines, in median use by the subjects. Thus, alcohol, secobarbital or both were implicated in 31 of the 36 episodes of drug-associated assaultive crimes; in five of these cases alcohol and secobarbital were reportedly combined. Although alcohol has often been linked with violence, the role of secobarbital is less well known; however, current investigations are assessing secobarbital-related violence (7). Many of our subjects reported the frequent party use of alcohol and secobarbital together in dosages of three or four secobarbital capsules and variable amounts of wine or other alcoholic beverages.

Marihuana, alone or in combination with other drugs, was associated with six serious assaultive offenses including one death. It should be noted that marihuana was reported as the most frequently used drug among the assaultive group. The relative underrepresentation of marihuana use in violent crime has been described in other studies (8). In contradiction to reports suggesting close ties between amphetamines and violence, the use of amphetamines was reported in only two violent crimes (2, 9, 10). Again, one should note that assaultive subjects reported using amphetamines more frequently than secobarbital. If each episode of drug intoxication is viewed as an "at risk" episode one could argue that the individuals in our study were at greater risk of involvement in crimes with marihuana and amphetamines than with secobarbital, yet secobarbital is implicated in more instances of assault.

The totals in Table 10.4 indicate that assaultive crimes were more often linked with drug states than with non-drug states. In contrast, the non-drug state was more frequently implicated than drug states for sexual offenses. As has been previously reported, alcohol was the only drug associated with a substantial number of sexual offenses (11).

SUMMARY

In summary, our findings concerning the interrelationship between drugs and crime are as follows. Alcohol was the drug most likely to be associated with serious assaultive and sexual offenses. In proportion to overall drug use and compared to other drugs, secobarbital was overrepresented in violent crimes. In addition, it was overwhelmingly selected by these pharmacologically experienced delinquents as the drug most likely to *increase* aggression. Marihuana was relatively underrepresented in serious assaultive or sexual crimes and was generally touted as the drug which *decreased* aggressive tendencies. More frequent or multiple drug use *per se* did not positively correlate with assaultive or sexual offenses; on the contrary, extensive previous drug use was more frequently reported by delinquents who had never been charged or convicted of assaultive or sexual crimes. Assaultive offenders described no clear correlations between drug preference and expectations of drug effects on assaultiveness; however, both nonassaultive and sexual offenders definitely preferred drugs which they expected to decrease assaultiveness, a fact which suggests that among these adolescents drugs may be used in an effort to control their aggression.

ACKNOWLEDGMENTS

Without the cooperation of Mr. Richard Kolze, Mr. Lloyd Bennett and others at the California Youth Authority, this study could not have been done. We are indebted to Dr. Helena Kraemer for her statistical assistance and to Dr. Donald Goodwin for his helpful comments. We are also appreciative for the technical support provided by Caroline Bowker, Fran Elgan, Vernon Gates, Patricia Murphy and Peggy Murphy.

REFERENCES

1. The National Commission on the Causes and Prevention of Violence: To Establish Justice, To Insure Domestic Tranquility. New York, Bantam Books, 1970.
2. ECKERMAN, WC, BATES, JD, RACHEL, JV, POOLE, WK: Drug Usage and Arrest Charges, A Study of Drug Usage and Arrest Charges Among Arrestees in Six Metropolitan Areas of the United States. Washington, D.C., U.S. Government Printing Office, 1971.
3. ALLEN, JR, WEST, LJ: Flight from violence: Hippies and the green rebellion. Am J Psychiatr 125: 364, 1968.
4. WOLFGANG, ME: Patterns in Criminal Homicide. Philadelphia, University of Pennsylvania Press, 1958.
5. GOODWIN, DW: Alcohol in suicides and homicides. Q J Stud Alcohol 34: 144, 1973.
6. TINKLENBERG, JR: Alcohol and violence, in Alcoholism: Progress in Research and Treatment, edited by Bourne, PG, Fox, R. New York, Academic Press, 1973.
7. United States Senate Report of the Subcommittee to Investigate Juvenile Delinquency Based on Hearings and Investigations 1971–1972: Barbiturate Abuse in the United States, 1972.
8. TINKLENBERG, JR, MURPHY, P: Marihuana and crime. J Psychedelic Drugs 5: 183, 1972.
9. TINKLENBERG, JR, STILLMAN, RC: Drug use and violence, in Violence and the Struggle for Existence, edited by Daniels, DN, Gilula, MF, Ochberg, FM. Boston, Little, Brown & Co., 1970, p. 327.
10. ELLINWOOD, EH: Assault and homicide associated with amphetamine abuse. Am J Psychiatr 127: 1170, 1971.
11. AMIR, M: Patterns in Forcible Rape. Chicago, The University of Chicago Press, 1971.

DISCUSSION

DR. FRANK OCHBERG (San Francisco, California): When you began your work in this field in 1968, there was no clear relationship shown between the particular drug of abuse and the specific violent process. Are you finding any correlation now?

DR. JARED TINKLENBERG (Stanford, California): Although we do not have firm, systematic data, my clinical impression from interviewing a large number of people is that there may be differences. It seems to me that the process of violence under the influence of alcohol or secobarbital tends to be, at least in the adolescent age group, a process of enhanced irritability and indiscriminant assaultive tendencies directed toward anyone who might happen to be present. When an individual commits violence while under the influence of amphetamines, the process seems to more often follow a defensive, self-protective pattern that could be characterized in paranoid terms. In these situations, the individual may explain that his assaultive behavior seemed necessary for self-defense. One might use the Pentagon term of "preventative retaliation": Hit the guy before he hits you! Occasionally this happens with marihuana or the psychedelics, especially LSD, although much more rarely than with the amphetamines.

DR. JEROME FRANK (Baltimore, Maryland): I realize that the sample is too small to reach any conclusions, but in view of the fact that child molesters are considered to be psychologically very different from people who commit forcible rape, I wonder if you looked at these two groups separately to see if there were any differences.

DR. TINKLENBERG: As you suggest, the sample size of 28 subjects was too small to make definitive conclusions. There seemed to be no marked differences in drug use patterns between subjects who admitted committing forcible rape and those who admitted to pedophilia. Both groups, the forcible rapists and the pedophiliacs, tended to use drugs less extensively than the nonassaultive or the assaultive group. When a drug was involved in a sexual episode, it was almost always alcohol.

DR. DAVID HAMBURG (Stanford, California): Did you find a distinctive pattern of secobarbital use associated with violent behavior?

DR. TINKLENBERG: Part of the process, again at a clinical level, seems to be diffuse irritability with indiscriminate violence. For example, if I were under the influence of secobarbital right now and I didn't like the way you asked that question, I might attack you or perhaps someone else in the front row. I would be inclined to act out my extreme irritability in an assaultive way.

These young subjects do not use secobarbital—Seconal or "reds"—the way they are used in a treatment situation. These adolescents take more than one capsule or tablet at a time—as many as 3, 4 or 5—and then attempt to stay awake, to stay, as they say, on top of the drug by keeping themselves physically active. Often they deliberately seek excitement which frequently culminates in violence.

DR. SALEEM SHAH (Rockville, Maryland): Two questions: The person who examines large numbers of offenders frequently hears that the person was under the influence at the time of the offense. You mentioned some indices of alcohol involvement. Were you able to assess the extent of exaggerated use of alcohol as opposed to just the presence or absence?

My second question is this: When you ask an individual about his expectancy of whether a certain drug would tend to increase or decrease aggressive or deviant sexual behavior, to what extent is his response determined by the social set? He cannot on the one hand admit to taking drugs that he knows will increase antisocial behavior, and then expect lenient judicial handling.

DR. TINKLENBERG: As for your first question on concentrations of drugs, we did not systematically look at concentrations of alcohol in body tissues in relationship to these crimes. The only investigator that I know to have done this was Shupe back in the 1950's. His findings suggest more assaultive crimes in the higher blood alcohol range, from 0.10 up to about 0.25. Of course in the very high ranges, assaultiveness drops off, as you would expect, because of incoordination. Although we were unable to systematically investigate drug concentrations, self reports indicated that in most cases there was a significant level of intoxication.

As for the second question, on expectation, I can only say that we thought the subjects were exceedingly frank about both their deviance and their drug use. We were Stanford investigators, in no way affiliated with the California Youth Authority, who interviewed these subjects at least 6 months after incarceration when most were scheduled for parole and had already passed their board review. There was no reason for them to bias their answers to us one way or another.

MISS MATHEA FALCO (Washington, D.C.): Were the juveniles who were secobarbital users just sporadic spree takers or were they more chronic abusers or, in fact, addicted?

DR. TINKLENBERG: Most of them were sporadic users of barbiturates, just as they were sporadic users of most drugs, including alcohol. They used drugs primarily on weekends, although not exclusively so. These are young people, most in their late adolescence, and they had not yet acquired any marked drug dependencies, at least not in a physiological sense.

Chapter 11

ALCOHOL, AGGRESSION AND ANDROGENS[1]

JACK H. MENDELSON AND NANCY K. MELLO

INTRODUCTION

There is abundant evidence that consumption of large quantities of alcohol may facilitate and perhaps induce violent and aggressive behavior (40). Studies of criminal homicides indicate that more than half the offenders had ingested large quantities of alcohol before commission of the crime (47). Similar findings have been obtained in studies of assaultive behavior, armed robbery with aggravated assault and a variety of other crimes of violence (38, 40). Drunk and disorderly conduct accounts for over half the arrests reported annually in the United States (42). The high concordance between automobile accidents and alcohol abuse is well known (2, 44), and traffic fatalities associated with alcohol abuse seem to involve not only enhanced risk taking, but also an overt expression of anger and violence.

Over the past 15 years, there has been increasing concern with study of the possible biological concomitants of aggressive behaviors (4, 8). Testosterone levels have been implicated in the expression of both sexual and aggressive behaviors. Most studies which have attempted to examine the relationship between aggression and testosterone levels in man have relied on instruments which assess feelings of hostility and aggression (29) or a past history of aggression and violent crimes (15). Findings from these studies have not yielded any simplistic correlations between plasma testosterone levels and current or past history of aggression.

The amount of ongoing physical aggression in young prisoners was found to be unrelated to plasma testosterone levels (15). However, prisoners with a history of violent crimes during adolescence did have significantly higher testosterone levels than prisoners without such a history. It was suggested that certain individuals may be at high risk for the commission of violent crimes if they are predisposed to aggression as a function of high androgen levels during adolescence (15).

In normal young men, psychometric indicators of hostility and aggres-

[1] Collection of these data was supported by the Intramural Laboratory of Alcohol Research, NIAAA, National Institute of Mental Health. The analysis of plasma testosterone samples was supported by the Insurance Institute of Highway Safety Research and by Grant MH-20551 from the National Institute of Mental Health. Part of these data were reported at the 1973 meeting of the American Psychiatric Association.

sion were significantly correlated with testosterone production rate (29). It has also been reported that psychological stress may be associated with suppression of plasma testosterone levels in healthy young men (16). During the early phase of officer candidacy training, plasma testosterone levels were significantly lower than during the later and relatively non-stressful period of training. Recruits observed during the 1st month of basic training and special forces personnel awaiting combat in Vietnam also showed lower excretion of urinary testosterone (32). These data support the idea that testosterone levels may be an important psychoendocrine correlate of stressful environmental stimuli (31).

Data obtained on experimental animals present a more consistent indication that androgen levels can modulate and influence aggressive behaviors in several species (12). Rose and his associates have shown that plasma testosterone is correlated with rank in a dominance hierarchy and with aggression frequency in male rhesus monkeys (33). More recently, Rose and co-workers reported that changes in the social environment change plasma testosterone levels (34). Male rhesus monkeys, given individual access to a group of receptive females, became dominant, copulated frequently and showed a 2- to 3-fold increase in plasma testosterone levels within the 2-week exposure period. Subsequent exposure to and defeat by a group of males was associated with a precipitous fall in plasma testosterone levels to 80 per cent below base line. Plasma testosterone levels increased above base line upon re-exposure to receptive females (34). These data were interpreted to suggest that social variables may influence plasma testosterone levels, which may subsequently affect behavior in an adaptive way—i.e., high testosterone levels support sexual activity with receptive females and low testosterone levels are consistent with submissiveness in a group of dominant and aggressive males (34). Although the sexual and aggressive components of dominance hierarchies are multiply determined, the dramatic changes in testosterone levels observed in primates suggest the importance of the relationship between the expression of aggression and sexuality.

It is well known that testosterone is the most active and potent androgen in human males. The relative levels of plasma testosterone significantly affect libidinal function and influence the intensity of sexual desire. The literature on alcoholism has consistently protrayed the male alcohol addict as experiencing diminished heterosexual desire and activity (18) and sexual impotence (17). However, exceptions to this general impression have also been noted. Clinical interviews with 16 alcoholics and their wives indicated essentially normal sexual behavior and good communication about sexual attitudes (3).

The effect of alcohol on sexual function has been the subject of many anecdotes in the nonscientific literature which usually concur with the classic observation that intoxication evokes desire but compromises sexual performance (37). The experimental literature has shown that moderate to high doses of ethanol (2.4 to 3.2 mg. per kg.) may abolish the ejaculatory reflex in dogs (11, 13). These behavioral observations are consistent with biological data which indicate that chronic alcohol abuse may impair sexual function through a disruption of gonadal function. In 1926, Silvestrini (39) reported the occurrence of testicular atrophy and gynecomastia in male alcoholics who also had evidence of liver disease. This observation has been confirmed by many other investigators and the most recent studies show that a derangement in androgen metabolism is the primary causal factor in the development of gynecomastia and testicular atrophy (10). However, abnormally high urinary testosterone excretion has been observed in alcohol addicts with no signs of gynecomastia, testicular atrophy or liver dysfunction (7).

These several threads of evidence from the experimental and clinical literature suggest the importance of trying to analyze the interrelationship between chronic alcohol intake, aggressive behavior and androgen function in adult male alcohol addicts. The present investigation differs from previous human studies in that concurrent measures of aggressive behavior and plasma testosterone levels were taken before, during and after a period of chronic intoxication. The purpose of this study was to determine if alcohol produced a consistent change in plasma testosterone levels in male alcohol addicts. A second goal of this study was to determine if the extent or direction of change in plasma testosterone levels was associated with observable changes in aggressive behavior. Finally, we were also interested in examining the distribution of testosterone level abnormalities in alcohol addicts during sobriety. Consequently, the chronic studies of alcohol addicts during sobriety and intoxication were supplemented by acute studies of alcoholics in a correctional institution during a period of sobriety.

METHODS

I. Chronic Studies of Alcoholics during Sobriety and Intoxication

Subjects

Nine male alcohol addicts were observed before, during and after a drinking period of 11 or 12 consecutive days. All subjects were volunteers, selected from the population of a local alcohol rehabilitation center. No subject was under any legal constraint during the course of this study. Subjects were told the details of the experimental procedures, and informed consent was obtained from each man. Each subject had abstained from alcohol for at least 6 days prior to admission to the clinical research ward of the NIAAA Laboratory of Alcohol Research at Saint Elizabeth's Hospital, National Institute of Mental Health.

These subjects ranged in age from 28 to 48 years ($\overline{X} = 39$) and had a history of alcoholism of 3 to 25 years' duration ($\overline{X} = 13.7$). Some of the subjects had completed high school and all had a recent work history of sporadic employment at a variety of semiskilled and nonskilled jobs. All subjects were spree drinkers, accustomed to consuming about 1 quart of whiskey each day. All subjects were alcohol addicts, physically dependent upon alcohol. Each subject reported that when he stopped drinking, withdrawal signs and symptoms ranging from mild tremulousness to overt delirium tremens occurred.

Each subject was given a complete physical examination and mental status assessment before his participation in these studies. All volunteers selected were in good health, and none had a history of neurological disease; seizure disorder; hepatic, renal, pulmonary, cardiac or gastrointestinal disease or nutritional or metabolic disorder. No subject showed evidence of alcohol-induced liver disease, as measured by serum enzymes (serum glutamic oxaloacitic transaminase) and a Bromsulphalein clearance test administered before, during and after the experimental drinking period. No subject had a history of opiate or barbiturate addiction or was using any form of medication at the time of the study. Inasmuch as the sleep patterns of these subjects were studied simultaneously, clinical screening EEGs were performed to rule out any focal or generalized abnormal EEG activity. A more complete description of the standard medical screening procedures used for subject selection is available in a previous report (23).

Ward Facilities

Subjects were studied in groups of four and five. Each subject had a private bedroom which contained cable connections for sleep EEG recordings. All subjects had access to a spacious dayroom which contained a variety of recreational facilities (*e.g.*, television, games, books, shuffleboard, and so forth) as well as a dining and kitchen area and an alcohol-dispensing machine. No other patients were present on the research ward and subjects were not allowed to have visitors. Subjects were fed a standard hospital diet with daily vitamins. This diet was supplemented with specialty foods which subjects could prepare for themselves.

Sequence of Procedures

The overall sequence of procedures for each group of subjects was as follows. A 6- to 9-day base line period preceded an 11- or 12-day spontaneous drinking period which was followed by a minimum of 7 nonalcohol recovery days. All subjects concurrently participated in studies designed to assess the effects of chronic alcohol intoxication on EEG sleep patterns and on serum lipids. Separate reports will describe the data obtained on sleep patterns (22, 48) and on alcohol-induced hyperlipidemia (25).

Experimental Procedures

ALCOHOL ADMINISTRATION. Subjects were given unrestricted access to alcohol over an 11- to 12-day period. A spontaneous drinking paradigm rather than a programmed drinking paradigm was used in an effort to simulate natural drinking patterns (20). During the alcohol-available period, each subject could earn approximately 32 tokens each day by cooperating with the several experimental procedures. He could spend these tokens whenever he wished during the entire drinking period. Each token purchased 1 oz. of alcohol which was directly dispensed from an alcohol dispenser located on one wall of the dayroom. Each subject was given a choice between two types of alcohol: 100-proof beverage alcohol (bourbon) and 100-proof grain alcohol. A variety of mixers were available and there were no constraints as to how much alcohol a subject could buy at any one time.

The alcohol dispenser was turned on at 9:00 a.m. on the 1st day of drinking. The alcohol withdrawal period began at midnight on the final day of drinking. Subjects were encouraged to sleep between about midnight and 7 a.m. to facilitate the recording of sleep EEGs. Upon awakening, subjects were vigorously discouraged from consuming food or alcohol until after collection of the morning blood samples at 8 a.m.

EXPERIMENTAL ASSESSMENTS. Throughout the course of the study, assessments involving EEG recordings, breathalyzer readings, neurological examinations and clinical interviews, collection of urines for catecholamine analysis and collection of blood samples for serum lipid and testosterone analyses were made each day. The details of the EEG recordings and clinical interviews are presented elsewhere (48).

BLOOD ALCOHOL DETERMINATIONS. Before, during and after the alcohol-available period, blood alcohol levels were determined every 4 hours (except during sleep) with an instrument designed to measure the concentration of ethanol in the breath (Breathalyzer, Stephenson Corporation, Red Bank, New Jersey). Breathalyzer values were recorded during the abstinent periods in order to insure that subjects had not obtained alcohol from some outside source.

NEUROLOGICAL EXAMINATIONS. A neurological evaluation of the occurrence of tremor, nystagmus and disorientation was completed 3 times daily on each subject by the attendant staff before, during and after the drinking period. This procedure was intended to permit detection of partial with-drawal signs and symptoms which frequently accompany an abrupt fall in blood alcohol levels (*e.g.,* from 200 to 100 mg. per 100 ml.) (21). Upon cessation of drinking, daily neurological examinations were conducted by the resident physician.

TESTOSTERONE ANALYSIS. Fasting blood samples were collected for the analysis of plasma testosterone levels at 8:00 a.m. each morning. This sampling time was chosen because there is a small diurnal variation in plasma testosterone, and levels tend to be highest in the morning upon awakening (35). On the 1st day of drinking, plasma testosterone samples were taken *before* subjects began drinking.

Plasma testosterone levels were determined by a radioimmunoassay technique which has a high degree of precision, specificity and accuracy (9). The range for normal adult male testosterone levels observed in our laboratory, and in other laboratories employing this method, is 400 to 650 ng. per 100 ml.

BEHAVIOR RATINGS. Subjects were asked to complete two self-report scales, the Monroe Scale and the F-A-V Questionnaire Scale daily through-out the study. Both of these self-report scales focus upon feelings of anger and acts of violence. An aggression checklist, recently developed at the Boston City Hospital, was completed 3 times a day, once on each shift. This checklist described the subject's overt behavior. In addition, staff were encouraged to keep careful notes concerning all aspects of a subject's behavior.

In the final data analysis, the various rating scales proved to be far less accurate reflections of actual behavior than the staff's observations and detailed notes. Consequently, data presented in Figure 11.1, A through D, are based upon observed behaviors rather than self-report data. The observed aggressive behaviors were assigned to a 3-point scale from least (+1) to most(+3) extreme. One point was given for any verbal or gestural indication of aggressivity. Two points were assigned for verbal aggression, mild tantrums or any derivative acting out behaviors. Three points were assigned for direct physical assault on another subject or staff member or deliberate self-injury.

II. Acute Studies Of Alcoholic Addicts During Sobriety

Two studies were conducted with sober alcohol addicts, and either *single* or *repeated* blood samples were taken for the analysis of plasma testosterone levels. The *repeated* sample study was conducted on eight subjects who had been admitted to the clinical research ward of the NIAAA Laboratory of Alcohol Research for participation in the chronic studies. In each instance, the subject was discharged during the base line screening procedures because he was found to be medically or emotionally unsuitable. Three of these subjects had a history of violent aggressive behavior, including convictions for major felonies. This information was obtained during intensive clinical screening interviews following admission. Any subject with a history of felonies is automatically excluded from our clinical research program.

These eight subjects ranged in age from 27 to 52 years ($\overline{X} = 39.5$) and had a history of alcoholism of 6 to 15 years ($\overline{X} = 12.4$). Testosterone values obtained on these sober alcohol addicts were compared with values obtained from six control males with an age range of 23 to 51 ($\overline{X} = 34.8$). The control volunteers were members of our ward staff.

A second study was carried out with sober alcohol addicts who were residents of a local correctional and rehabilitation facility. Single blood samples were obtained from 34 male alcohol addicts between the ages of 20 and 36. A standardized clinical interview was conducted with each subject prior to obtaining a blood sample and subjects were paid for their cooperation with cigarettes.

Three categories of past history of violent behaviors ranging from most to moderate to least violent were established on the basis of clinical interviews. The least violent category included 11 persons who reported engaging in occasional fighting while intoxicated. The moderate violence category included nine persons who had reported arrests for drunk and disorderly conduct associated with aggressive acting out. The category of most violent consisted of 14 persons who had been arrested and sentenced for assault and aggressive behavior during intoxication. Some of these individuals admitted to being poly-drug users and their data are coded separately from men who reported exclusive addiction to alcohol.

The 14 subjects categorized as most violent reported a 2- to 18-year history of problem drinking ($\overline{X} = 8.9$). All except one subject reported signs of physical dependence (tremor, nausea, sweating, vomiting, insomnia) upon cessation of drinking. Most of these subjects had been in the correctional institution for 1 or 2 weeks at the time samples were collected. Only three subjects had been institutionalized for periods of 2 months or more.

The nine subjects in the moderate violence group reported a 3- to 12-year history of problem drinking ($\overline{X} = 6.3$). Each of these subjects reported signs of physical dependence upon cessation of drinking. Eight subjects had been abstinent from alcohol for periods of 2 weeks to 3 months at the time of sampling. One subject had been abstinent for only 4 days.

Subjects in the least violent group reported an average history of alcoholism of 9 years' duration with a range of 2 to 23 years. All subjects except one reported evidence of physical dependence upon cessation of drinking. Nine of the eleven subjects had been abstinent from alcohol for periods of 1 to 6 months at the time of sampling. One subject had been abstinent for 18 days and a second subject for only 4 days at the time of sampling.

RESULTS

I. Chronic Studies of Alcoholics during Sobriety and Intoxication

Suppression of plasma testosterone levels occurred in 8 of the 9 subjects during chronic alcohol intoxication (Table 11.1, column 2). The one subject (RB) who did not show any significant change in plasma testosterone levels drank very little alcohol. A statistically significant suppression of plasma testosterone was observed in six subjects (Table 11.1, column 2). The decrease in plasma testosterone levels seem to be largely independent of the range of testosterone levels observed during base line. In Table 11.1, subjects are grouped according to testosterone levels recorded during base line, i.e., normal, high or low. Although the magnitude of fall was greatest in those subjects with abnormally high testosterone levels during base line, significant decrements occurred even in one subject (DB) with abnormally low testosterone levels during base line.

Following cessation of drinking, 6 of the 9 subjects showed an increase in testosterone levels over that observed during the alcohol period, and this increase was statistically significant in 4 of the 6 cases (Table 11.1, column 4). However, the increased plasma testosterone levels seen during withdrawal were significantly higher than base line only in two subjects (RM and DB) (Table 11.1, column 5). Both JH and HC showed slight increases in plasma testosterone levels during alcohol withdrawal, but these levels remained significantly lower than their base line values.

Data for four individual subjects, for consecutive days of the pre-drinking base line, the 11- or 12-day alcohol-available period and the post-alcohol withdrawal period are presented in Figure 11.1, A through D. The severity of aggressive behavior ($+1$, $+2$ or $+3$) is presented at the top of each figure. Plasma testosterone levels are shown as histograms in the second row of each figure. The daily mean and range of blood alcohol levels are shown in the bottom row of each figure. The types of withdrawal signs and symptoms exhibited by each subject are shown at the far right of the lower half of each graph.

Subjects RM and HC each showed abnormally high testosterone levels during the base line period (Fig. 11.1, A and B). Subject RM (Fig. 11.1A) maintained blood alcohol levels of above 150 mg. per 100 ml. for 10 of the

TABLE 11.1

Direction and significance[1] of changes in plasma testosterone levels between base line, drinking and alcohol withdrawal

Base Line	Alcohol Available[2] (Change from Base Line)	Blood Alcohol Level ($\bar{X}$ and Range) mg./100 ml	Alcohol Withdrawal[2]	
			Change from Alcohol	Change from Base Line
Normal range (ng/100 ml)				
LB (463–637)	↓ P < 0.05	144 (0–320)	= N.S.	= N.S.
JH[3] (530–539)	↑ + P < 0.01	138 (0–360)	↑ N.S.	→ P > 0.01
JR (408–694)	→ P < 0.01	74 (0–230)	= N.S.	= N.S.
DP (540–617)	→ N.S.	100 (0–260)	↑ P < 0.05	= N.S.
TR (443–498)	→ N.S.	207 (30–310)	↑ N.S.	= + → N.S.
Normal to high (ng/100 ml)				
RM (545–855)	→ P < 0.05	180 (20–310)	↑ P < 0.01	← P > 0.01
HC (659–1048)	→ P < 0.01	105 (0–250)	↑ P < 0.05	→ P > .05
Normal to low (ng/100 ml)				
DB[3] (287–324)	↓ P < 0.01	167 (40–400)	↑ P < 0.01	↑ P < 0.01
RB[3] (277–446)	= N.S.	33 (0–150)	= N.S.	= N.S.

[1] Mann-Whitney U test (1-tailed). [2] ↓, decreased; ↑, increased; =, equivalent; N.S., not significant. [3] No aggressive behavior observed.

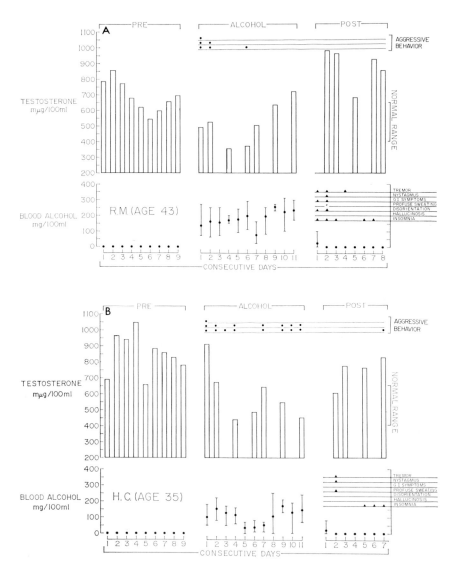

Fig. 11.1, A–D. Each figure presents data for an individual subject during the pre-drinking base line period, the alcohol-available period and the postalcohol withdrawal period. The severity of aggressive behavior is shown at the top of the figure for each consecutive day. One dot indicates minimal agressivity and 3 dots indicates overt assaultive behavior. Plasma testosterone levels (ng. per 100 ml.) are shown as histograms for each consecutive day. The normal range of testosterone levels is indicated at the far right of the upper portion of the graph. The daily mean and the range of blood alcohol levels (mg. per 100 ml.) obtained between 8 a.m. and 4 a.m. of the following day are shown in the lower portion of the graph. The type and time course of withdrawal signs and symptoms are indicated at the far right of the lower portion of the graph.

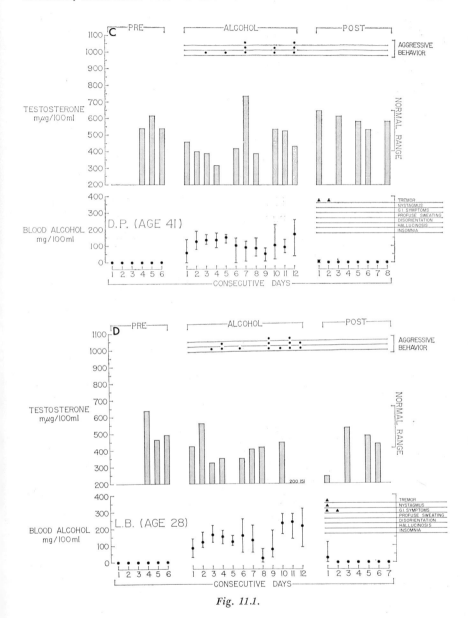

Fig. 11.1.

11 days of drinking and peak blood alcohol levels reached above 250 mg. per 100 ml. During the withdrawal period, subject RM showed an increase in serum testosterone levels which was significantly above base line or drinking levels (see Table 11.1).

Subject HC maintained blood alcohol levels between 100 and 150 mg. per 100 ml. for 8 of the 11 days of drinking (Fig. 11.1B). Peak blood alcohol levels exceeded 200 mg. per 100 ml. on 4 of the 11 days of drinking. Although HC drank less alcohol on the average than subject RM, his plasma testosterone levels were more significantly depressed during the alcohol available period. HC's plasma testosterone levels increased significantly during alcohol withdrawal, but this increase was significantly lower than the prealcohol base line levels (see Table 11.1).

Despite high testosterone levels, neither HC nor RM engaged in verbal or overt aggressive behaviors during the base line period. Indeed, subject RM was an exceptionally quiet and passive individual. Subject HC was somewhat more outgoing and conveyed an impression of joviality. On the 1st day of drinking, both RM and HC became aggressive and physically assaultive. At about 10:00 p.m., HC and RM began to fight with one another and exchanged blows. It is important to note that HC's plasma testosterone level on the 1st day of drinking had been taken at 8 a.m., 1 hour before the alcohol dispenser was turned on. Subject RM's aggressive behavior associated with intoxication occurred hours after a somewhat lower plasma testosterone level recorded at 8 a.m.

Throughout the remainder of the drinking period, subject HC frequently was verbally aggressive and given to mild tantrums and acting out behavior. However, he never again assaulted another patient or staff member. His intoxication-related aggression was associated with lower testosterone levels than were observed during the base line or the post-alcohol withdrawal period. After the initial episode of aggression associated with intoxication, subject RM returned to his former compliant and docile state. Despite the dramatic increase in plasma testosterone levels during alcohol withdrawal, subject RM was never verbally or physically aggressive.

Data for two subjects (DP and LB) with *normal* plasma testosterone levels during the prealcohol base line are presented in Figures 1, C and D. Subject DP showed a significant alcohol-related suppression of plasma testosterone levels initially, with a somewhat erratic pattern thereafter. He was consistently irritable throughout the drinking period. On the 7th evening of drinking, subject DP became violent and attacked members of the staff, hitting, kicking, biting, punching and throwing things. This dramatic acting out behavior was associated with an increased testosterone level, although blood alcohol levels were slightly lower than during the previous several days. On the 12th day of drinking, subject DP's blood alcohol levels increased to above 200 mg. per 100 ml., and shortly after noon he had a major temper tantrum which involved hitting staff and patients, kicking, spitting, throwing objects, cursing, stamping feet, tearing off his clothes and threatening to injure himself and others.

Subject LB was pleasant and cooperative throughout the base line period and during the first 2 days of drinking (Fig. 11.1D). By the 3rd day of drinking, he became demanding of staff and verbally threatening. On the evening of the 9th day of drinking, subject LB became heavily intoxicated and was verbally threatening and assaultive. He tore off his EEG electrodes, woke up other patients, yelled and had temper tantrums. Unfortunately, no testosterone sample was obtained on the morning preceding this late evening outburst, but the 8:00 a.m. value on the following day (day 10) was only slightly increased. On day 11, subject LB's average blood alcohol level was above 250 mg. per 100 ml. and the morning testosterone value was very low (200 ng. per 100 ml.). By nighttime, LB became physically and verbally assaultive, tried to stab subject DP with a fork and was placed in a seclusion room. In the course of having a temper tantrum in the seclusion room, he broke his right hand by smashing it into a door. The testosterone sample on the following morning was 151 ng. per 100 ml. and blood alcohol levels exceeded 300 mg. per 100 ml. During the withdrawal period, LB returned to his previous pleasant and cooperative mode of relating and there were no further incidents until his discharge.

In general, evaluation of dose-response relationships between alcohol and plasma testosterone levels is complicated by what seems to be an adaptational effect which occurred during the course of drinking. In four subjects whose blood alcohol levels remained reasonably stable over the 11- to 12-day drinking period, an initial suppression of plasma testosterone levels was followed by a gradual return to the predrinking base line range.

At present, it is not possible to establish a simplistic dichotomy between high and low plasma testosterone levels and similar parameters for describing aggressive behavior. Although it seems that plasma testosterone levels are associated with alterations in mood states, the various mood changes may either facilitate or suppress overt aggressive behaviors. Of the six instances of 3+ aggression observed in these nine subjects during the course of drinking, two were associated with suppressed testosterone levels and three were associated with increasing or elevated plasma testosterone levels. It is important to recognize that many of these subjects showed no significant changes in aggressive behavior during drinking when plasma testosterone levels were suppressed.

II. Acute Studies of Alcohol Addicts during Sobriety

Figure 11.2 presents a comparison between single testosterone samples taken from six normal control subjects and multiple samples taken from eight alcohol addicts during a period of sobriety. Seven of the eight alcohol

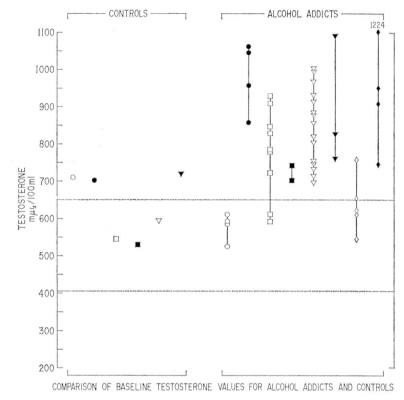

COMPARISON OF BASELINE TESTOSTERONE VALUES FOR ALCOHOL ADDICTS AND CONTROLS

Fig. 11.2. Single testosterone samples for six control subjects are compared with repeated testosterone levels obtained from eight alcohol addicts during sobriety. Testosterone values are presented in nanograms per 100 ml. and the normal range of values using this radioimmunoassay technique is between 400 and 650 ng./100 ml.

addicts had several plasma testosterone values which exceeded the normal range. These data are consistent with the previous findings of Fabre and associates (7).

Only three of the alcoholic subjects reported a history of aggression during intoxication. One subject (solid circles) reported that he had last been arrested after "busting up" all the furniture in a girl friend's apartment. Another subject (open squares) had a history of juvenile delinquency and had been placed in a corrective school between the age of 13 and 18, because he had broken into his grade school and committed vandalism. He reported frequent fights during drinking. A third subject (solid triangles) reported a history of "blackouts" during intoxication which were associated with multiple arrests, fighting and traveling long distances in stolen cars.

Subjects with no history of aggressive behavior during intoxication included one individual (solid squares) who was discharged because of medical problems. Another subject (open triangles) did not report any history of arrests or aggressive behavior. The subject with the highest testosterone levels (solid diamonds) had no history of aggression or arrests during intoxication. Finally, the single subject whose testosterone values were always within the normal range (open circles) had a history of intermittent overt homosexual behavior.

Figure 11.3 presents data for 34 male alcohol addicts who were in residence at a local correctional and rehabilitation institution at the time of sampling. These subjects were categorized according to their reported history of aggressive behavior. Data shown in Figure 11.3 indicate that plasma testosterone values were equally distributed in the abnormally low and abnormally high range within each of the three groups. Most of these subjects fell within the normal range. These data support the impression derived from the chronic data reported in study 1, that there is no compelling relationship between plasma testosterone levels and observed or reported violent behavior in male alcohol addicts.

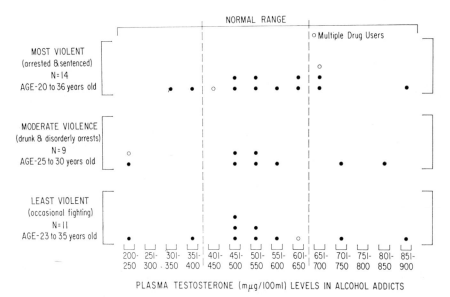

PLASMA TESTOSTERONE (mμg/100ml) LEVELS IN ALCOHOL ADDICTS

Fig. 11.3. Plasma testosterone values are presented for 34 individual alcohol addicts grouped according to their history of violent and aggressive behavior during intoxication. The normal range of serum testosterone levels is indicated in the middle section of the graph between the dotted lines. Subjects who admitted to use of drugs other than alcohol are shown as open circles. Single samples were obtained from each subject during a period of sobriety.

CONCLUSIONS

Plasma Testosterone Suppression

The major finding of this study is that chronic ethanol intake is associated with decreased plasma testosterone levels in male alcohol addicts. This finding is consistent with data recently obtained by Fabre and his associates (1973) (7). Earlier studies by Williams and co-workers (46) demonstrating decreased 17-ketosteroid excretion in male alcoholics have been reconfirmed by Fabre and associates (6, 7). These data converge to suggest that chronic alcohol intake may be associated with a decrease in androgen secretion.

Suppression of plasma testosterone levels observed in alcohol addicts during intoxication is also consistent with the recent findings that other centrally acting depressant drugs, which have addictive potency, also suppress levels of this hormone. Narcotics addicts on heroin maintenance in treatment facilities in England had significantly depressed plasma testosterone levels in comparison to healthy adult male controls (27). It has also been reported that barbiturates suppress circulating androgen levels as a function of alterations in biotransformation of these steroids (30). Finally, high dosage methadone maintenance is also associated with a high probability of depressed plasma testosterone levels in otherwise healthy narcotics addicts. A progressive increase in plasma testosterone levels was found in narcotics addicts during methadone detoxification while methadone dosage was progressively reduced (27).

There are three basic mechanisms which may underly alcohol-induced suppression of plasma testosterone levels. One would involve a direct effect on the hypothalamic-pituitary gonadal system resulting in decreased testosterone secretion. It is possible that ethanol may inhibit the secretion of pituitary gonadotrophins. Narcotics have been shown to inhibit pituitary gonadotrophin secretion in experimental animals (12). Ethanol is known to inhibit pituitary secretion of hormones such as the antidiuretic hormone, but it will be necessary to analyze pituitary gonadotrophins after ethanol intake to determine if this aspect of pituitary function is also effected by alcohol.

It is also possible that ethanol may have a direct effect on gonadal secretion without a primary effect on the hypothalamus or pituitary. There is evidence that ethanol may directly effect adrenal secretion of cortisol (24) and a similar phenomena may obtain *vis à vis* ethanol effects on the testes. Confirmation of this hypothesis would require detailed assessments of testosterone production rates in experimental animals and man after acute and chronic ethanol administration.

A third mechanism which may account for decreased plasma testosterone levels after alcohol intake is related to the effects of ethanol on metabolism in the liver. There is abundant evidence that alcohol has significant effects on metabolic processes in the liver as a consequence of ethanol-induced alterations of oxidation-reduction states (14, 19, 24). During ethanol catabolism, there is a shift in the ratio between nicotinamide adenine dinucleotide and its reduced form, and there is a preponderant diversion of catabolism from oxidative to reductive pathways. This is dramatically reflected in the biotransformation and catabolism of catecholamines (28), and it is likely that biotransformations of steroids are similarly effected. Therefore, it may be postulated that decreased plasma testosterone levels during chronic ethanol consumption may be attributable in part to enhanced and altered catabolism of androgens. Examination of this hypothesis would require study of degradation rates of isotopically labeled testosterone administered to alcoholics during acute and chronic ethanol ingestion.

Whatever the mechanism of alcohol-induced suppression of plasma testosterone levels, dose-response relationships have not been clarified in the present study. Single blood samples were collected upon awakening when testosterone levels are highest (35). However, blood alcohol levels are usually lowest after a night's sleep. The cumulative effects of alcohol probably influence both the production and catabolism of androgens during the course of chronic drinking. In order to establish alcohol-testosterone dose-response relationships, multiple blood samples for testosterone analysis would have to be collected each day. Such studies are currently feasible with techniques which require small volume blood samples for testosterone and ethanol analysis.

The free choice alcohol consumption paradigm used in this study also precluded obtaining orderly dose-response relationships. Although administration of programmed doses of alcohol over fixed intervals of time would facilitate study of dose-response relationships, we have previously found that programmed alcohol administration limits the generality of biological and behavioral data (20). Inasmuch as this study was designed to explore alterations in androgen function and aggressive behavior which would be consistent with real life situations, subjects were allowed to drink in a spontaneous and unrestricted manner.

Chronic Effects of Alcohol Abuse on Testicular Function

The relationship of chronic alcohol abuse to gynecomastia, testicular atrophy and decreased sexual desire in alcoholics has not been determined. It has been assumed that the deranged hepatic function associated with cirrhosis causes disturbances of estrogen metabolism which in turn are related to testicular atrophy and gynecomastia (1). It has also been found that cirrhotic males have lower than normal mean plasma testosterone levels (5) and reduced testosterone production rates (43). Most recently, Galvao-Teles and his associates (10) have reported that plasma testosterone levels were significantly lower than controls in patients with chronic liver disease and lowest in patients with cirrhosis. These investigators concluded that decreased 17-β-hydroxyandrogen in combination with normal unbound plasma estradiol levels may lead to the development of gynecomastia and testicular atrophy in men with chronic liver disease (10). The data obtained in the present study indicate that suppression of plasma testosterone levels, in alcohol addicts without evidence of cirrhosis, may further contribute to the pathophysiological processes underlying these disorders.

Aggression and Testosterone

Although it is unlikely that any single biological variable will prove to be a significant determinant of behaviors as complex as the expression of aggression in man, there have been many efforts to correlate androgens and aggression. The results of this study indicate that there is no invariant relationship between aggressive behavior and plasma testosterone levels in alcohol addicts. Alcohol-induced expression of aggression and violent behavior was not correlated with elevations in testosterone level as might be predicted from human data obtained by Persky and his associates (29) and the animal studies of Rose and co-workers (33, 34). These investigators found that dominance, aggression and hostility were related to testosterone levels with a suggestion that the higher the level, the greater the probability of aggressive behavior (29, 33, 34). Aggressive behavior observed in our subjects was associated either with a fall or an elevation in testosterone levels. However, it is important to note that an initial change in testosterone levels from base line values during alcohol ingestion was often associated with overt expression of aggression. This finding suggests that change *per se* and magnitude of change (rather than direction of change) may be the crucial variable in relating testosterone levels to aggression. But it is also important to recognize that direction and magnitude of change may only be associated with intoxication or with aggression during intoxication and not have any direct causal links to either.

Testosterone Levels as a Predictor of Aggressive Behavior

Kreuz and Rose (15) found that prisoners with documented histories of violent crimes committed during adolescence had significantly higher plasma testosterone levels than prisoners without such histories. These data were interpreted to suggest that testosterone levels might have predictive value for identifying individuals who were either at high risk or had been at high risk for commission of violent crimes (15). Data obtained on sober alcoholics in this study does not support this contention. The range of testosterone values observed in individuals who reported committing violent acts was not different from those who reported no such past history (see Fig. 11.3). Moreover, in the chronic studies, subjects who had high base line testosterone levels did not exhibit more aggressive behavior than subjects whose testosterone levels were within the normal range before drinking. Those subjects with abnormally high testosterone levels did not show any inclination to aggression or violence during the base line or withdrawal phase of the study. It is of interest that the two subjects with subnormal testosterone levels during base line did not express aggression when they were intoxicated. However, one of these subjects consumed very little alcohol during the alcohol available period.

Possible Changes in Testosterone Levels as a Function of Nonspecific Psychopathology or Stress

It could be argued that the observed suppression of testosterone levels during intoxication was not related to the pharmacological action of alcohol but rather was associated with alterations in mood and thought processes caused by intoxication. It is unlikely that thought disorders induced by alcohol would indirectly contribute to a depression in plasma testosterone level. Tourney and Hatfield (41) have found no abnormalities in plasma testosterone levels of acute schizophrenics, chronic institutionalized schizophrenics and chronic noninstitutionalized schizophrenics. Evidence that plasma testosterone levels are not significantly altered in severe affective disorders has been presented recently by Sachar and his associates (36). A very wide range of testosterone levels was observed in adult males during depressive illness and following recovery. No systematic changes in the testosterone levels occurred as a function of changes in the severity of the affective disorder (36). These findings would argue against the interpretation that an alcohol-induced mood change could account for depression or elevation in plasma testosterone levels.

Finally, it is possible that suppression of plasma testosterone levels could occur as a function of psychological stress associated with prolonged drinking. Kreuz and his associates (16)[2] have reported that plasma testos-

---

[2] It should be noted that the base line testosterone values obtained by Kreuz and his associates for army volunteers, prison volunteers and officer candidates during the later phase of training were higher than the normal range of values for adult males observed in our laboratory. It is possible that this difference was attributable to differences in technique for measuring plasma testosterone, *i.e.*, competitive protein binding versus radioimmunoassay.

terone levels were significantly lower in young adult males during the early and presumably most stressful phase of officer candidate training as contrasted with values observed during the latter less stressful phase of the program. However, the major argument against a stress-induced suppression of testosterone in our subjects is the observation that plasma testosterone levels were not suppressed during alcohol withdrawal, despite the occurrence of severe withdrawal signs and symptoms (see Table 11.1). Alcohol withdrawal states are usually associated with significant increases in serum cortisol levels and catecholamine excretion in comparison to base line and intoxication levels (26, 28). In addition, elevation of cortisol and catecholamines are usually accompanied by stress-related phenomena during chronic ethanol consumption. Therefore, it seems that stress-induced depression of plasma testosterone during alcohol ingestion is not the most parsimonious interpretation of these data.

Summary

The effects of 11 or 12 days of spontaneous drinking on plasma testosterone levels and aggressive behavior were studied in nine chronic alcohol addicts. Intoxication was associated with suppression of plasma testosterone levels in eight subjects. The suppression seemed to be independent of base line testosterone values. During alcohol withdrawal, plasma testosterone levels returned towards base line levels. There was no systematic relationship between testosterone levels and aggressive behavior during base line, intoxication or withdrawal.

Single or multiple samples for plasma testosterone analysis were also collected from 42 alcohol addicts during a period of sobriety. Thirty-four subjects were categorized according to their reported history of violence which ranged from occasional fights during intoxication (+1) to arrest and sentence for assaultive behavior (+3). Most subjects' plasma testosterone levels were within the normal range, but 14 subjects (41 per cent of this sample) had abnormally low or high values. The distribution of plasma testosterone values was comparable in each of the three violence history categories.

ACKNOWLEDGMENTS

We are grateful to Miss M. Sellers and Mrs. E. Taylor for their many contributions to all phases of data collection and analysis. We thank Dr. John Kuehnle for assistance in collection of samples from the institutionalized population. We are grateful to Dr. John Sokolowitz and Dr. Steven Wolin for medical management of these research subjects.

REFERENCES

1. ALDERCREUTZ, H: Oestrogen metabolism in liver disease. J Endocrinol 46: 129, 1970.
2. BACON, SD, ed: Studies of drinking and driving. Q J Stud Alcohol suppl. 2, 1964.
3. BURTON, G, KAPLAN, HM: Sexual behavior and adjustment of married alcoholics. Q J Stud Alcohol 29: 603, 1968.
4. CLEMENTE, CD, LINDSLEY, DB, eds: Brain Function, Vol. 5: Aggression and Defense: Neural Mechanisms and Social Patterns. Berkeley, University of California Press, 1967.
5. COPPAGE, WS, COONER, AE: Testosterone in human plasma. N Eng J Med 273: 902, 1965.
6. FABRE, LF, BROWN, JH, HOWARD, PY, FARMER, RW: Abnormal androgen metabolism in male alcoholic subjects, in Proceedings of the Fifth International Congress on Pharmacology. Abstr. 390, 1972, p. 65.
7. FABRE, LF, PASCO, PJ, LIEGEL, JM, FARMER, RW: Abnormal testosterone excretion in male alcoholic subjects, 1973, in press.
8. FREEMAN, D: Aggression: instinct or symptom? Aust NZ J Psychiatry 5:66, 1971.
9. FURUYAMA, S, MAYES, DM, NUGENT, CA: A radioimmunoassay for plasma testosterone. Steroids 16: 415, 1970.
10. GALVAO-TELES, A, ANDERSON, DC, BURKE, CW, MARSHALL, JC, CORKER, CS, BROWN, RL, CLARK, ML: Biologically active androgens and oestradiol in men with chronic liver disease. Lancet (No. 7796) 1: 173, 1973.
11. GANT, WA: Effect of alcohol on the sexual reflexes of normal and neurotic male dogs. Psychosom Med 14: 174, 1952.
12. GEORGE, R: Hypothalamus: Anterior pituitary gland, in Narcotic Drugs, Biochemical Pharmacology, edited by Clouet, DH. New York, Plenum Publishing Corp., 1971, p. 283.
13. HART, BL: Effects of alcohol on sexual reflexes and mating behavior in the male dog. Q J Stud Alcohol 29: 833, 1968.
14. ISSELBACHER, KH, GREENBERGER, NJ: Metabolic effects of alcohol on the liver. N Eng J Med 270: 351, 402, 1964.
15. KREUZ, LE, ROSE, RM: Assessment of aggressive behavior and plasma testosterone in a young criminal population. Psychosom Med 34: 321, 1972.
16. KREUZ, LE, ROSE, RM, JENNINGS, JR: Suppression of plasma testosterone levels and psychological stress. A longitudinal study of young men in officer candidate school. Arch Gen Psychiatr 26: 479, 1972.
17. LEMERE, F, SMITH, JW: Alcohol-induced sexual impotence. Am J Psychiatr 130: 212, 1973.
18. LEVINE, J: The sexual adjustment of alcoholics—A clinical study of a selected sample. Q J Stud Alcohol 16: 675, 1955.
19. LIEBER, CS: Alcohol and the liver, in The Biological Basis of Medicine, Vol. 5, edited by Bittar, EE, Bittar, N. London, Academic Press, 1969, p. 317.
20. MELLO, NK, MENDELSON, JH: Experimentally induced intoxication in alcoholics: A comparison between programmed and spontaneous drinking. J Pharmacol Exp Ther 173: 101, 1970.
21. MELLO, NK, MENDELSON, JH: Drinking patterns during work-contingent and non-contingent alcohol acquisition. Psychosom Med 34: 139, 1972.
22. MELLO, NK, BLUM, R, WOLIN, S: EEG sleep patterns in alcohol addicts during intoxication and withdrawal. 1974.
23. MENDELSON, JH, ed: Experimentally induced chronic intoxication and withdrawal in alcoholics. Q J Stud Alcohol suppl. 2, 1964.

24. MENDELSON, J. H: Biological concomitants of alcoholism. N Eng J Med 283: 24, 71, 1970.
25. MENDELSON, JH, MELLO, NK: Alcohol-induced hyperlipidemia and pre-beta serum lipoproteins, Science 1973, in press.
26. MENDELSON, JH, OGATA, M, MELLO, NK: Adrenal function and alcoholism: I. serum cortisol. Psychosom Med 33: 145, 1971.
27. MENDELSON, JH, MENDELSON, JE, PATCH, VD: Plasma testosterone levels in heroin addiction and during methadone maintenance. 1973.
28. OGATA, M, MENDELSON, JH, MELLO, NK, MAJCHROWICZ, E: Adrenal function and alcoholism: II. Catecholamines. Psychosom Med 33: 149, 1971.
29. PERSKY, H, SMITH, KD, BASU, GK: Relation of psychologic measures of aggression and hostility to testosterone production in man. Psychosom Med 33: 265, 1971.
30. RESAN, TK, SHAHIDA, NT, KORST, DR: The effect of phenobarbital on testosterone-induced erythropoiesis. J Lab Clin Med 79: 187, 1972.
31. ROSE, RM: Androgen responses to stress. I. Psychoendocrine relationships and assessment of androgen activity. Psychosom Med 31: 405, 1969.
32. ROSE, RM, BOURNE, PG, POE, RO, MOUGEY, EH, COLLINS, DR, MASON, JW: Androgen responses to stress. II. Excretion of testosterone, epitestosterone, androsterone and etiocholanolone during basic combat training and under threat of attack. Psychosom Med 31: 418, 1969.
33. ROSE, RM, HOLADAY, JW, BERNSTEIN, IS: Plasma testosterone, dominance rank and aggressive behavior in male rhesus monkeys. Nature 231: 366, 1971.
34. ROSE, RM, BORDON, PP, BERNSTEIN, IS: Plasma testosterone levels in the male rhesus: Influences of sexual and social stimuli. Science 178: 643, 1972.
35. ROSE, RM, KREUZ, LE, HOLADAY, JW, SULAK, KJ, JOHNSON, CE: Diurnal variation of plasma testosterone and cortisol. J Endocrinol 54: 177, 1972.
36. SACHAR, EJ, HALPERN, F, ROSENFELD, RS, GALLAGHER, TF, HELLMAN, L: Plasma and urinary testosterone levels in depressed men. Arch Gen Psychiatr 28: 15, 1973.
37. SHAKESPEARE, W: Macbeth, Act II, Sc. 3, e. 1606.
38. SHUPE, LM: Alcohol and crime. A study of the urine alcohol concentration found in 882 persons arrested during or immediately after commission of a felony. J Criminal Law Criminol 44: 661, 1954.
39. SILVESTRINI, R: Gynecomastia Reforma Med 142: 701, 1926.
40. TINKLENBERG, JR: Alcohol and violence, in Alcoholism: Progress in Research and Treatment, edited by Fox, R, Bourne, P. New York, Academic Press, 1973, in press.
41. TOURNEY, G, HATFIELD, LM: Androgen metabolism in schizophrenics, homosexuals and normal controls. Biol Psychiatr 6: 23, 1973.
42. U.S. Federal Bureau of Investigation: Uniform Crime Reports for the United States—1965. U.S. Dept. of Justice, Washington, D.C., 1966.
43. VERMEULEN, A, MUSSCHE, M, VERDONCK, L: Testosterone and estradiol production rates, an inter-conversion in normal males and male cirrhotics. Excerpta Med Int Congr Ser No. 256, Abstr. 305, 1972.
44. WALLER, JA: Factors associated with alcohol and responsibility for fatal highway crashes. Q J Stud Alcohol 33: 160, 1972.
45. WIELAND, WE, YUNGER, M: Sexual effects and side effects of heroin and methadone, in Proceedings of the Third National Conference on Methadone Treatment. Washington, D.C., U.S. Government Printing Office, 1970, p. 50.
46. WILLIAMS, TL, CANTAROW, A, PASCHKIS, KE, HAVENS, WP: Urinary 17-ketosteroids in chronic liver disease. Endocrinology 48: 651, 1951.
47. WOLFGANG, ME: Patterns in Criminal Homicide. Philadelphia, University of Pennsylvania Press, 1958.

48. WOLIN, S, MELLO, NK: A study of altered states of consciousness and hallucinations during alcohol intoxication and withdrawal. Ann NY Acad Sci 215: 266, 1973.
49. ZONDAG, HA, VAN BOELZLELER, GL: A rapid modification of the Pearson Reaction for total serum cholesterol. Clin Chim Acta 5: 943, 1960.

DISCUSSION

DR. SALEEM SHAH (Rockville, Maryland): From the literature that I have seen, it may not perhaps be accurate to characterize the 27 XYY group as more frequently involved in violent behavior. The early literature has given this impression in part, I think, because of some rather premature conclusions. All those which I have seen suggest that if anything, compared to 46 XY criminals, the 47 XYY patients have somewhat less violence. Price, Watmo, Jacobs, and Hope and his group in England found that on psychological test indices, they were certainly not more violent. It may be that the XYY has been somewhat stigmatized. They have other problems, but I do not think they are necessarily more violent.

DR. JACK MENDELSON (Boston, Massachusetts): We appreciate receiving that information. The major focus of our presentation was the relationships between alcohol ingestion and aggressive behavior. If the situation with the 47 XYY's is as complex as it is with the ethanol problem, there are going to be many equivocal findings before the issues are resolved.

DR. JOHN RAINEY (Nashville, Tennessee): O'Malley has shown that estrogen acts at the molecular level on RNA and the nucleus of chick oviduct cells. The mechanism seems to be on the operant controlling protein synthesis by messenger RNA. Would Dr. Mendelson comment on the possibility that estrogens and/or androgens act on nuclear RNA of neurons in a similar manner, perhaps controlling synthesis ration of significant enzymes in neurotransmitter metabolic pathways in adults?

DR. MENDELSON: I am not able to answer that question. It has been raised in a number of different ways, such as: What influences do sex steroids have on rather crucial neurochemical processes? Do they involve protein synthesis or transmitter reuptake? How do receptor sites respond to such transmitters?

DR. SHERVERT FRAZIER (Chairman) (Boston, Massachusetts): Dr. Rainey goes on to say that this is an alternative to direct androgen enzyme allosteric interactions in the control of catecholamines synthesis, as suggested by Dr. Kety to explain central nervous system testosterone-related aggressive phenomena. Further, the demonstration of chick oviduct estrogen RNA interactions suggest that androgens and estrogens may be involved in a similar manner in neurons in the developing central nervous system. If present, this might be related to the phenomenon discussed earlier by Dr. Raisman in neonatal rats.

DR. RONALD REIS (New York, New York): Dr. Pfaff can corroborate that there is no evidence of any uptake of estrogen into the neurons which synthesize the catecholamines.

DR. MENDELSON: I believe that we did hear that there was some rather selective uptake of labeled estradiol. These are not the neurons that synthesize catecholamines, however.

DR. REIS: That is correct.

Chapter 12

BEHAVIORAL AND COGNITIVE EFFECTS OF VIOLENT STIMULI[1]

RUSSELL G. GEEN

To most people, aggression is something that happens because of what goes on inside a person. One man strikes another "because he is angry." A child smashes a toy because he "feels frustrated." A woman snaps at her friend because she is upset over being snubbed by the other woman. In each case, naive psychology tells us that some event creates a condition inside the person and that aggression is an outcome of that condition. Such a conclusion is supported by common sense and everyday experience. Many experimental studies of human aggression have likewise examined or manipulated conditions leading to an "instigation to aggression," often defined in terms of some state of the person such as anger, hostility or emotional arousal. Among the conditions examined, the most common have been frustration (1), interpersonal attack (2) and real or imagined threat to the self (3). Similar explanations are frequently offered for collective violence. Urban revolts are commonly thought of as mass outbursts brought on by accumulated frustrations and anger that builds up over many incidents. The Watts riot of 1965, for example, has been described by one analyst as ". . . not a race riot in the traditional sense, but an outpouring of tremendous aggression and emotional feeling, much of which had been pent up for some time" (4).

Whereas organismic factors undoubtedly have some influence on human aggression, theories that rely on them alone overlook a growing body of evidence from experimental psychology showing that aggression is often a reaction to stimuli external to the organism, especially stimuli having strong associations with aggression and violence. For example, observing aggressive acts carried out "live" by another person may produce a spreading effect, so that one person's aggression becomes another person's stimulus to respond and a spiraling escalation of violence may follow. Such a phenomenon has long been familiar to students of collective behavior and probably forms the basis for some of the violence often manifested by crowds. Furthermore, Berkowitz (5) has cited evidence that major crimes

---

[1] The author's research reported in this paper was supported by Research Grant GS-2748 from the National Science Foundation.

of violence tend to cluster in time, and has suggested that crimes occurring early in the clusters may help create the stimulus conditions for the later ones. Nor does violence need to be observed live to elicit aggression in the viewer. Numerous experimental studies have been reported relating aggression to the viewing of aggressive stimuli through movies and television (6, 7).

THEORETICAL EXPLANATIONS FOR ELICITED AGGRESSION

Why the observation of violence, either live or symbolically portrayed, should bring about aggression in the observer is a question that has engaged the attention of many psychologists and led to several theoretical explanations. One possible mechanism for such aggression is simple imitation, a process usually demonstrated in small children (7), but also found in young adults (8). Another possibility is that aggression may be a learned response elicited by stimuli that have become conditioned to violence in the person's past through either classical or instrumental processes (5, 9). Still another possibility is that the witnessing of aggression produces a general increase in the observer's level of emotional arousal (10, 11). The perception of a violent event may arouse a person to the extent that any response he is ready to perform becomes greatly intensified. If the person has a reason to express hostility and aggression at the time of observing such an event, aggressive responses are likely to be energized by the increased arousal. Finally, elicited aggression has been described as a result of reductions in restraints against aggression acquired through the process of socialization. Observing violence may inform a person that aggression is permissible or even desirable under certain circumstances. If the observer is prepared to aggress for some reason but is inhibited in acting out his desires, such information may lower his remaining restraints (12).

All of these explanations emphasize that aggression may be a reaction to stimuli external to the person rather than a necessary outcome of the person's internal state. Some investigators have shown that such aggression can occur even when the person has not been aggressively aroused in any obvious way (13, 14). Furthermore, by paying attention to external stimuli we are often able to resolve some of the problems that arise in studies of internal causes of aggression. For example, many attempts to show that frustration is an antecedent of aggression have ended in failure (2), leading some observers to reject the frustration-aggression hypothesis entirely. However, several years ago Geen and Berkowitz (15) showed that when a violent movie is shown to a person after he has been frustrated, he becomes more aggressive than a nonfrustrated person who sees the same movie. Such a finding may indicate that frustration raises an individual's level of arousal and that increased arousal activates aggressive responses elicited by the film. In a later study, Geen and O'Neal (16) found that subjects who were stimulated by noise failed to manifest more aggression than subjects given no noise when an exciting but nonviolent motion picture was shown to them. When a movie depicting a prizefight was shown, however, subjects stimulated by noise were considerably more aggressive in attacking an experimental accomplice than those given no noise. Still another example of the function of aggressive stimuli in eliciting aggression from aroused subjects has been provided by Baron and his colleagues. Noting that civil unrest usually occurs in summer months, Baron (17) proposed that high ambient temperature might lead to aggression by making people irritable and prone to outbursts of temper. At first his data failed to support his contention. High temperatures (95 to 100° F) in and of themselves did not facilitate aggression; if anything, they tended to inhibit aggressive behavior. In a second study, however, Baron and Lawton (18) manipulated not only ambient temperature but also the presence or absence of an aggressive model. The results of the second experiment again failed to support the idea that temperature by itself facilitates aggression, but did show that subjects who observed an aggressive model under conditions of high temperature were more aggressive than similarly overheated subjects who did not observe a model. We may conclude from these studies that heat, noise and frustration—three conditions commonly thought to be among the main causes of stress in urban surroundings—may not in and of themselves lead to violence, but rather may interact with effects produced by aggressive stimuli in the environment.

COGNITIVE PROCESSES IN ELICITED AGGRESSION

To this point nothing has been said concerning cognitive processes that occur between the perception of violence and the aggressive behavior that observed violence elicits. The importance of such processes, however, has been shown in several studies. Several years ago Berkowitz and Rawlings (19) showed that when persons who have been made angry see a fight that is described as morally justified, they subsequently behave more aggressively than similarly angry people who regard the same fight as less justified. More recently, Hoyt (20) has shown that the perceived reasons for justification of violence exert different amounts of restraint on aggressive behavior. In his experiment, angry subjects who saw a movie of a fight in which the winning boxer was said to be seeking revenge later acted more aggressively than angry subjects who regarded the fight as an instance of self-defense.

In the two experiments described here the internal representation of the observed violence formed by subjects who regarded the action as justified differed from the representation formed by subjects who perceived the same action as less justified. The question we must ask is why these two different cognitive representations produced differential amounts of aggression. One possible reason is that disinhibition of aggression is involved: the interpretations that a person places on observed violence determine whether the violence leads to a reduction of restraints against aggressing (19).

Recently David Stonner and I conducted two studies that further support the disinhibition hypothesis. In the first experiment (21) each subject, a college-age male, interacted with another man who was actually an experimental confederate. In the course of the interaction, the confederate deliberately provoked and angered the subject in half the conditions whereas he treated him in a more neutral manner in the other half. Every subject then saw a short movie of a prizefight in which one man savagely beats the other. One-third of the subjects were simply shown the film without comment. Another third were presented a short narrative before the film describing the fight as a grudge match motivated by a desire for revenge on the part of the winning boxer. The final third were told that the fight was a match between two professionals who bore no animosity for each other but were simply boxing for money. Later, the subject was given an opportunity to deliver some electric shocks to the confederate with whom he had interacted earlier. The subject could use 1 of 10 buttons for shocking, supposedly to punish the confederate for making errors on a task. The 10 buttons were said to govern 10 increasing intensities of shock. Actually no shocks were given, and the subject's choices of the intensity of each of the shocks that he thought he was giving were monitored electronically. The shock intensities chosen by the subjects in each of the six experimental conditions are shown in Figure 12.1. When the subject had been attacked by the confederate he counterattacked most intensely after observing violence that had connotations of vengeance. However, when the subject had not been attacked previously, he reacted most aggressively to what was described as professional violence. In order to assess the possible reason for this finding we included a questionnaire containing several self-report items. One item asked the subject to describe the degree to which he had "held back" in shocking the confederate, and was included as a direct measure of the subject's feelings of restraints against aggressing. The ratings of restraint, shown in Figure 12.2, indicate that angry subjects felt least restrained against aggressing after witnessing vengeful aggression, whereas nonangered subjects experienced the lowest restraints after ob-

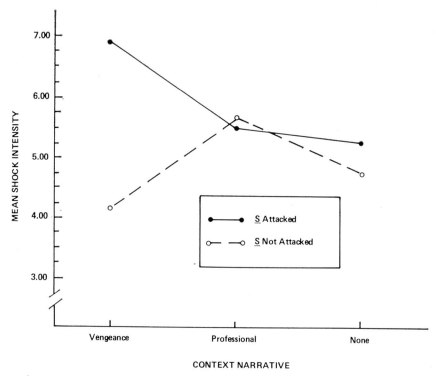

Fig. 12.1. Mean intensities of shocks given by subjects after seeing boxing movie. Each point represents average numerical value of button chosen by subject (1 to 10) to deliver shocks. Reproduced by permission from *Aggression* by Russell Geen. © General Learning Corporation, 1972.

serving nonhostile professional violence. Moreover, when we analyzed the aggression data with expression of restraints against aggressing as a covariant, the interaction between anger and film interpretation was found to be not significant. In other words, the variance in aggression found in this experiment can be attributed largely to variance in restraints against aggressing.

Our second experiment (22) provided more support for our conclusion that placing differing interpretations on observed violence leads to different levels of inhibition against aggression and that these differences are correlated with levels of aggressive behavior. In the first study we had told some of the subjects that the man who eventually wins the fight had been seeking to avenge himself against the loser. The film then showed him to be successful. In the second study we not only repeated this condition but also added another in which we explained that the man who eventually

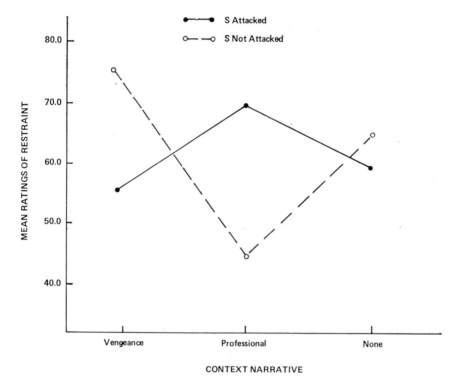

Fig. 12.2. Mean reported degree subject held back in shocking. Scale is 100-mm. line anchored by "did not hold back" (0) to "held back very much" (100). Reproduced by permission from *Aggression* by Russell Geen. © General Learning Corporation, 1972.

loses the fight had been the one seeking revenge. We found that angered subjects in this latter group were subsequently less aggressive in shocking the confederate than others who had witnessed a successful attempt at revenge, and also significantly more inhibited, according to self-reports. Thus, when observed violence is placed in an explanatory context that produces increased, rather than lowered, restraints against aggressing, the result is a lowered intensity of aggression.

Another dimension along which people may interpret observed aggression, especially that seen in movies and television, is that of reality versus fictionality. Studies by Feshbach (23) with children as subjects, and by Berkowitz and Alioto (24) with young adults, have shown that violent films tend to elicit less aggressive behavior when they are explicitly described as fiction than when they are offered as representations of real violence. The reason for this finding is not obvious, but one recent study from our laboratory (25) suggests that violence described as fiction may be less arousing

than that which is presented without an explicit reminder of its fictionality. In this study we showed the boxing movie to several groups of subjects, introducing it in each case with a narrative that supplied the context
in which the fight supposedly occurred. Some subjects were told that the
fight was motivated by the winner's desire for revenge, others that it was a
professional aggression and still others that it was a beating justified by
the loser's bad character. Another group of subjects was told that the film
depicted revenge but was in addition reminded that the violence was just
being acted and was patently fictitious. During the film the subject's heart
rate and skin conductance were continuously monitored. The results
showed that subjects who had been reminded of the fictitiousness of the
fight emitted significantly fewer galvanic skin responses (GSRs) than subjects given one of the introductory narratives without any reminder of
fictionality. We cannot conclude, of course, that attributions of fictionality
to observed violence affect subsequent aggressiveness solely through their
influence on emotional arousal. Fictional violence may also have less of
a tendency to lower inhibitions against aggressing than realistic violence;
further experimentation is required to test this possibility. Nevertheless,
we do have some evidence that arousal differences are correlated with descriptions of the observed violence as real or fictional.

In another experiment just completed in our laboratory, Stonner and
I found that the interpretations a subject places on observed violence may
affect not only the amount of restraint he feels over aggressing but also his
level of physiological arousal. In this experiment we showed each subject a
5-minute sequence from a western film in which a group of gunmen fight
and eventually defeat a band of outlaws. Some of the subjects were told
that the gunfighters fought because they wanted to avenge the murders of
some of their men at the hands of the outlaws. Others were told that the
gunmen had been hired to fight the bandits and therefore fought for professional reasons. Other were told that the gunmen were fighting for
altruistic motives, to protect the citizens of a village from the outlaws. The
film itself was ambiguous enough to make any of these three interpretations plausible. Finally, a fourth group of subjects saw the film without an
introduction. Half the subjects in each condition had previously been
made angry by a confederate and a half had not. All subjects were then
allowed to give electric shocks to the confederate.

The results of the experiment bore out our expectation that the context
in which observed violence is judged to occur affects the amount of aggressive behavior it elicits (see Table 12.1). Angry subjects gave shocks of
greater intensity after they had seen violence supposedly motivated by
revenge than after seeing the same bloodshed prompted by professional or
altruistic motives. They also gave slightly stronger shocks than subjects

TABLE 12.1

Mean intensities of shocks given by angered and nonangered subjects after seeing western film

Explanation of Film Violence	Treatment of Subject[1]	
	Angered	Not angered
Vengeance....................................	5.53	3.38
Professional.................................	3.98	3.88
Altruism.....................................	3.85	3.57
No story.....................................	4.15	3.22

[1] Results represent average numerical value of button chosen by subject (1 to 10) to deliver shocks.

who merely saw the film. Also as expected, angry subjects expressed weaker restraints against aggressing after seeing vengeful violence than after witnessing professional or altruistic aggression. Subjects who had not been angered were less aggressive across all conditions of interpretation than angered subjects and did not react to any of the film's interpretation with differential levels of aggression.

In addition to measuring aggressive behavior and self-reports of restraint, we also took measures of both systolic and diastolic blood pressure at several times during the experiment. Although these data have not been completely analyzed at this time, one important finding has emerged. Following the manipulation of anger and just before the film began, angered subjects showed a significant increase in mean arterial pressure not shown by nonangered subjects. At the conclusion of the film subjects who had seen altruistic and professional violence had significantly lower blood pressures than subjects who had seen vengeful aggression. The difference was attributable to differential rates of return to base line levels: the blood pressures of angry subjects tended to remain high when they watched vengeful aggression whereas the blood pressures of subjects who saw altruistic or professional aggression tended to return to pre-anger levels. The blood pressure of nonangered subjects was not affected by the interpretation they placed on the film; in all of the conditions nonangered subjects tended to become somewhat aroused by the film itself. We thus have some evidence that the interpretations people have on witnessed violence have an effect on physiological reactions to such violence.

CONCLUSIONS

The following conclusions seem warranted by our findings to date.

1. Observation of violence, such as that shown in motion pictures and on television, can, under some conditions, lead to aggressive behavior in the observer. Several reasons for this have been offered such as prior learn-

ing, imitation, lowering of restraints against aggressing and heightened arousal produced by the violent stimuli.

2. The interpretations that the observer places on the violence he witnesses have effects on the degree to which aggression is elicited. Violence that is obviously fictitious elicits less aggressive behavior than that which is perceived as more realistic. Violence that is regarded as revenge seems to elicit more aggression in angry people than that to which other motives are imputed.

3. Different interpretations of observed violence produce varying feelings of restraint against aggressing and also lead to different levels of autonomic arousal. Either or both of these effects may be involved in the aggressive behavior that is sometimes elicited by displays of violence.

The general conclusion we have reached regarding our own research is not at all remarkable. It is simply the old principle that when one wishes to gauge the impact of a stimulus upon an organism he must consider the subjective value of the stimulus to the organism, or, to put it another way, he must consider the proximal representation of the distal event. If we have learned nothing else, we have at least learned to be cautious in forming answers to the question of whether observation of violence leads to aggression. It may or it may not, and the context in which it is presented will do much to determine the outcome.

REFERENCES

1. DOLLARD, J, DOOB, L, MILLER, NE, MOWRER, OH, SEAR, RR: Frustration and Aggression. New Haven, Yale University Press, 1939.
2. BUSS, AH: Instrumentality of aggression, feedback, and frustration as determinants of physical aggression. J Pers Soc Psychol 3: 153, 1966.
3. FESHBACH, S: The function of aggression and the regulation of aggressive drive. Psychol Rev 71: 257, 1964.
4. PLOG, SC: Rebellion in Los Angeles: The Watts riots, in Brain Function. Vol. 5: Aggression and Defense: Neural Mechanisms and Social Patterns, edited by Clemente, CD, Lindsley, DB. Berkeley, University of California Press, 1967, p. 297.
5. BERKOWITZ, L: The contagion of violence: An S-R mediational analysis of some effects of observed aggression, in Nebraska Symposium on Motivation, Vol. 18., edited by Arnold, WJ, Page, MM. Lincoln, University of Nebraska Press, 1970, p. 95.
6. BERKOWITZ, L: The concept of aggressive drive: Some additional considerations, in Advances in Experimental Social Psychology, edited by Berkowitz, L. New York, Academic Press, 1965, p. 301.
7. BANDURA, A: Principles of Behavior Modification. New York, Holt, Rinehart, & Winston, 1969.
8. BARON, RA: Reducing the influence of an aggressive model: The restraining effects of discrepant modeling cues. J Pers Soc Psychol 20: 240, 1971.
9. GEEN, RG, STONNER, D: The effects of aggressiveness habit strength upon behavior in the presence of aggression—Related stimuli. J Pers Soc Psychol 17: 149, 1971.
10. ZILLMAN, D: Excitation transfer in communication-mediated aggressive behavior. J Exp Soc Psychol 7: 419, 1971.

11. Tannenbaum, PH: Studies in film- and television-mediated arousal and aggression: A progress report, in Television and Social Behavior: V. Television's Effects—Further Explorations, edited by Comstock, GA, Rubinstein, ES, Murray, JP. Washington, D.C., U.S. Department of Health, Education and Welfare, 1972, p. 309.

12. Wheeler, L, Caggiula, AR: The contagion of aggression. J Exp Soc Psychol 2: 1, 1966.

13. Walters, RH, Llewellyn, TE: Enhancement of punitiveness by visual and audio-visual displays. Can J Psychol 17: 244, 1963.

14. Hartman, DP: Influence of symbolically modeled instrumental aggression and pain cues on aggressive behavior. J Pers Soc Psychol 11: 280, 1969.

15. Geen, RG, Berkowitz, L: Some conditions facilitating the occurrence of aggression after the observation of violence. J Pers 35: 666, 1967.

16. Geen, RG, O'Neal, EC: Activation of cue-elicited aggression by general arousal. J Pers Soc Psychol 11: 289, 1969.

17. Baron, RA: Aggression as a function of ambient temperature and prior anger arousal. J Pers Soc Psychol 21: 183, 1972.

18. Baron, RA, Lawton, SF: Environmental influences on aggression: The facilitation of modeling effects by high ambient temperatures. Psychonom Sci 26: 80, 1972.

19. Berkowitz, L, Rawlings, E: Effects of film violence on inhibitions against subsequent aggression. J Abnorm Soc Psychol 66: 405, 1963.

20. Hoyt, JL: Effect of media violence "justification" on aggression. J Broadcasting 16: 455, 1970.

21. Geen, RG, Stonner, D: Context effects in observed violence. J Pers Soc Psychol 25: 145, 1973.

22. Geen, RG, Stonner, D: The context of observed violence: Inhibition of aggression through displays of unsuccessful retaliation. Psychonom Sci 27: 342, 1972.

23. Feshbach, S: Reality and fantasy in filmed violence, in Television and Social Behavior: II. Television and Social Learning, edited by Murray, JP, Rubinstein, ES, Comstock, GA. Washington, D.C., U.S. Department of Health, Education and Welfare, 1972, p. 318.

24. Berkowitz, L, Alioto, JT: The meaning of an observed event as a determinant of its aggressive consequences. J Pers Soc Psychol 28: 206, 1973.

25. Geen, RG, Rakosky, JJ: Interpretations of observed violence and their effects on GSR. J Exp Res Pers 6: 289, 1973.

DISCUSSION

Dr. John P. Spiegel (Boston, Massachusetts): I have two questions with regard to this excellent presentation. One has to do with using the electric shock to deliver an attack. Isn't there some possibility that this remote and depersonalized way of expressing the aroused anger might have, in itself, an inhibiting effect because it interposes a machine between the aggressor and the object of the attack?

In Stanley Milgram's experiments on what he called "authoritarianism," in which subjects were instructed to deliver a shock to someone else, the subjects had some resistance toward using this sort of mechanism because it seemed rather cruel and unnatural and, in any event, was a way of averting a direct interpersonal relationship. The fact that the results you obtained moved in the right direction tends to diminish my question, but I wonder if your results might not have been more prominent if there had been some more human way of delivering the aggression.

My second question has to do with the function of revenge, and whether or not it would be possible to discover, through a questionnaire or some other way, exactly how revenge fits into the subject's system of rationalization. Might this be seen as justified aggression?

DR. RUSSELL GEEN (Columbia, Missouri): Answering the second question first, the hypothesis is that when a subject is angered by the other person, he seeks revenge. To show him an example of someone else obtaining revenge actually gives him a sort of model for social comparison. This is facilitated by the great similarity between his own situation and the one he sees in the movies. We have research under way now that is systematically investigating this possibility of social comparisons. I think what you say is correct. We are predicting that that is what we are going to find.

With regard to the distance between the attacker and his victim, as I recall Milgram's work, he found that bringing the victim closer to the attacker tended to decrease the amount of aggression. He found the least aggression when the attacker had to grab the victim and force him onto the shock electrode. Although this may be a problem in our research, I think it is at least a constant problem because in every one of our studies so far we have maintained exactly identical conditions of distance and separation. The two persons are in separate cubicles out of sight of each other. You are right that the aggression they commit is done in an impersonal way. This may account for much of the lack of restraint we find.

DR. SALEEM SHAH (Rockville, Maryland): When I try to conceptualize the experimental situation and the paradigm implicit in your discussion and explicit in a lot of the social-psychological research, I see three sets of variables which have, in turn, subcategories. These may be biochemical or cognitive or they could be stimulus-control elements. The modality may be physiological, biochemical or psychological. The third major factor is situational, as in your point about context. It is very complicated to consider all of these three sets, yet unless one does so, and looks at the context, one might attribute different kinds of meanings to some single relationship between variables.

My question pertains to a criticism made in the past about the experimental paradigm that you used, namely, the lack of a control. I am curious to know whether you used another film as a control. When Berkowitz used both a violent and a nonviolent film, the nonviolent film was rather boring; and it is difficult to compare a boring, nonviolent film with an exciting, violent one. You would need an exciting nonviolent film.

DR. GEEN: In a number of studies prior to these, we showed the violent films along with films that we had scaled and prejudged for nonviolent arousal, mainly of sporting events. This has also been done by Tannebaum and his group at Berkeley who have, in fact, worked with a number of the same films we used. We found that the arousing violent film elicits more aggression than the arousing nonviolent film, so we have control in our previous work. Because of design demands, we have not been able to have control in all these subsequent studies.

DR. DONALD REIS (New York, New York): How long does the effect last after the termination of the experience? Secondly, is there any evidence that seeing a revengeful film somehow has a cathartic effect, that some time after the experience an individual is less prone to violence than he would be otherwise?

DR. GEEN: Essentially everything I have told about here is very short term, a matter of minutes. We have the aggressive act take place 5 to 10 minutes after showing the film. Anthony Doob of the University of Toronto extended his investigations from several minutes to an hour after the film was shown and found a decrement in aggression taking place after 5 to 10 minutes. He proposes that the arousal effects are chiefly short term. Everything I have shown so far has been effective up to about 6 or 7 minutes. We have never studied the question of catharsis.

DR. PAUL D. MACLEAN (Bethesda, Maryland): I would like to ask Dr. Geen what is the basis for your statement that adults are less imitative than children?

DR. GEEN: First, there is voluminous evidence on imitation in children but very little on adults. The second factor, I must admit, is more prejudice than scientific judgment. I think children have greater suggestibility, although maybe I am overstating the case.

DR. JEROME FRANK (Baltimore, Maryland): In all experiments with college students, as Orne has pointed out and also Rosenthal and a few others, the student may not be defining the situation the way the experimenter thinks he is. One has to be very cautious about what the student thinks, and what he thinks the experimenter wants, and so on. This can be asked, of course, about any research; and this is an excellent piece of research. I wonder whether you use the safeguard of questioning the students afterwards as to what they thought you wanted, or as to what they made of the experiment. It would be especially valuable in a highly artificial situation like this.

DR. GEEN: Yes, we do even more than that. First of all, the experimenter interviews the student quite rigorously to get at the demand characteristics. Then, after he leaves, we have him meet another person sitting out in the hall who is supposedly the next subject waiting to come in, who asks him very confidentially what is going on inside. If the subject is able to give to fairly good rundown on what it is, we throw that data out.

DR. JOSEPH M. FOLEY (Cleveland, Ohio): How do social psychologists get informed consent for experimental studies on humans without losing the purpose of the experiment?

DR. GEEN: Of course we cannot get fully informed consent from these people because we are using deception. If we told them what is really going on, we would be measuring their theories of behavior rather than their actual behavior. We attempt to overcome the deception, to make the experience as meaningful for the subject as we can, by fully informing him after it is over. We tell him what we have done and what his role in the research has been. Then, at the end of the semester, we give him a report of the findings of the experiment, so that it becomes for him, I think, a fairly important learning experience. Most of our subjects have told us that they greatly appreciate this sort of treatment. Also, we do not inveigle anyone into this work without at least uninformed consent. Anyone can leave whenever he wants to and, as you might expect, a number of people have walked out on us.

Chapter 13

THIRD-PARTY INTERVENTION IN COMMUNITY CONFLICT

JOHN P. SPIEGEL

It is perhaps ironic that just as public concern over collective violence is diminishing, techniques for coping with or even preventing violence are becoming crystallized. Race-related community disturbances, campus disorders and ghetto uprisings are rarely front-page items, although they still occur with sufficient regularity to place considerable strain on local authorities. One has only to recall Attica, the trashing and tear gassing on the last night of the Republican Convention in Miami Beach last summer, the shooting at Southern University in Baton Rouge 2 weeks ago and the recent inter-racial disturbances among naval personnel aboard the carriers Kitty Hawk and Constellation, to realize that group aggression, with often fatal consequences, is still a troubling phenomenon in our society. And the cases that come to national attention are only a small proportion of those that occur on an endemic basis.

Nevertheless, as the reports of the Lemberg Center have demonstrated (1), the annual levels of collective violence are much reduced from the peaks reached in the 1967 to 1970 period. The reasons for the reduction are complex and I do not have time to consider them this afternoon. What I propose to concern myself with is one factor among the many that are correlated with the reduced frequency of disorder events, namely, the influence of third-party intervention on potentially violent confrontations. Third-party intervention consists of a series of conflict-shaping and conflict-reducing inputs that have emerged over the past 3 years from efforts to cope with the wildly escalating, chaotic events of naturally occurring disorders.

Interventions of this sort are largely unreported and are therefore relatively unknown, both to laymen and to scientific audiences. The procedures involved are not well understood even by those who practice them because they are too new, too subject to change, too much a response to intense practical needs growing out of evanescent circumstances. To capture and report the circumstances of the kaleidoscopic, emotionally heated disorder of events is a triumph in itself. Therefore, codification of these practices is just getting underway. But there is another reason for the lack of reporting of intervention procedures. As we all know, it is dangerous to intervene in a fight between two other people. They can both easily turn on the third person. Accordingly, the interveners are reluctant to present themselves as experts, feeling especially at this early stage that they might elicit more hostility than acceptance, more doubt than credibility. In the tenuous, delicate situation in which intervention takes place credibility depends more on word of mouth reports of past behavior than on scientific reputation or professional standing.

For these reasons, my paper this afternoon will differ from the usual scientific contributions characteristic of the meetings of the Association for Research in Nervous and Mental Disease. It constitutes a field report from the fighting front. More seriously, it can be regarded as an attempt to organize and codify a set of social procedures—social engineering, if you will—which promise to be helpful in the reduction of levels of collective violence. I should also like to state that my discussion, although varying in some respects, is derived from the previous work of Dr. James Laue and his associates at the Community Crisis Intervention Project, Social Science Institute, Washington University, St. Louis (2).

To begin with, I have to point out some of the issues relevant to my topic that I won't be able to deal with today. I will not touch upon the general theory of conflict behavior because it is too diffuse and in any event needs to be specified for system levels, such as personality, small group, wider community, the nation state or the international system (3). Second, so far as the community level is concerned, which is the focus of today's discussion, I shall not discuss either the remote or underlying causes of civil disorders nor theories of the riot process and the escalation of violence. These are matters, currently, of vigorous debate (4). Nevertheless, because it is necessary to impose some sort of time frame upon the phenomena of community conflict in order to explain third-party interventions, I shall propose a rather *ad hoc* set of states of conflict which may characterize the community situation at any one moment of time.

Let us assume that the conflict in the community occurs between two parties. The first consists of a set of "aggrieved" groups, such as racial or minority, student or political protesters who believe their goals have not been met, or even listened to, and that they do not have the power to effect change through the ordinary political process. The second group consists of local authorities who have three not always compatible responsibilities: to deal with the demands of the protesters, to keep the peace and to punish wrongdoing. It is generally assumed that the authorities always have the power, if not necessarily the inclination or the capacity, to meet these responsibilities.

In the context of this two-party conflict, there is always the possibility of intervention by a third or outside party. What can be done, however, depends upon the state of the conflict at the time. The relevant states referred to above are the following. The conflict may be: 1) *dormant,* that is, not only quiescent, but unrecognized or its symptoms denied by the authorities; 2) *escalating,* that is, giving rise to demonstrations, protest meetings, confrontations or minor scuffles whose significance can no longer be denied; 3) *in crisis,* that is, characterized by intense confrontations in streets, school buildings, prison yards and other localities which threaten to or actually become violent; 4) *stalemated,* that is, unresolved and characterized by alternating periods of quiescence and flare-ups, a chronic state that leaves no one's mind really at rest; 5) *resolving,* where the issues at conflict are being solved through compromise by means of negotiation or the use of normal political channels and 6) *relapsed,* that is, after a course of apparent resolution the whole structure of compromise breaks down and the situation returns to escalating or crisis states.

Third-party interveners enter the situation and perform roles, or functions, adapted to the prevalent state of conflict. I will now describe these roles, but I must first say that I am not altogether comfortable about using the word "role." In standard usage, role describes a conventionalized behavior pattern associated with the function, position or title a person holds within a group or organization. The behavior patterns I shall describe are not yet sufficiently conventionalized nor is there complete agreement on what role term to assign to the various functions (5). There are other reasons for questioning this usage, such as their lack of clear differentiation from each other (6), but since role terms—like names for hurricanes—are convenient devices, I shall overlook the objections. In describing the application of the roles to concrete situations I shall refer frequently to the conflict between protesters and authorities during the Democratic and Republican Conventions in Miami Beach last summer. The staff of the Lemberg Center had the opportunity to study the entire sequence of events from June through September, including the prior planning for the confrontations and the aftermath of the violence on the last day of the Republican Convention. Since this represented what collective violence researchers call a "scheduled event"—as opposed to an unexpected, spontaneous disorder—it was possible to collect more systematic data on the planning and the outcome of plans than is usually the case.

The first of the intervener roles is that of the *advocate.* He represents a person, or group, entering a conflict situation during the dormant state or when escalation is just beginning as an adviser or consultant to the aggrieved group. Unlike all the other interveners to be discussed, he is unabashedly *not* neutral, being pledged to support and facilitate the goals of just one party to the conflict (7). He lends his skills as an organizer to the group, helping it to create a structure capable of taking action, advising the group on the formulation of its demands and on sources of financial or political support. Inasmuch as he is not a part of the group but enters from the outside, he is presumably cooler and more objective, more capable of creating an effective strategy of protests, demonstrations and confrontations than indigenous members of the group. He may be committed to nonviolent techniques or he may be willing to risk violence in pursuit of the groups' goals, depending on his moral values and his previous strategic experience.

A decade ago the advocate would probably have been called an "outside agitator," and he may still receive this label in some parts of the country today. To be sure, his function is to heighten a dormant conflict or to escalate one in progress in order to bring the issues to a head and to achieve change. But, as a result of the disorders of the 1960's, public attitudes toward collective violence have become more sophisticated. In metropolitan areas especially, the focus is on conflict management in order to avoid violence while preserving the possibility of peaceful change. There is a general consensus that the more highly organized and successfully led the protest group, the greater the opportunity to avoid the irrationality and chaos that breed violence. Although the advocate would usually prefer change without violence if this is possible, he is increasingly perceived as playing a part in the complex maneuvers involved in conflict management.

Although the advocate contributes to conflict regulation, human relations in extreme and emotionally laden circumstances are inevitably unpredictable, and the conflict may still mount to the crisis stage. Crowds assemble on the streets, hostages are taken in prisons, face-offs occur in which the atmosphere of impending violence is reinforced by rapid, physical motion, confusion and the possibility of an impulsive, aggressive act. The prime characteristic of a community disorder in the crisis stage is the possibility of surprise—the unexpected act which precipitates the violence. It is at this stage that the second intervener role, the *conciliator*, makes its appearance. The conciliator attempts to cool inflamed tempers by creating physical and emotional distance between adversaries and by suggesting temporary expedients to resolve the crisis.

For example, you may recall the incident at the Washington, D.C. jail, Wednesday, October 11, 1972, when the enraged inmates, largely black, seized Correction Director Kenneth Hardy hostage and were ready to die when told that 100 riot-equipped police were prepared to rush Cell Block 1, which they were holding. Aggression arousal was so high that they were scarcely able to articulate the demands or grievances underlying their uprising. Washington lawyers Julian Tepper and Ronald Goldfarb appeared, and, reinforced by the presence of Representative Shirley Chisolm, managed to calm the inmates and obtain the release of the hostage by arranging for the inmates to appear in court to plead their case before Judge Bryant (8).

The actions of the conciliators in this case were impromptu. If they had not happened to show up after hearing about the incident on the radio, another Attica might well have occurred, and this illustrates the lack of conventionalization of intervener roles. But, in other instances, particularly at Miami Beach for the conventions, conciliator roles were planned months ahead. An organization called Religious and Community Leaders Concerned (with the Conventions—R.C.L.C.) arranged to bear witness to nonviolent confrontation for the greater Miami community by training neutral observers, setting up a rumor-control and reporting service, and by offering to serve as go-betweens for the authorities and the protesters. For example, they negotiated a campsite at Flamingo Park for the nondelegates, as the protesters were called. Another organization, the National YMCA Outreach Program, arranged for medical and legal services for the nondelegates and provided communications equipment for the not always congenial groups, the Yippies, the Zippies, the S.D.S., the Women's Lib, the Gay Organizations and the Viet Nam Veterans Against the War, to name a few, who planned to participate in street theater, sitdowns and demonstrations against the Nixon war policy.

The actions of conciliators are distinguished from the functions of the advocates because they are taken only after consultation with the authorities—or, at least, with their sanction. Conciliators represent the interests of both sides in an emergency situation. Although they may be closer to one than another side, they cannot function unless they have credibility with both sides. For example, during the boycott of the John Wilson Junior High School in the Canarsie section of Brooklyn by a group of white parents protesting the transfer of black students from the Brownsville area, street confrontations took place featuring rock and egg throwing and the hurling of racial epithets. From October 31 to November 8, 1972, violence was averted in this tinderbox situation to a large extent by on-the-spot conciliation conducted by the Community Relations Service (CRS), which is an official arm of the federal Justice Department. That a government agency could obtain credibility with both racial groups during this crisis is testimony to the careful cultivation of human relations with individuals and groups residing in the area on the part of the CRS far in advance of the crisis itself. This is only one example of the many crisis events in which the Community Relations Service has been quietly involved. But inasmuch as it seduously avoids publicity, its activities are relatively unknown and unappreciated.

The third type of intervener is the *mediator*. The Community Crisis Intervention Project at Washington University has defined the functions of mediators in this fashion: "Mediation is the process by which a third party who is acceptable to all conflicting parties in a dispute helps them in reaching a mutually satisfactory settlement of their differences." One might also say that if advocates generate a situation in which mediation may be necessary to avoid violence, conciliators produce the situation, in the midst of crisis, in which mediation is possible. However, it is important to point out that if mediators enter the conflict situation during escalation and before a crisis occurs, the crisis may be altogether avoided.

Mediators not only have to be acceptable to both sides but may also have to do a great deal of legwork and perform psychological feats of interpretation in order to get each side to be willing to sit down and talk together. For this reason, mediators are sometimes called negotiators. As I said previously, there is some disagreement about role terms. However, there is a growing consensus that negotiations can only take place between the two parties—the adversaries—who are in direct conflict with each other. Mediators can prepare the way for negotiations by offering neutral ground for a meeting place, by interpreting each side's position to the other, by carrying messages back and forth and, above all, through their steady and optimistic attitudes that compromise and peace is possible. A noncontroversial, anxiety-reducing, problem-solving and yet realistic and tough orientation is an essential part of the mediator's equipment.

In Miami Beach, because it was a well advertised event and because both the protesters and the police, plus other local authorities, had indicated well in advance their desire to avoid violence, would-be mediators offered their services by the dozens. However, only a few groups managed to obtain the confidence of both sides. Their activity, particularly during the planning process before and between the conventions, generated the spirit of trust between the police and the protesters which was instrumental in avoiding violence during all but the last day of the Republican Convention. On that day the carefully nurtured trust broke down. Unfortunately time is too short to review here the reasons for the breakdown of trust and the emergence of trashing, tear gassing, injuries and arrests that marred the otherwise successful conflict management.

The fourth of the intervener roles is that of the *arbitrator*. This is the newest and perhaps the most promising of all the community conflict intervener roles. In many neighborhood conflicts, for example, between tenants and landlords or housing authorities, or between hospital boards and administrators, on one side, and patient groups or health care consumers on the other, specialists who have had much experience in mediation are beginning to be given legal authority by the courts to settle the dispute. The arbitrator must, of course, again be acceptable to both sides. Arbitrators can also function without such formal, legal authorization. For example, in Miami Beach a mediator representing the Religious and Community Leaders Concerned organization was given responsibility, for the Republican Convention, of obtaining a park permit on behalf of the protesters, enabling them to occupy Flamingo Park as a campsite. The City Council was not willing to give the park directly to the protesters because the various groups were too antagonistic to each other to be responsible for governance of the campsite. As the responsible holder of the permit, this mediator had then to arbitrate the various disputes that erupted on the campsite between the rivalrous groups of nondelegates. If this sounds like an impossible assignment, it should be considered that the arbitrator has the advantage (or disadvantage, depending upon one's view) of being blamed by each side for the settlement he imposes. To be sure, he would rather obtain an agreement than impose a settlement. But if he is forced to be arbitrary, the leaders of the various factions can minimize the disappointment and resentment of their followers by blaming the arbitrator. This enables them to preserve their leadership position. Rapid leadership turnover, which is characteristic of most dissident groups, is dysfunctional from the point of view of conflict management.

The fifth and final intervener role is that of the *research evaluator*. This is the role that my colleagues and I assumed in Miami Beach. As with the other roles, the researcher must be acceptable to all sides or he will not be permitted access to the data he needs. If he is not careful he may even be chased off the premises, as most participants easily adopt the attitude, "Who needs research?" Protesters resent the money that goes to research rather than to their needs, whereas authorities fear that they will be portrayed in a damaging light. Therefore, the researcher does his best to behave in an impartial, objective and helpful way while minimizing any direct intervention in the event he is observing, lest he influence the very process he is studying. At the same time, the researcher must be clear concerning his own sympathies, attitudes and values and be prepared to articulate them if requested. His direct effect on the conflict should thus be minimal, subject only to the possibility that people may behave differently if they know they are being observed. However, the ultimate impact of his work on future conflicts through the writing and dissemination of his research reports may be more substantial.

In conclusion, I would like to report our impression that these intervener roles represent a valid contribution to the reduction of collective violence. Only future events and the study of more cases will determine whether this impression will stand up over time and be supported by firmer empirical evidence than is now available. In the meantime, however, the effectiveness of such intervention is dependent on two concepts which have been introduced into this paper without the extended discussion they deserve: "conflict management" and "conventionalization." Conflict management (9) is proposed as an alternative to the expression "conflict resolution" on the grounds that conflict over important social issues is seldom completely resolved. It can, nevertheless, be made manageable—that is, violence within the community can be averted—through the process of conventionalization, or, as the anthropologists would suggest, ritualization (10). Given the innate aggressiveness of human beings, it would seem that conflict management through ritualization of hostile encounters accompanied by problem-solving procedures offers the best hope of keeping levels of intergroup violence within acceptable limits of tolerance.

DISCUSSION

DR. FRANK OCHBERG (San Francisco, California): Are you evaluating the methodological issues that arise when the evaluator is interested in outcome measures pertaining to the avoidance of violence and helping both factions achieve their goals?

DR. JOHN P. SPIEGEL (Waltham, Massachusetts): We make it very clear that we are researchers studying the processes which can be invented to reduce violence. It's very complex to be an evaluator: one has to evaluate each side, and some of the sides have multiple parties. In addition, if the evaluator is not careful to state his own values and his own goals, he could seem to be an agent of one side, particularly of the government. The evaluator has to take the position that the situation is being studied in an overall and complex way.

DR. DAVID HAMBURG (Stanford, California): You touched on the fact that a number of these roles borrow something from the labor-management field. That is very interesting since this is one area of intergroup conflict in which there is a lengthy experience, both in the United States and Western Europe, moving from a rather high level of violence to a relatively low level of violence. There has not been much systematic research on how that conflict resolution was achieved. Do you think there are promising lines of inquiry for learning more from the labor-management field about handling community conflicts and other intergroup disputes?

DR. SPIEGEL: Yes. That is being intensively studied now, particularly by two groups, not for research purposes but to train interveners. The staff of these training centers are mostly lawyers from the management field who are trying to adapt their techniques to community situations. One group is the National Center for Dispute Settlement in Washington, and the other, the Institute for Mediation and Conflict Resolution, is in New York.

DR. MURRAY GLUSMAN (New York, New York): Yesterday, in the animal studies, note was made of the very close relationship of fight and flight or, in subjective terms, fear and anger. Yet this morning, in the discussion of violence, no special mention has been made of fear. I wonder to what extent fear goes hand-in-hand with anger and collective violence.

DR. SPIEGEL: Certainly the conciliator, insofar as he can reduce aroused levels of aggression, is operating simultaneously on the interaction between fear and anger. In that interaction, each increases the other. The more frightened a person becomes, the easier it is for him to defend himself against his fear by aggressing before he is attacked; and the more he is inclined to attack, the more frightened he becomes about the consequences of attack.

When the conciliator produces emotional distance, he reduces the possibility of direct aggression. "Step back five paces and you can't hit each other." He reduces the component of fear by interjecting reassurances into the situation. "We're doing our best to see a) that you are protected and b) that some of your demands can be met, or at least c) that the situation can be resolved."

DR. SALEEM SHAH (Rockville, Maryland): John's excellent discussion points up the fact that as one moves from the laboratory into the social situation, some concepts from political science and political sociology and some considerations of public policy become important. There is also the crucial question of the distribution of power. Who defines whether the deviance is crime or violence? Who has the power to make others agree with his definition? Who can define the violence as legitimate or illegitimate? Who has the power to enforce sanctions?

This relates to Dr. Hamburg's point. In a mediation or collective bargaining situation, isn't it essential that there be some equitable distribution of power? Without some balance of strength, there is no way to bargain. This has obvious implications for the necessity of providing more access to power. It could be done through mediation agencies for those who are typically rather powerless, like prison inmates.

DR. SPIEGEL: When I talked about the advocate, I was alluding to this matter of the distribution of power. The advocate enters the situation on the side of the aggrieved group, who define themselves and are usually seen by others as having lesser power than the authority. With less power, they have to use nonpolitical confrontation in order to get power and have their goals met. Conflict resolution has always depended on a better distribution of power. For example, the protesters in Miami Beach were eminently successful in meeting their immediate goals, even though by their self-definition, they failed because they did not make the slightest difference to the Republican Convention or alter Nixon's war policy. Nevertheless, through the operation of both the advocates and the mediators, they got Flamingo Park. They determined their own procedures and negotiated them with the police, which did not happen in Chicago.

DR. PAUL D. MACLEAN (Bethesda, Maryland): If I understood correctly, you said that the more highly organized the demonstration, the better the chances to avoid violence. It seems to me that one could substitute the word *ritual:* the more highly ritualized the demonstration, the better the chances to avoid violence. Animals seem to have learned this very well. Going back at least to the reptiles, any infractions of the rules leads to violent behavior.

Dr. Spiegel: The crucial factor is preventing surprise, and ritualization is one of the ways to do it. I would say to the protesters who questioned the need for research that written reports promote ritualization, which is now dependent upon word of mouth, a very unreliable mechanism.

Dr. Leo Alexander (Boston, Massachusetts): What differentiates the crowds at Miami from the crowds that stormed the Tuilleries?

Dr. Spiegel: Ritualization varies with time and culture. Without going back to the 18th century, one can say that the ritualization of confrontation between students and police in New York and Paris is quite different. The Paris police are quite prepared to use their lead-lined capes which can also decapitate. The students know this, and know when to run.

REFERENCES

1. Race-Related Civil Disorders, 1967–1969. Report No. 1, Lemberg Center for the Study of Violence, Brandeis University, Waltham, Mass., 1971.
    The Long, Hot Summer? Report No. 2, Lemberg Center for the Study of Violence, Brandeis University, Waltham, Mass., 1972.
2. Crisis and Change: Intervener Roles I, The Mediators. Volume 2, No. 1, and Intervener Roles II, The Community Advocates. Volume 2, No. 2. Community Crisis Intervention Project, Social Science Institute, Washington University, St. Louis, Mo., undated.
3. For general theories of conflict behavior, see:
    Bernard, J: The sociological study of conflict, in The Nature of Conflict: Studies on the Sociological Aspects of International Tension. Paris, International Sociological Association, 1957.
    Coser, LA: The Function of Social Conflict. New York, Free Press, 1964.
    Deutsch, M: Toward an understanding of conflict. Int J Group Tensions 1: 42, 1971.
    Boulding, KE: Conflict and Defense: A General Theory. New York, Harper Torchbacks, 1962.
    Markus, GB, Tanter, R: A conflict model for strategists and managers. Am Behav Scientist 15: 809, 1972.
4. Spiegel, JP: Theories of violence: an integrated approach. Int J Group Tensions 1: 77, 1971.
    Firestone, JM: Theory of the riot process. Am Behav Scientist 15: 859, 1972.
    Bowen, PR, Masotti, LH: Civil violence: a theoretical overview, in Riots and Rebellion: Civil Violence in the Urban Community, Beverly Hills, Sage, 1968.
5. For a more generalized view of the intervener role than that presented here, see:
    Fisher, RJ: Third party consultation: a method for the study and resolution of conflict. J Conflict Resolution 16: 67, 1972.
6. The problem of determining the actual versus the perceived amount of role differentiation in closely related tasks is not easy to solve. For a review of this literature, see:
    Lewis, GH: Role differentiation. Am Sociol Rev 37: 424, 1972.
7. Whether an intervener who is not neutral can legitimately be designated a "third party" is still an open question. However, most authors accept the inclusion. For a discussion of this point and of the issue of "neutrality," see:
    Young, OR: Intermediaries: Additional thoughts on third parties. J Conflict Resolution 16: 51, 1972.

8. Osnos, P: Guards air grievances; jail is calm. The Washington Post, Friday, October 13, 1972.

Claiborne, WL: Tragedy averted by talks. The Washington Post, Friday, October 13, 1972.

9. Fink, CF: Conflict management strategies implied by expected utility models of behavior. Am Behav Scientist 15: 837, 1972.

10. Nieberg, HL: Agonistics—rituals of conflict, in Collective Violence, edited by Short, JF, Wolfgang, ME. Chicago, Aldine Press, 1972.

Chapter 14

TELEVISED VIOLENCE: RECENT RESEARCH ON ITS EFFECTS

ALBERTA E. SIEGEL

Technological change alters the fabric of our social life. Often this social alteration is a side effect of the technological innovation, not its intended purpose. As an example, new modes of transportation—the automobile and the jet airplane—have enlarged our socially significant peer groups, enabled us to remove our homes considerable distances from our places of work, enabled our children to attend schools and colleges far distant from their homes and perhaps remote from their parents' alma maters, and so forth. Similarly impressive effects on our social life could be cited as stemming from changes in the technology of warfare, of healing, of food manufacture, of construction. The ways human beings relate to each other, in families, at work, in communities, are altered by technology.

My concern here is with yet another set of technological innovations: modern means of communication. At the same time that psychiatric theorists are concentrating on communication between people as a central issue in both normal and psychopathological development, electronic engineers have devised new technologies for communication. I believe that these have profound implications for our social system, including our socialization of the young.

The higher primates communicate primarily by visual signals: gestures, postures, expressions. The visual display is supplemented by auditory signals: grunts, calls, murmurs, smacks, howls. Usually these two forms of signaling are to convey emotional meanings, and usually they are redundant.

Man uses these same communication modalities. In the human infant, in fact, they constitute his total communicative repertoire. In older children and adults, visual and auditory signaling continue to be important, but speech is the central communication modality, the most sophisticated and the most differentiated. Washburn estimates that man has had speech for the last 40,000 years. It is during the years that man has had speech that most of the distinctively human social institutions have emerged.

Written language is much newer. Although early man may have communicated with his fellows by pictures, the earliest evidence of a written language meeting minimal linguistic criteria appears only about 5000 years ago, with the Sumerian lexigraphic systems.

Written communications were not mass communications until the development of printing. Forms of printing existed in China and Korea at least 2000 years ago, but the ideographic scripts of the Oriental languages did not lend themselves to mechanization. The same limitation did not constrain the European alphabet of the 15th century, with its 23 letters, so that when printing and moveable type were developed in the West 5 centuries ago, they found ready use.

With the advent of printing, nonverbal communication and speech and writing were supplemented by books, newspapers, journals and even comic books and penny dreadfuls. Our modern systems of education—with their textbooks, libraries, lectures, assigned reading—are based on a combination of face-to-face speech and printed communications, as is our system of scientific discourse, based on professional meetings plus printed journals.

In the last 100 years, a panoply of new communications media has been developed. We may expect them to alter our social arrangements just as profoundly as printing has done over the past 5 centuries. In fact, the alterations may be more fundamental, for these new media reach all humans, whereas the print media reached only those who were literate. Until very recently the literate have been only a small minority of the human population.

The phonograph was developed in the final quarter of the 19th century, and its commercial heyday was the initial decades of our own century. Commercial radio broadcasting followed in the 1920's. Here were mass media of communication which did not require the audience to be able to read. Small children as well as adults could be reached. And the technique spanned both time and space: a radio listener in Oregon could hear the President speak in Washington, a housewife in Nebraska could hear a gramophone record preserving Caruso's performance years earlier in a New York concert hall.

Motion pictures were developed during the same era. Film appealed to the eye whereas the phonograph and radio were beamed to the ear. Film technology was more complex, so that whereas radios and gramophones were home equipment, the movies were shown in nickelodeons during the 1st decade of our century and in vaudeville houses and cinema theaters thereafter. The audience paid for each sitting. No special training was required to enable a child to comprehend film material, and by the 1920's most American children spent most of their cash on movie tickets.

When sound was synchronized with visual image, it seemed that the pinnacle had been reached in the development of techniques to communicate with the illiterate. With the talkies, eye and ear received an integrated message. Al Jolson's *The Jazz Singer* was screened late in 1927, and by 1930 the silent movies were a thing of the past. Children and adults flocked to American movie theatres in the 1930's as do children and adults today in underdeveloped nations, where movies are still the most advanced medium of communication. When color was introduced (the first commercially successful color film, *Gone With The Wind*, appeared in 1939) it seemed that man had bridged both time and space with a totally effective communications technology, one attuned to the primate's keenest senses—vision and audition—and capable of transmitting gestural, spoken and written communication to these senses, with a musical soundtrack thrown in at no extra charge.

From the vantage point of 1972, we see this past as merely prologue. We recognize how movies were circumscribed by the walls of the movie theatre, their impact blunted by the barrier of the box office. We remain at home with today's medium of eye and ear; we pay no admission fee to watch *Hawaii Five-O* or *Mod Squad*. And the TV receiver brings us events the moment they occur. No longer must we wait until the film is processed, printed and transported to the movie house. As we watch the political conventions and football games live on TV, we wonder how we could have been so patient with those quaint newsreels and their week-old "news."

The first regular program of entertainment offered on TV was in London in 1936. Three years later, regularly scheduled telecasting was initiated by NBC in the United States. World War II interrupted the commercial development of this new device, but when wartime manufacturing restrictions were lifted the TV broadcasting industry grew very rapidly. By 1949, there were 1 million TV receivers in use in the United States. Two years later that figure had increased 10-fold. Well before 1960, there were 50 million receivers in use here, a number close to the saturation point. Today, over 60 million homes in the United States receive television, and more than one-third of U.S. families own more than one TV set. All but about 4 per cent of American homes have TV, more than have refrigerators or indoor plumbing. The Kerner Commission report called television "the universal appliance of the ghetto." In 1971, Americans shelled out $3.8 billion for new radios and TV sets. In the same year, advertisers spent $3.5 billion to support radio and television broadcasting.

The other media remain onstage in America, but frequently, like aging actors, their assigned role is that of the supporting player, enhancing the glamour of the new young star, television. Among magazines, for example, the one with the largest readership today is *TV Guide*. Here we see the 500-year-old art of printing being used to guide the literate in their attention to a nonprint medium. Newspapers remain an important medium, and the TV page is one of the best read of their features. A survey was conducted among 300 students at the University of Oregon shortly after Governor Wallace was shot. All had heard the news, but only 3 per cent had learned it from a newspaper. About 60 per cent had first learned of the event from radio or TV, whereas more than 33 per cent did so from another person. The aristocrats of the print media are books. Today, many books become best sellers when their authors are featured on TV talk shows. Movies continue to be important, of course, but when Hollywood produces a film today it is with an eye to the TV audience, for profits come from selling the Hollywood products to the TV stations for airing to the home viewer.

In the average American home, the TV set is turned on over 6 hours a day. No one person in the home is watching throughout that period, but most Americans watch TV at least 2 hours a day.

American children become TV watchers at a very early age, just about as soon as they can toddle over to the set and turn the knob. In interviews with mothers of preschool children in Los Angeles, Lyle and Hoffman (1) learned that the majority reported their children were singing TV jingles by age 2, and over 90 per cent had joined this youthful chorus by age 3. Of these mothers, many from poor and welfare families, 87 per cent reported that their preschool children asked for food items they had seen on TV, and 91 per cent said the preschoolers asked for toys seen on TV. The preschoolers themselves were interviewed individually. Although they could not express themselves very well, the 3-year-olds made it clear that they watch TV regularly on a daily basis. Viewing was particularly heavy during afternoons and on Saturday mornings, but the majority also indicated that they watched on weekday mornings and in the evenings. Many of the 3-year-olds could state what their favorite program was. Almost 9 out of 10 of them could identify Fred Flintstone from a photograph. Seven out of ten could identify Big Bird (from *Sesame Street*). Among the 4- and 5-year-olds, recognition of various TV characters was much higher.

It is not only Los Angeles toddlers who watch a lot of TV. Stein and Friedrich (2) studied 97 4- and 5-year-olds in a university community in central Pennsylvania. Detailed interviews with their mothers revealed that these preschoolers watched TV an average of 30 hours a week. This means they are in front of the set well over $\frac{1}{3}$ of their waking hours.

In Washington, D.C., Murray (3) observed in the homes of 27 black male children, ages 5 and 6. All were TV watchers. Viewing hours per week were highly variable, ranging from 5 to 42, but on average these young boys spent half of an adult's work week—21 hours—watching TV. About half of the programs they watched were adult shows: situation comedies and action dramas.

One might think that children would have fewer hours to watch TV at home after they begin attending school. The facts show the opposite. School-age youngsters watch more TV than do preschoolers. Lyle and Hoffman (4) studied TV-watching hours over the week among well over 1000 first graders, sixth graders and tenth graders. The weekly averages were: 23 hours, 31 hours and 28 hours. These results are similar to those of several other studies, showing a buildup of viewing time during the school years, then a drop in viewing time during adolescence.

Time does not permit my reviewing the extensive data on adult viewing. Suffice to say that teen-agers and college students are light watchers, viewing becomes heavier during young adult years when more time is spent at home and heavy viewing is characteristic of the middle-aged and even more characteristic of the elderly.

To the child psychologist, what is of interest is that the average American child spends more time watching TV than he spends in school, for TV engages his attention 7 days a week, 52 weeks a year, and TV recruits his attendance several years before he begins attending public school.

I am offering this capsule history of the mass media and this commentary on how the newest medium is especially attuned to the receptive sensibilities of the human young in order to dramatize my point that in attempting to evaluate the far-reaching effects of TV we are faced with the same difficulties that face those attempting to evaluate any technological revolution.

The worst mistake is to take the new technology at its face value. From the vantage point of 1972, what can we say about the effects of the automobile on human social organization? No exhaustive list of those effects could be offered, but surely they already exceed anything dreamed of by the social scientists of Mr. Ford's era, and we are far from seeing their end—only now is mass use of autos taking hold in the European nations, and the technological revolution has not even started in Asia except in Japan. Those who produce and market a new technology have in mind a particular purpose. In the case of the car, it was transportation. But to think about the car's effects only within the domain of transportation is simply to miss the boat.

With American television, there are two avowed purposes: entertainment and advertising. Social scientists cannot ignore these purposes, but it would be folly to limit our attention to them.

The nervous system of the immature primate is adapted for learning. This learning occurs not only through direct reinforcement of acts, but also, and I think more importantly, through observation. The child does not need to be rewarded for learning to occur; reward bears on the probability that he will perform what he has learned and maybe on the probability that he will attend to certain stimuli from which he might learn. Attention and observation are sufficient for new learning to be stored by the child. Practice and imitation perfect his acquisitions from observation.

To my mind, the most brilliant research on television's effects on young children is that pioneered by my colleague at Stanford, Professor Albert Bandura, in the early 1960's. He demonstrated that preschool-age children imitate the aggressive behavior they observe on film and TV. In his experiments, he devised several TV sequences in which adults performed novel aggressive acts. Young children who observed these sequences subsequently performed the same aggressive behaviors. Bandura's findings have now been replicated by many psychologists, and their limits are currently being explored. When the *Report* to the Surgeon General was being prepared by his Scientific Advisory Committee on Television and Social Behavior, we were able to list about 20 references to scientific papers on children's imitation of TV aggression (5). The fact that the television industry appreciates the implications of these findings is reflected in their successful efforts to blackball Professor Bandura for membership on the Advisory Committee.

Although the media men would have us think that their electronic wonder is simply a method of entertaining the public and selling soap to them, as behavioral scientists we ought to be thinking of television as a teacher, a source of information, a form of cultural transmission, an agency for socializing the young, a technique of displaying behavior that children will observe and imitate.

The learning need not be antisocial. Stein and Friedrich (2) conducted a careful study in which children in a nursery school had one of three possible TV "diets" in school: aggressive, neutral or prosocial. The prosocial series were episodes from *MisteRogers' Neighborhood,* with themes of cooperation, sharing, sympathy, affection and friendship, understanding the feeling of others, verbalizing one's own feelings, delay of gratification, persistence and competence at tasks, learning to accept rules, control of aggression, adaptive coping with frustration. The children's behavior in play in the nursery school was observed before, during and after their 4-week exposure to these three diets. Among lower socioeconomic children, those who had the prosocial diet on TV increased markedly in prosocial interpersonal behavior in the nursery school: there were no changes in such behavior for lower socioeconomic children having other TV diets. This finding awaits replication, but it is in accord with certain laboratory experiments on the modeling of prosocial behavior in suggesting that young children can learn prosocial as well as aggressive behavior from watching TV.

What do American children watch on TV? This has been widely studied, and the findings are fairly consistent.

Only the very youngest children spend the preponderance of their viewing time with so-called "children's" shows. (These have the derogatory label of "kid vid" in industry circles.) Four-year-olds have well established program preferences. Cartoons are their favorites, *e.g., The Flintstones.* Situation comedies also rank high: *The Courtship of Eddie's Father, Here's Lucy, Bewitched.* In some communities, *Sesame Street* and *Miste-Rogers' Neighborhood* attract some of the very young viewers; in others, these noncommercial shows are not available or not widely watched. Middle-class children are among the most loyal viewers of the public television shows designed for the disadvantaged.

By the time they are in first grade, children have family situation comedies as their favorites. More adult shows and fewer children's shows appear on their lists of TV programs regularly watched.

When a child reaches sixth grade, cartoon shows and "kiddie" shows no longer attract him at all. He watches family situation comedies, other situation comedies, and "hip adventure" shows like *Mod Squad, It Takes A Thief* and *Star Trek.*

The preferences of tenth graders are dominated by adventure programs—those already mentioned, *Dark Shadows, Highway Patrol,* and so forth. Music and dramatic shows also rank high.

Adolescents and adults are more favorably disposed to very violent shows than are school-age children. Men watch more violence than women. Blacks watch more violence than do whites. The poor and less educated watch more violence than do white collar workers and the college educated. Violence viewing is especially high among adult males who were high school dropouts.

Young children see a great deal of violence on commercial TV not because they seek it out or prefer it, but rather because commercial programming is so saturated with violence and children watch so much television. Also significant is the cartoon-maker's regular recourse to aggression as a method of conflict-resolution, inasmuch as cartoons are favored by young children.

As a child psychologist with a special interest in the social psychology of childhood, I am impressed by two facts about television. The first is that it is a superb technique for communicating with children. It reaches the home, the child's ecological niche. It brings vivid visual and auditory images to children, requiring no ability to read or write. That is, it speaks their language. Young children learn primarily by observation and imitation. TV presents them with behavior to observe and imitate, in a form which they can assimilate. The second fact which impresses me is that there is simply no social institution to govern television as a socializing agency for America's next generation: no board of TV education, no professional school to train the television socializers and child care workers, no textbook commission to screen, evaluate and upgrade the contents of the TV curriculum.

The work of the Surgeon General's Scientific Advisory Committee on Television and Social Behavior was initiated because of concern among some U.S. Senators about TV violence and its possible social consequences. The Committee was organized by U.S. Surgeon General William H. Stewart in 1969. Funds and organizational support were made available through the National Institute of Mental Health (NIMH), under the experienced and very capable leadership of its Assistant Director for Behavioral Sciences, Eli Rubinstein. Twenty-three research projects were supported by NIMH contracts after the proposals had received approval under review procedures modeled on the peer review system which has been so effective in assuring quality control of extramural research. These investigations, in various parts of the nation, concentrated on the violent and aggressive content of entertainment materials presented on commercial TV; this is the material which has been the focus of public and Congressional concern. Although adults were studied in some of the investigation, children were the subjects in most. The research is reported in five volumes of articles spanning almost 2500 pages. In these volumes, the authors of the research speak in their own words. The Advisory Committee's words appear in a separate volume, offering a cautious interpretation of the new studies as well as some consideration of earlier research on the topic (5). These materials appeared in print early in 1972, and at that time they were the subject of 4 days of hearings by the Senate Subcommittee on Communications under the Chairmanship of John O. Pastore (6). A capsule summary of the research findings was published simultaneously in a scholarly journal (7) by NIMH staff members who had earlier published a very useful annotated bibliography on the entire previous research literature (8). We are now seeing scholarly reviews of the whole effort (9) and a book is in press which will offer an independent assessment of the research sponsored by the Program (10).

Over the years since the advent of TV, many investigators have analyzed the content of TV drama, repeatedly demonstrating the preponderance of violent themes on American mass entertainment. George Gerbner is among the most original, thoughtful and persuasive of these investigators. He has surveyed the contents of TV dramatic shows on prime time in 1967, 1968 and 1969, making detailed content analyses of 281 programs appearing over 182 hours in these 3 years (11). His materials reveal that about 8 out of every 10 TV programs contain violence. Incidents of violence occur at the rate of about 8 per hour during prime time. Saturday morning cartoons have the heaviest saturation of violence on all television, with one violent episode every 2 minutes. The incidence of violence in cartoons beamed to child viewers increased from three times the level in programming for adults in 1967 to six times that level in 1969.

The world of TV drama is a mythical world with its own social rules, norms and mores. It is peopled by persons who may look and talk like our neighbors and friends, so that children and foreign viewers may confuse them with America's citizens, but their lives follow a script which in some ways mirrors American social realities and in some ways diverges radically from those realities. In TV drama, law enforcement agents are involved in only one-tenth of all violent episodes. In those episodes in which they are involved, law enforcement agents are themselves violent more often than not. Weapons, most commonly guns, are used in about one-half of all violent episodes on TV. TV violence is eerily vacuous. In one-half of all of the violent episodes chronicled by Gerbner's painstaking observers, no painful effect of any kind was discernible, whereas in the other one-half it was often difficult for the observers to agree whether any pain at all had been shown, or indeed any consequence. In only one-third of the violent episodes does the viewer see either death or injury as a result. The long term disabling effects of violence, so familiar to the physician and the nurse, are almost never evident to the observer of TV drama. Nor does he see the emotional and social effects of violence. He is spared any exposure to the bereaved: the children who are left fatherless, the widow left to mourn her husband's loss and to attempt creating a life for herself and his family without him. This "sanitizing" of violence is but one way in which TV drama differs from life as we know it. There are other ways. In TV dramas, the leading character is typically male, American, middle or upper class, unmarried and in the prime of life. Of all the TV dramatic characters we see on prime time, only one-half are gainfully employed, and their work is usually not central to the dramatic portrayal. Those who do have visible means of support are typically in high status jobs. Gerbner suggests that his fascinating ethnography of the TV culture, in some ways so similar to American culture and in some ways so different, is to be understood as a description of a mythology which functions to convey values and norms about power and influence to the TV viewers who fall under its spell.

Gerbner's social anthropological view of the societal implications of the contents of TV entertainment is not congenial to many psychiatrists. Instead, psychiatrists have commonly spoken of TV watching as an essentially harmless opportunity for emotional catharsis of unacceptable impulses, including aggressive and sexual impulses. Freud followed Aristotle in his view that vicarious participation in dramatic themes allows an emotional purging in the audience. Most psychiatrists follow Freud and Aristotle, and whereas one must admire their fastidious good taste in selecting such intellectual leadership, one must also note that neither of these men based his work on observing children and that both were discussing serious drama presented by living actors and were not in a position to comment on entertainment in the modern commercial electronic media.

Investigators of TV's effects have found it difficult to get a handle on the catharsis notion in its psychoanalytic form. When it is formulated in behavioral terms, it becomes amenable to experimental test. The results of the many experiments on catharsis in the past 2 decades are not terribly clear-cut and are hardly satisfying to the research purist. But at least one can say that the evidence does not favor the emotional catharsis theory. Where it has been possible to isolate emotional effects of viewing violence on film or TV, usually it is an increase in aggressiveness which has been found. The catharsis notion would predict a decrease. In our 1972 report, the Surgeon General's Advisory Committee reported that the weight of the evidence is against the catharsis notion (p. 65 to 67). I have commented elsewhere (12) on the one major investigation which has yielded findings dissonant with the dominant trend.

Many psychiatrists have not stayed in close touch with the relevant research, and their thinking has been relatively uninfluenced by the results that emerged in the late 1950's and the 1960's. Unfortunately, the television industry's leadership has exploited statements by psychiatrists expressing the catharsis notion, inasmuch as these statements seem to provide expert opinion in support of the industry's position that TV violence has no appreciable antisocial consequences. A notable and admirable exception to the general trend of psychiatric opinion has been the views of Dr. Frederic Wertham (13). The respect which the public extends to psychiatric opinion and the concern which parents and other citizens feel about TV violence is reflected in the wide and sympathetic hearing which Dr. Wertham has gained for his incisive statements.

In their preoccupation with the significance of early experience in the family in shaping the level and the expression of a person's aggressiveness, many psychiatrists have seemed to imply that other influences are negligible. As a child psychologist, I quite agree that the family's influence is central, but I disagree that we can afford to minimize or dismiss the effects of other influences in a child's life, especially those that reach into the family home and intrude on family life (14, 15). I have been delighted to see efforts toward increased communication between psychiatrists and behavioral scientists, and I am hopeful that the public pronouncements of members of the psychiatric profession will increasingly reflect knowledge of contemporary research findings as well as personal clinical observations and psychodynamic theory.

Among the seven distinguished social scientists who were blackballed by the TV industry from membership on the Surgeon General's Committee, only one was a psychiatrist, Dr. Leon Eisenberg, Professor at Harvard and editor of the leading journal of child psychiatry. It is hardly an accident that the blackball was reserved for a specialist in child behavior, a scholar who is notable in his profession for his cordial familiarity with social scientific research and his ability to synthesize and integrate clinical and research findings, for his thoughtful dissent from tired psychoanalytic cliches and for his personal qualities of leadership, articulateness and social vision. It is especially to be regretted that the Committee was denied the benefit of his participation.

In brief, then, the new research confirmed that children and adults watch a lot of TV, that TV entertainment is dominated by themes of violence, that young children can and do imitate the aggression they observe on TV and that there is no convincing evidence of any cathartic or purging effect of TV viewing. What else did we learn?

Both short term experimental studies and long term correlational field studies yielded evidence that watching TV violence instigates or arouses aggressive emotions and behavior. This finding holds for preschoolers, school-age children and teen-agers.

There is one longitudinal study of TV viewing, conducted in upstate New York (16). Among boys, those who preferred aggressive TV material when studied in the third grade were rated higher in aggressiveness by their peers 10 years later. This correlation holds up after the obvious statistical correctives are applied.

We found that both children and their parents think of TV as providing information on how to behave, how to speak, how to dress, what to eat, and so forth. As a social institution, commercial television provides a definition of what's new, what's important and who's who. Because the contents of TV are widely thought of as defining "what's happening," the violent content of TV is a special cause for concern.

Research on the effects of movies on children has been conducted since the late 1920's, and TV research got underway in the 1950's. Why have results been so slow in coming, and why must our statements be so cautious even though we base them on literally hundreds of investigations? In the first place, we have no animal model for media use. Only human beings serve as our subjects. This limits the interventions we may envisage. Second, aggressive tendencies and proclivities are not easy to measure. Aggression, like homosexuality or drug use, is a taboo behavior, and the difficulties in studying taboo behaviors accurately are well known. Many of our studies rely on self-report or parental report, and there is convincing research evidence that both forms of reports are frequently distorted. Third, the research designs of social psychology are best suited to the study of explosive events. In the before and after experiment, conducted over a short period of time, we can study dramatic single events which have a strong impact. But TV violence may have effects more like corrosion than explosion. The effects may be subtle and continuous, chronic rather than acute, insidious rather than blatantly overt. I suspect they are. If so, short term experiments will not reveal the full measure of the effects.

We are left with evidence which gives some cause for concern, plus common sense which tells us that any activity occupying so many hours in a person's life must have lasting significance for him. Both the evidence and common sense converge to suggest that TV's continuous preoccupation with stereotyped violent conflict and its resolution through violence can hardly be constructive and healthful for the child viewer.

REFERENCES

1. LYLE, J, HOFFMAN, HR: Explorations in patterns of television viewing by preschool-age children, in Television and Social Behavior, Reports and Papers, Vol. IV. Television in Day-to-Day Life: Patterns of Use, edited by Rubinstein, EA, Comstock, GA, Murray, JP. Washington, D.C., U.S. Government Printing Office, 1972, p. 257.
2. STEIN, AH, FRIEDRICH, LK: Television content and young children's behavior, in Television and Social Behavior, Reports and Papers, Vol. II. Television and Social Learning, edited by Murray, JP, Rubinstein, EA, Comstock, GA. Washington, D.C., U.S. Government Printing Office, 1972, p. 202.
3. MURRAY, JP: Television in inner-city homes: Viewing behavior of young boys, in Television and Social Behavior, Reports and Papers, Vol. IV. Television in Day-to-Day Life: Patterns of Use, edited by Rubinstein, EA, Comstock, GA, Murray, JP. Washington, D.C., U.S. Government Printing Office, 1972, p. 345.
4. LYLE, J, HOFFMAN, HR: Children's use of television and other media, in Television and Social Behavior, Reports and Papers, Vol. IV. Television in Day-to-Day Life: Patterns of Use, edited by Rubinstein, EA, Comstock, GA, Murray, JP. Washington, D.C., U.S. Government Printing Office, 1972, p. 129.
5. Surgeon General's Scientific Advisory Committee on Television and Social Behavior: Television and Growing Up: The Impact of Televised Violence. Washington, D.C., U.S. Government Printing Office, 1972, p. 159.
6. Committee on Commerce, Subcommittee on Communications, United States Senate, Ninety-Second Congress, Second Session. Hearings on the Surgeon General's Report by the Scientific Advisory Committee on Television and Social Behavior. March 21–24, 1972. Serial Number 92-52. Washington, D.C., U.S. Government Printing Office.
7. ATKIN, CK, MURRAY, JP, NAYMAN, OB: The Surgeon General's research program on television and social behavior. J Broadcasting 16: 21, 1972.
8. ATKIN, CK, MURRAY, JP, NAYMAN, OB: Television and Social Behavior: An Annotated Bibliography of Research Focusing on Television's Impact on Children. Public Health Service Publication No. 2099. Bethesda, Md., National Institute of Mental Health, 1971.

9. Bogart, L: Warning: The Surgeon General has determined that TV violence is moderately dangerous to your child's mental health. Pub Opinion Q 36: 491, 1972–73.

10. Liebert, RM, Neale, JM, Davidson, ES: The Early Window: Effects of Television on Children and Youth. New York, Pergamon Press, 1973.

11. Gerbner, G: Violence in television drama: Trends and symbolic functions, in Television and Social Behavior, Reports and Papers, Vol. I. Media Content and Control, edited by Comstock, GA, Rubinstein, EA. Washington, D.C., U.S. Government Printing Office, 1972, p. 28.

12. Siegel, AE: Can we await a consensus? A review of S. Feshbach and R. D. Singer's Television and Aggression, Jossey-Bass, 1971. Contemp Psychol 18: 60, 1973.

13. Wertham, F: A Sign for Cain: An Exploration of Human Violence. New York, Macmillan, 1966.

14. Siegel, AE: Statement before the Senate Subcommittee on Communications of the Committee on Commerce of the United States Senate, Ninety-Second Congress, Second Session, March 21, 1972. Hearings. Washington, D.C., U.S. Government Printing Office, Serial No. 92-52, p. 62.

15. Siegel, AE: Educating females and males to be alive and well in century twenty-one, in Changing Education: Alternatives from Educational Research, edited by Wittrock, M. Englewood Cliffs, N.J., Prentice-Hall, 1973.

16. Lefkowitz, MM, Eron, LD, Walder, LO, Huesmann, LR: Television violence and child aggression: A follow-up study, in Television and Social Behavior, Reports and Papers, Vol. III. Television and Adolescent Aggressiveness, edited by Comstock, GA, Rubinstein, EA. Washington, D.C., U.S. Government Printing Office, 1972, p. 35.

DISCUSSION

Dr. David Hamburg (Stanford, California): Dr. Siegel highlights the enormity of the social change brought about by the widespread availability of TV. As to whether children's behavior is really affected, her reference to the Lyle and Hoffman study, that the food preferences of about nine-tenths of the Los Angeles preschoolers were affected by TV advertising, makes one wonder whether there are other impacts as well. It seems to me that the Report of the Surgeon General's Advisory Committee gives a very cautious interpretation of the data. I feel that Dr. Siegel's somewhat stronger interpretation is well justified.

It is important to remember that the recent empirical studies which show some effect on children's behavior have dealt largely with short term exposure, whereas in real life we are concerned with massive, long term exposure during the highly formative years of growth and development. It seems to me that the modest effect demonstrated from brief exposure raises very serious questions about the long term impact.

I wonder if there is a way to maintain an objective scrutiny of the level of violence presented, with adequate feedback to the public and the regulatory bodies. Such a scrutiny might also cover other questions, for instance, the way in which certain racial and ethnic groups are portrayed, or other issues pertinent to hostility and violence in our society.

I would also like Dr. Siegel's comment about the prosocial aspects. If TV can be a school for violence, it can also presumably be a school for skills and problem-solving attitudes. The follow-up study on *Sesame Street* by the Educational Testing Service shows not only considerable acquisition of cognitive skills but also some modest evidence of changing intergroup attitudes in the direction of less hostility.

DR. ALBERTA SIEGEL (Stanford, California): I will start with the question of what ought to be done in response to the Report to the Surgeon General. In the last few years, three major bodies, the Eisenhower Commission, the Kerner Commission and now the Surgeon General's Committee, have all called attention to TV violence, echoing what social scientists were saying years before. They have all, I think, issued the same recommendation: that there should be some kind of standing organization to monitor television and provide violence ratings as feedback to the television industry. Several of us recommended this to Senator Pastore's Committee. The ratings would be a kind of continuation of the work that Gerbner has done at the University of Pennsylvania, coding the themes and the emphases of TV dramatic content. I think that such a body should be independent of the government in order to speak effectively.

With regard to prosocial teaching, as *Sesame Street*, which was aimed at teaching cognitive skills to disadvantaged children, there have been several assessments showing that although it is especially successful with the middle class children of normal and high intelligence who watch it the most, there has also been good effect for those disadvantaged children who see it. We need more evaluation of shows like MisteRogers Neighborhood which are aimed at teaching not so much cognitive abilities as social and interpersonal skills.

DR. JOHN P. SPIEGEL (Boston, Massachusetts): Some years ago my colleagues and I were doing a study of family interactions in Irish, Italian, Puerto Rican and Greek working class families. We did our observations in the home and were interested in the relation of the interaction in the home to the mental health of the children. As an incidental observation, we found that when an aggressive interaction was about to take place, someone would usually turn up the television set. It did not seem to matter very much what the program was, although an aggressive program most particularly helped avert what might have erupted into a real quarrel. I am wondering if it would not be important to conduct, at least as a supplement to well controlled experimental procedures, a certain amount of naturalistic observation in the home to see how TV programs actually affect family life.

DR. SIEGEL: As you know, invading the privacy of the home is not easy. Bechtel has done some pioneering work which shows that self-report about television watching is sometimes wildly erroneous, and that older individuals, that is, 7 years and up, often divide their attention, watching television while eating or engaging in conversation. There is no reason why the kind of observation you mention couldn't be done.

DR. SEYMOUR S. KETY (Boston, Massachusetts): It is interesting that attention has been focused on neurophysiological technology and psychosurgery as threats to the manipulation of human behavior rather than on the press or television. I wonder whether there is any sociological explanation for this choice.

DR. SIEGEL: The people who were here yesterday to protest psychosurgery would be extremely cynical about television as an institution but would not have a comparable attitude toward the medical profession. The communications industry does not pretend to be working for the welfare of other people, whereas the medical profession does aspire to do just that. Therefore, it is especially vulnerable to criticism by idealistic people. Those people have already written off commercial television.

DR. PAUL D. MACLEAN (Bethesda, Maryland): I would like to focus on what Dr. Geen and Dr. Spiegel said about imitation. Because of the mass media, the matter of imitation looms more important than ever in human affairs, not only as it applies to fads, fashions and drug cultures, but more significantly to mass hysteria and violence. There is now abundant evidence from the animal studies of John B. Calhoun, Kenneth Meyers and others that the conditions of crowding lead to increased aggressive behavior in animals. In addition to bringing out the aggressiveness, the conditions of crowding also increase the opportunities for imitation. I think it is therefore possible that violent behavior, when seen on television, can lead to a kind of vicious circle through the positive feedback of imitation. It is a perversity, of course, that television brings violence, crowding and imitation right into the living room.

It is curious that we know almost nothing about the neural mechanism underlying imitation. Some of our recent work on squirrel monkeys would suggest that the striatal complex, or what I would call the major mammalian counterpart of the reptilian forebrain, is basic for species, typical forms of behavior and the associated imitation factors.

DR. DOMINICK PURPURA (Bronx, New York): We are concerned about the young child watching 30 hours a week of cartoons and other shows loaded with aggression and violence, but if we get the kids away from the television sets, what are they going to do with the 30 hours? Couldn't there be social programs which would allow more effective utilization of that enormous amount of a child's waking hours?

DR. SIEGEL: I do not see TV as necessarily a vicious institution. At the Pastore hearings, FCC Comissioner Johnson referred to television people as "child molesters." I would think "child neglecters" is the more appropriate term. The industry simply has no concern for children, and the effects on children are side effects of its functioning.

We have developed nothing for television comparable to the elaborate social organization which governs public education—the professional schools to train teachers, the state certification, the local school boards, the committees which review texts, and so forth. Yet I suspect that television now is a prepotent educational medium.

MR. HENRY GREEN (Washington, D.C.): Have there been any studies to determine the extent to which television has had an impact on people who have engaged in violent acts or criminal behavior?

DR. SIEGEL: There have been several case studies which do suggest some connection but are not completely convincing. For example, in upstate New York a group of young people 1 year out of high school were rated by their peers as to how aggressive they were. The more aggressive were heavy violence watchers in the third grade. But what makes the research a problem is that, in general, highly aggressive males are heavier violence watchers.

Dr. Susman (Washington, D.C.): What can be done about the lure and the problem of the pleasure element in aggression and violence?

Dr. Siegel: I don't know that anything can be done about it. It has to be noted. Cartoons are the most violent shows for young children and also the most popular with young children. I suppose the whole task of teaching is to make prosocial behavior at least as attractive as antisocial behavior.

Eleanor Rieger (Producer of Tomorrow Entertainment, New York, New York): As a TV producer attempting to improve children's programs, I'm faced with the demonstrated preference for action, violent or otherwise. Could child psychologists contribute their knowledge of what interests children so that improved programs which will attract the audience could be made?

Dr. Siegel: I suggested to the Pastore Committee that some foundation should fund travel fellowships for TV producers so that they could travel to see the excellent prosocial programming for children that is done in other countries.

Dr. Fred Plum (New York, New York): The Swedes are clearly less violent than we are. The only movies which are censored in Sweden are those which deal with aggressive violence. Only those who are over 18 may see such movies. This means that they can never appear on television.

Chapter 15

CROSS-CULTURAL ASPECTS OF DELINQUENT AND CRIMINAL BEHAVIOR[1]

FRANCO FERRACUTI AND SIMON DINITZ

The need for interdisciplinary research (and for fusion and cross-communication) in the study of deviant and criminal behavior is an article of faith for most professionals in the field. Unfortunately, the call for a multidisciplinary perspective usually remains only a statement of principle and an exercise in wishful thinking. For this reason, any research effort which promotes interaction between disciplines is, regardless of specific results, an important achievement. It is all too obvious that future progress in our field depends primarily on teamwork and communality of concepts.

In this context, we intend to discuss some general points related to cross-cultural or comparative work in delinquency and then to relate some recent findings from an interdisciplinary study on delinquents and controls from the metropolitan area of San Juan, Puerto Rico. This paper will not deal directly with violence, even though a large group of our delinquents were violent, but may serve the purpose of illustrating some selected general methodological problems, which have a bearing also on the study of violent criminal behavior.

It is self-evident to all professionals in the field of criminology that the major obstacles to the development of comparative research consist of: a) a lack of available reliable data, b) national legal differences, c) differences in methodology and in methodological emphasis and d) cultural variations in the identification and handling of offenders.

Similar difficulties, of course, exist in any kind of comparative work. For example, cultural differences in the definition and handling of schizophrenia still delay the development of valid cross-cultural concepts of psychosis, and the World Health Organization is slowly and painfully struggling with the task of developing a valid international classification of mental diseases.

The situation is even more complicated in the field of crime and de-

---

[1] Data presented in this paper are abstracted from a book in press: F. Ferracuti, S. Dinitz, E. Acosta de Brenes, *Puerto Rican Juvenile Offenders,* prepared under the joint sponsorship of the University of Puerto Rico, Social Science Research Center and United Nations Social Defense Research Institute.

287

linquency. Normative differences which derive from variations in legal definitions of offenses and offenders are so great that, in the case of homicide, murder in the first and second degrees and manslaughter, for example, no exact counterparts are found in non-Anglo-saxon criminal codes.

These cultural variations, on the other hand, also modify the perceptions by the public, no less than by the professionals involved, of the functioning of the criminal justice system. The perception of violence is a very different thing, indeed, in a country where civil protest and revolution are endemic, or under war conditions or where a subculture of violence prevails, than in a peaceful, traditional Swiss or midwestern village. A Pennsylvania Dutch rural adolescent will give a very different definition of violence-eliciting behavior from that offered, verbally or behaviorally, by a culturally deprived black youngster in an urban ghetto in a major U.S. city.

Yet, because of these obstacles, the need for comparative work is such that an effort must be made to overcome the existing difficulties inhibiting comparative research.

Criminal behavior, as a sociopsychological phenomenon with occasional biological determinants or facilitating factors is, in essence, defined by legal and social norms. We consider criminal a behavior which is either a) so defined by the law, b) so defined by the prevailing social norm or c) frequently, but not always, both. Since legal and sociocultural elements are fundamental to the definition of crime and delinquency, cross-cultural, comparative research is essential to our understanding to the etiology of the phenomenon of crime.

Existing etiological theories, particularly when single discipline oriented, have conspicuously failed to achieve a level of "proof" that we can consider satisfactory for explanation, prediction and, more dramatically, for prevention and control. As in other behavioral fields, the question of "why," implied in explanatory and etiological studies, does not overlap exactly with the question of "how," implied in prediction, prevention and control. Also, a basic fallacy led early criminologists to study crime as if they were dealing with a physical phenomenon and not with a legally or socially defined behavior which cannot be framed into our existing biological science-oriented nosographies. There is no valid reason why crime and delinquency should follow the distribution, the etiological aspects and the normal-abnormal dichotomies of, say, mental deficiency or epilepsy.

Cross-cultural research cannot but facilitate a sharing of concepts, data and experiences which will allow theory testing and validation of tactics, results and programs. Just to cite one example, the assessment of the incidence of crime and delinquency in countries at different points of the developed-underdeveloped continuum will permit the testing of theories which relate crime to socioeconomic development and to urbanization and industrialization.

Confrontations between Western and Soviet data (when and where available) will in the light of the convergence theory make it possible to assess factors, such as level of expectations and anomie, in a context where such concepts are sharply defined and reasonably different.

Replication in different legal settings and in contrasted cultural milieux will allow us to focus on these factors which constitute the essential, hard-core set of cross-culturally valid crime related variables.

It is, therefore, in this direction that our efforts should be directed. An interdisciplinary comparative criminology is a major priority in our research efforts.

In this context, we will present some interesting findings from our recently completed Puerto Rican study. The milieu under study was the San Juan metropolitan area, a large, rapidly increasing Latin (and yet North American in laws and partially in culture) megalopolis which has a serious crime and delinquency problem. Yet, even though criminality, especially by juveniles, is a major concern in San Juan, many of the characteristics associated with juvenile delinquency in U.S. mainland cities are absent. To cite the two most evident differences, gangs as a way of life and gang warfare are almost totally unknown in San Juan, and the color problem has not poisoned the atmosphere in the San Juan slums. The population of the slum areas is composed, of course, of multiproblem families, but color-determined isolation is not a factor for entering, or remaining, in the slum culture. Economic and mobility factors prevail in assigning a subject or a family into a caserio (low income public housing quarter) or arrabal (natural slum area, Latin style), the Puerto Rican equivalents of the inner city ghetto. Consequently, our delinquency data are "color-free" and may provide an interesting element of comparison with similar studies in the "non-color-free" mainland high delinquency areas.

THE RESEARCH DESIGN

As in many projects which originate out of a variety of inputs and expectations, several design and methodological decisions were made which did not necessarily optimize the feasibility of this investigation. Inasmuch as so little was known of Puerto Rican delinquency, for example, the research strategy employed was to use a multifactor approach in designing the study and collecting data.

Within the range of possibilities which existed for a multifactor approach, we decided to start with the work of Sheldon and Eleanor Glueck (1950). Their work provided an eclectic research model which, in its scope, remains unparalleled in delinquency research. Consequently, the decision was made that all data (or as many as possible of the data) collected by the Gluecks in the original Boston study would be included in the Puerto Rican study, with those modifications and additions made necessary by one of the following rationale:

1. Revision of a technique, subsequent to the Glueck study, which provided a more reliable, less expensive and more meaningful assessment.

2. Nonfeasibility, in practical terms, of obtaining reliable data (*e.g.*, somatotyping was out in Puerto Rico because juvenile law specifically forbids the photographing of delinquents for any purpose).

3. Specific differences which warranted the inclusion of data not collected in the original Boston study or in similar research efforts (*e.g.*, the high rate of addicts in the Puerto Rico population warranted the inclusion of more data on addiction than the original Glueck study which was conducted when the use and abuse of drugs was not yet a problem of epidemic proportions).

The research design was therefore limited to an operational plan for data gathering on matched pairs of delinquents and nondelinquents. Our design included careful checking of the delinquency and nondelinquency status of the matched subjects. This made our nondelinquents as free as possible from hidden delinquency involvement.

The following general objectives were accepted as basic in our study: a) to assess the medical, neurological, psychiatric, psychological and social patterns prevailing in Puerto Rican juvenile delinquents as compared to nondelinquents; b) to establish the relationship, if any, between these factors and antisocial behavior and c) to draw from the analysis indications for control and treatment policies to be based simultaneously on general theoretical knowledge about juvenile delinquency in other cultures and on specific data on Puerto Rican delinquency.

The total group of subjects included in the study was composed of 202 males varying in age between 11 and 17 years, all resident in one of the several slum areas in the city of San Juan. Of the 101 pairs, 20 percent were living in arrabales and the remainder in caserios. The subjects were divided into two groups. Each subject in the delinquent group was carefully matched with a nondelinquent subject. The delinquent group was composed of 101 juveniles with a case pending in the juvenile court in San Juan. They were selected from all cases on the court list, year by year, between 1966 and 1969. Each year a certain number of cases were selected, following the procedure of choosing every 25th name from the court listing until the predetermined number of cases for that year had been reached. If for any reason the 25th, 50th, etc, subject was not available, the preceding or following name was chosen.

The control group was composed of a number of juveniles equal to that of the experimental group. Each member of the control group was individually matched with a member of the experimental group on the following variables: sex (all males), area of residence, socioeconomic level, family income and age (with a 6-month tolerance margin in both direction). Each member of the control group had no known criminal history. This was checked not only in the court records, but also in the police records for "police contacts" which might have occurred without leading to court proceedings. If any evidence of criminal behavior appeared subsequently while taking the social history of the case, the subject was dropped and replaced with another one. The controls were located by the social workers attached to the project from the universe of juveniles attending public schools in the areas where the experimental group subjects were residing. Whenever possible, they were attending the same class as the delinquent match. In many cases the delinquents were not attending school, and in these instances the control group subjects were selected from the classes that the delinquents would have been attending had they not dropped out. Automatically, this meant that no control group subject was a dropout. The population characteristics are presented in Table 15.1.

For each subject the following data were collected: a) social history, in-

TABLE 15.1

Population characteristics: subjects selected from San Juan, Puerto Rico metropolitan area

Item	Delinquent Group	Nondelinquent Group
No. of subjects...	101	101
Sex.............	Male	Male
Age range		
11–14 years....	43%	43%
15–17 years....	57%	57%
Selected from....	1966–1969 Court list	Same neighborhood schools as delinquents
Type of residence		
Arrabales......	20%	20%
Caserios.......	80%	80%
Average height..	61.7 in.	62.8 in.
Average weight..	105.4 lb.	111.1 lb.
Skin color		
Light..........	49%	55%
Medium.......	25%	29%
Dark..........	27%	25%

cluding educational history and criminal history (for the experimental group); b) psychiatric examination; c) psychological test battery; d) physical examination, including laboratory tests; e) neurological examination and f) electroencephalogram.

The 42-page social history was taken from the subject himself, his available relatives and his neighbors; it was checked against available records from the school, courts, police and public welfare. Taking the social history involved a minimum of two to a maximum of eight visits by the social worker to the family.

The psychiatric examination was conducted in an interview which lasted approximately 1 hour. The interview was conducted in the psychiatrist's office and, as was the case in all other examinations, the subject was accompanied to the office of the examiner by the social worker. The psychiatrist was aware of the delinquent/nondelinquent status of the juvenile. The results of the interview were summarized in a psychiatric descriptive report and a final diagnosis was formulated following the American Psychiatric Association (APA) *Diagnostic and Statistical Manual of Mental Disorders,* 1968 edition.

The psychological examination consisted of the administration of a battery of tests over a period of two sessions. The battery included the following:

1. Wechsler-Bellevue Intelligence Scale for Children (WISC) or Wechsler Adult Intelligence Scale (WAIS), depending on the age of the subject (the cut-off point for using the WAIS was as usual 15 years of age and above). The Puerto Rican standardization of the WAIS was used; in the case of the WISC, the scores were adjusted for the Puerto Rican population.

2. Bender-Visual-Motor-Gestalt test.

3. Draw-a-person test.

4. Rorschach test.

5. Five plates from the Make-a-Picture-Story test. The five plates were the following: "Dream," "Street," "Bedroom," "Medical" and "Shanty."

The psychological tests were administered by a qualified psychologist who had knowledge of the delinquency/nondelinquency status of the subjects. However, the protocols were neither scored nor interpreted by him. They were sent to another clinical psychologist who interpreted them without any information on the subjects. The interpretation was scored on a psychological report blank which listed different areas of intellectual functioning, personality characteristics and modalities of reaction.

The physical examination was administered by a physician following standard procedures. The laboratory tests included the following: urinalysis, complete blood count, Venereal Disease Serology (VDRL) and stool examination for parasites. The neurological examination included standard testing of cranial nerves, motor areas, coordination, sensation, reflexes and station. The electroencephalogram was administered under standard conditions and included hyperventilation and photic drive.

The mountain of data yielded in these several protocols—medical, neurological, encephalographic, psychological and social history—were analyzed in two principal ways: by univariate and multivariate techniques. First, the two groups were compared on every variable in a straightforward χ^2 analysis. In general, the results supported the Gluecks' results in *Unraveling Juvenile Delinquency* in all important respects. Second, after eliminating all but 184 variables on statistical and theoretical grounds, each of the 101 delinquents was compared with his control across each variable in a sign test analysis. The purpose of the sign test was to address the question whether the *matched pairs* differed significantly from each other and, if so, on which items. In contrast, the χ^2 indicated whether the two groups differed from each other at an acceptable level of confidence. Third, all 184 items were subjected to a factor analysis, and seven separate clusters of variables emerged, accounting for more than a third of the total variance. Fourth, using a multidiscriminant function analysis approach, the identification of delinquents and nondelinquents in terms of small subsets of variables was compared with their actual status. Eventually, perfect discrimination was obtained using only 13 variables taken together and treated as one.

FINDINGS

The following results were obtained using the two univariate and two multivariate methods described briefly above:

1. Medical, neurological and encephalographic variables derived from physical examinations, laboratory tests and carefully taken histories generally failed to distinguish the delinquents from the nondelinquents. A few specific health findings did differentiate the two groups. There was, for example, a curious but explainable hematological finding. Our delinquents have more eosinophils (and consequently fewer neutrophils and basophils) than the nondelinquents. This seems to be related to chronic repeated, and more frequent parasitic infections in the delinquent group. More important than the specific items were the clinical impressions. On this grosser interpretive level, the nondelinquents predictably were rated as being in better overall health and having fewer organic signs and symptoms.

2. The psychological and psychiatric evaluations were highly discriminating. The data point to a rather serious degree of maladjustment in the delinquents. Whether antecedent, concomitant or consequence of delin-

quent behavior, interpersonal and emotional problems are clearly associated with delinquency in court-derived cases. This association, of course, tells us nothing very definite about the etiological implications of disturbance for delinquency (see Tables 15.2 and 15.3).

3. The major specific distinctions between the matched groups occurred on the family and school items. Interpolating from individual item differences, the families of the controls were more cohesive and stable in every respect. The economic aspirations were greater, the religious interests more firm (see Table 15.4).

TABLE 15.2

Significant psychological findings (χ^2 analysis)

Item	Delinquent Group	Nondelinquent Group
Verbal I.Q.		
Normal and above......................	24	40
Low-normal and above..................	77	61
Performance I.Q.		
Normal and above......................	37	58
Low-normal and above..................	64	43
Prognosis		
Unconditionally good....................	0	16
Conditionally good.....................	1	43
Uncertain..............................	45	39
Unfavorable............................	55	3

Significant traits

Creativity	Aggression (environment)
Other-oriented thinking	Capacity to relate (environment)
Reality orientation	Hostility (environment)
Fantasy control	Suspiciousness (environment)
Stereotyped thinking	Feelings of rejection
Perseveration	Overt homosexuality
Memory recall	Latent homosexuality
Speed of mental processes	Capacity for heterosexuality
Organic signs	Prognosis
Maturity	Assertiveness
Emotional instability and impulsivity	Defiance
Extroversion/introversion	Suspiciousness
Conformity (family)	Destructiveness
Aggression (family)	Emotional responsibility
Capacity to relate (family)	
Hostility (family)	
Suspiciousness (family)	

TABLE 15.3
Psychiatric diagnoses

Classification	Delinquent Group	Nondelinquent Group
1. Neuroses		
Anxiety	1	2
Obsessive-compulsive	0	1
Neurasthenic.	0	1
Hypochondriacal	0	3
Other	1	0
Subtotal	2	7
2. Personality disorders		
Cyclothymic.	0	1
Schizoid	2	2
Explosive	2	0
Hysterical	0	1
Asthenic	0	1
Antisocial	10	0
Passive-aggressive	16	5
Inadequate	2	1
Other (specified)	1	0
Subtotal	33	11
3. Homosexuality	2	0
4. Drug dependence (nonpsychiatric)		
Opium (heroin)	9	0
Other	2	0
Subtotal	11	0
5. Psychophysiologic disorders		
Cardiovascular	0	1
6. Transient situational disturbances		
Adjustment reaction of adolescence	18	24
7 Behavior disorders		
Hyperkinetic reaction	0	1
Overanxious reaction	0	1
Unsocialized aggressive reaction	1	0
Group delinquent reaction	3	0
Subtotal	4	2
8. Mental retardation		
Borderline	10	10
Mild	13	3
Moderate	6	1
Subtotal	29	14
9. Dyssocial behavior	2	0
Total impaired	101	59
Total no mental disorder	0	42

On nearly every major measure of school performance and attitudes toward school, the controls showed to great advantage. The policy implications here are evident (see Table 15.5).

With regard to the specific school, family and psychological-psychiatric variables, it is important to note that the results obtained in Puerto Rico

TABLE 15.4

Significant family items (χ^2 analysis)

Item	Delinquent Group	Nondelinquent Group
Size of household (not significant)		
5 or fewer persons	20	15
6–9 persons	63	70
10 or more persons	18	16
Mother's birthplace		
Rural	34	58
Urban	67	43
Father's birthplace		
Rural	37	65
Urban	64	36
Father's education		
None–9th grade	71	55
10th–12th grade	29	42
Vocational or other	1	4
Father's occupation		
Permanent	59	81
Temporary	13	6
Disabled, unemployed	29	14
Vertical mobility of family		
Rising	0	50
Stable	19	19
Declining	82	32
Mother's church attendance		
Never	54	26
Holidays	25	29
Weekly	22	45
Children's church attendance		
Never	61	2
Holidays	22	79
Weekly	11	20

TABLE 15.5

Significant school items (χ^2 analysis)

Item	Delinquent Group	Nondelinquent] Group
Dropped out of school....................................	63	N.A.
School conduct and learning problems (significant items)		
Fighting...	18	0
Lying..	13	0
Cheating...	10	0
Disrespectful...	26	0
General misconduct..	21	0
Domineering...	14	3
Temper tantrums..	21	0
Instigator/provoker.......................................	14	1
Too talkative..	20	14
Uncooperative...	13	1
Isolated...	38	26
Slow learner..	44	31
Inattentive..	20	2
Quiet..	19	69
Sensitive..	12	36
Attitudes of subject regarding school		
Like school to some degree.............................	28	98
Good relations with class mates........................	69	100
Good relations with teacher............................	65	99
Family encourages subject to stay in school.............	72	100
Mother wants subject in school.........................	72	100
Father wants subject in school..........................	52	89
Subject feels school important to life....................	57	98
Subject's peers feel school important to life.............	44	100
Truant..	17	7
Homework difficult..	95	50

corroborate the findings obtained in mainland city slums. This augurs well for comparative criminology in that intercultural generalizations may be possible under certain circumstances.

4. On the sign test, the matched pairs differed significantly on 29 of the 184 variables. Nearly all of these 29 differences occurred on the psychological and school behavior items. However, and at least as important, on 183 of the 184 items the matched pair difference fell in the expected direction. Thus, no matter what the items, the delinquents were not performing as well as their individually matched controls.

5. The principal axis factor analysis yielded seven clusters or patterns of variables which totally accounted for more than 34 percent of the vari-

ance. These seven patterns were named and identified as follows: a) personal and social pathology (34 items), b) psychological traits (12 items), c) school misconduct and problems (14 items), d) competent housekeeping (11 variables), e) broken home (11 items), f) interpersonal hostility and incompetence (17 items) and g) physical and intellectual maturity (11 items).

Weighted factor scores were computed on each of these seven clusters or patterns and an analysis of variance yielding F ratios was run on each cluster. All seven patterns of items significantly differentiated the delinquents from the controls. In addition, the 101 delinquents and 101 controls, as pairs, were compared on these seven factors with the result that the discrimination was even more pronounced within these pair sets than within the groups.

6. *The most significant achievement of this research was the retrospective identification of all 202 subjects as either delinquents or controls.* This altogether unique outcome was achieved in a stepwise multidiscriminant function analysis (Table 15.6).

It need only be noted here that the variables used in the univariate analyses and others, principally of a historical and clinical nature, were

TABLE 15.6

Classification after first 13 variables of SDFA

Actual Groups	Predicted	
	Delinquent	Nondelinquent
Delinquents....................................	101	0
Nondelinquents................................	0	101

$U = 0.12671$, degrees of freedom $= (14,1,20)$
$F = 99.67148$, degrees of freedom $= (13,188)$
$P \ll 0.001$

Optimal classification (with 39 variables)

Actual Groups	Predicted	
	Delinquent	Nondelinquent
Delinquents....................................	101	0
Nondelinquents................................	0	101

$U = 0.08412$, degrees of freedom $= (39,1,200)$
$F = 45.22392$, degrees of freedom $= (38,162)$
$P \ll 0.001$

grouped logically and theoretically into the following subsets of items: medical, psychological-psychiatric, home-family, school and other performances and electroencephalographic. Each subset was then used to retrospectively identify the subjects. The optimal medical subset misidentified 18 of the 202 boys, erring on 11 delinquents and 7 nondelinquents. The optimal clinical subset misclassified 12 boys calling 7 delinquents controls and 5 controls delinquents. The family variables subset was markedly more accurate. Only 3 of the delinquents and 1 control were mistakenly classified. The school subset was even more accurate. No controls were misidentified and 6 delinquents were called controls. In contrast, the EEG-neurological subset was of no use at all. Nearly as many subjects were misplaced as were identified correctly.

In view of the success with the first four subsets, a final analysis was done using as discriminators the first 10 variables from each of medical, psychological-psychiatric, home-family and school analyses. *Error-free classification of all 202 subjects was accomplished with only 13 variables including 2 from the medical, 3 from the clinical, 5 from the family and 3 from the school subsets.*

7. The stepwise discriminant function analysis (see Table 15.7) also yielded something never before reported in delinquency research: *a paradoxical effect phenomenon.* This phenomenon explains, in part at least, the seemingly erratic patterns obtained from social history data in previous prediction studies. The implications for diagnosis and outcome research are, therefore, of marked importance. In the paradoxical effect phenomenon, variables which operate in one direction when analyzed separately may reverse direction when included as part of a broader function. This reversal is reflected in the relative weight as well as the sign (direction) of the coefficient attached to the item. In our analysis, "father's church attendance" proved to be *paradoxical* in the context of children's church attendance and 11 other concurrent variables which resulted in perfect discrimination. These paradoxical items are footnoted in Table 15.7.

8. In the San Juan arrabales and caserios, juvenile delinquency in the index cases seems to be only one element of a multiproblem family syndrome. This is evident in the item clusters (broken home and competent housekeeping) obtained in the factor analysis. It is also evident in the lengthy case histories of each of the subjects. It is even more obvious in the repeated visits to the homes and in interviews with the parents or adults in the households. Of the three principal family patterns characteristic of mainland families—the truncated-extended (Jewish, Italian), the nuclear-atomistic and the mother-children—the latter, the female-based household, devoid of a significant father figure, or at least a stable one, best describes

TABLE 7

The best discriminators from the stepwise discriminant function analysis

Items

37. Subject is a truant   (yes)
39. Subject steals   (yes)
 7. Suspiciousness   (high)
14. Vertical mobility upward   (no)
28. Children's church attendance   (seldom)
27. Father's church attendance[1]   (often)
 3. Emotional instability   (high)
13. Birthplace of father   (urban)
21. Subject smokes   (yes)
 2. Complete blood count   (abnormal)
24. Home has dining room set   (yes)
33. Subject participates in social group activities   (yes)
12. Psychological diagnosis 318—no mental disorder   (no)

16. Family pays Social Security   (no)
30. Family encourages subject to stay in school[1]   (yes)
40. Subject's family members have police contact for type I offenses   (yes)
31. Subject likes school   (no)
38. Subject lies[1]   (no)
 8. Destructiveness   (high)
29. Teacher reports subject steals in school   (yes)
15. Subject has left home   (yes)
25. Subject's home has a television   (no)
 5. Guilt feelings   (low)

32. Subject is a dropout   (yes)
 4. Suspiciousness   (high)
22. Relatives had mental illness   (yes)
18. Subject has high blood pressure   (yes)
19. Subject has history of infections   (no)
26. Area surrounding the home was clean   (yes)
20. Subject has been treated for alcoholism   (yes, or needed but not obtained)
35. Subject's bedwetting   (less than age 3)
23. Subject has a mental defect   (yes)
17. Subject has ulcers   (yes)
 1. Health status   (fair)
11. Diagnosis 304.0—drug dependence[1] (opium)   (no)
 9. Diagnosis 300.1—hysterical neurosis   (no)
34. Subject participates in church group activities   (no)
10. Diagnosis 301.82—inadequate personality   (yes)
36. Subject sleeps out   (yes)

[1] Indicates paradoxical effect phenomenon.

the index families. This instability is coupled with a subsistence standard of living, physical and mental disabilities of every description and a retreatist philosophy which makes coping with external problems and realities difficult. Social agency intervention, geared to alleviating specific problems, has failed to enable these household units to reach the critical mass stage from which achievement and mobility are possible. The "Band-aid" approach has merely reinforced the coping inadequacies of these households and created hard-core families without the resources—inter or outer—to alter their destinies.

Thus, mainland and island are not so very different in respect to the multiproblem family origins of court-adjudicated delinquents.

9. A very careful analysis of police and court records and the 42-page social history suggests that mainland and island patterns of delinquency do differ in two very important respects. First, *Puerto Rico delinquent index cases are largely loners; gang involvement is minimal.* Second, *the personal violence so endemic in Hispano-American culture is effectively reflected in the aggravated assaults and simple assaults which dot the records of the index cases.* This propensity to violence, some 33 violent episodes resulting in court action were found, may well account for the deaths of 11 of the 101 index cases since the study was completed just a few years ago. This extraordinarily high mortality rate among the delinquents—now 21 years of age or under—deserves and will receive additional investigation. This is one area of research which will be explored in our future work.

10. Although Puerto Rico has very high rates of heroin use and addiction, the data regarding drug use in the delinquent group are still astonishing. *A careful check of police and court records revealed that 11 delinquents were either hard drug users or addicts. Interviews revealed 15 others who were also hooked—26 out of 101 cases in all.* Three observations are in order on this matter. First, official records grossly underestimated the problem of hard drug use. Clearly there is need for other procedures to estimate the prevalence of the problem in order to determine the effectiveness of drug prevention and control programs. Second, the 26 delinquents with serious drug problems were found to be even more seriously disadvantaged and impaired, in relation to their controls, than the other 75 delinquents studied. Whether cause or effect, this special group, aged 11 to 17 at the point of study, needs something more than the present institutions can offer if they are to survive and settle down. Third, no nondelinquent subject was even suspected—officially or in the interviews—of experimenting with narcotics. What more can be said of the "goodness" of these deprived youth?

Cross-cultural studies such as the one herein presented hopefully will do much to encourage better designed and better aimed prevention and treatment programs.

DISCUSSION

Dr. Saleem Shah (Rockville, Maryland): Studies in the States, as well as in the Scandinavian countries, show that when you compare the official delinquency and crime statistics with data derived from the South Report studies, you invariably find that the official statistics confound the behavior of the individual with the behavior of the decision maker. Studies like the one by Gold show a much smaller difference between lower and upper social class youngsters. Whether or not there is a formal charge against the youngster can be a matter of police handling and discretion. From your knowledge of San Juan, is there a differential decision maker effect?

Dr. Franco Ferracuti (Rome, Italy): Of course, but in our study, every nondelinquent was tested for delinquency, in that we examined both the court records and the unofficial police records. Also, if at any point during the social interview we found evidence of delinquency, we eliminated the subject. We wanted our nondelinquents as free as possible of delinquency. Our subjects were deliberately selected at the two extremes in order to study the contrasts.

Dr. Kenneth Livingston (Toronto, Canada): On the significant variable of school performance, do you have any information on the reading ability of the delinquent as compared with the nondelinquent child? Is dyslexia a factor?

Dr. Ferracuti: We have no direct information on dyslexia or reading ability, only general information on school performance. We regretted that we were not able to test for dyslexia or for minor motor disturbances. The EEG didn't pick up anything; but the Rorschach did pick up organic signs in approximately 15 to 16 percent of the delinquent group. One difficulty in Puerto Rico, as elsewhere, is getting established norms for this kind of examination. Misbehavior and poor performance in school is a constant characteristic in delinquents.

Dr. Weinstein (Discussant from the Floor): Would Professor Ferracuti comment on the discriminating value of the diagnosis "hysterical neurosis?"

Dr. Ferracuti: I leave that question to those who formulated the APA manual. I would question the validity of that diagnosis at that age which was, incidentally, 15 to 17.

Dr. Shah: There are matters of the selection factor and the sample. When you use the bottom of the barrel group, of course you will find a lot of signs of deviance, whether they are school or reading disabilities or medical or other complications. This population group also has the highest rate of malnutrition, rat bites, unemployment and mortality. It is hardly surprising if that population shows a very high incidence of whatever type of problem is being measured. This also accounts for some of the findings that institutionalized offenders in certain categories have lower I.Q.'s or, perhaps, some chromosomal abnormalities or abnormal EEGs.

I would like to comment also about the definitional issue as it relates, for instance, to the term "aggression." We have heard discussions on subjects ranging from laboratory paradigms of "sham rage" to the behavior of Iko children. The aggression may be playful or homicidal, or everything in between. We are dealing not only with behavior that has considerable complexity and plasticity, but with a definition which is also very plastic. I have some concern whether our understanding of the phenomena may be confounded when we use the same word to describe such a motley array of behavior. It might be desirable, at least for research purposes, if there could be more specificity on the varying degrees. There should be some attention to the social context in which the behavior occurs and the extent of the expectancy of the examiner. For example, with the film on the Iko children, it would be nice if someone with no theoretical interest, merely a professional photographer, photographed all the behavior of the youngsters without being interested in indices of aggressive behavior.

DR. FERRACUTI: I entirely agree with your comments on definitions. We were interested not so much in what we found as in what we did not find, what did not come out, even though we contrasted the cases so sharply. The points which most clearly emerged were that color and gross biology are not relevant factors. On education, the relation is not necessarily causal. Delinquency is a multiprob-lem-family phenomenon which does not come out of the blue sky. It appears in families which have to cope with such a fantastic range of other troubles that it is not surprising when they cannot cope with delinquency.

Chapter 16

MURDER—SINGLE AND MULTIPLE

SHERVERT H. FRAZIER

Murder as a human action state does not allow simple reductionistic conclusions about the "cause or causes." Action states require conceptual models, methods of definition, and definition of coexisting, so-called etiological forces—which are essentially descriptive.

This paper will review a series of murderers of individual and numerous persons in four perspectives:

1. Premurder personality of the murderer.
2. The buildup state or state of readiness.
3. The action state—the event or events of murdering a person or persons.
4. The alternative state—in which nonmurdering behavior releases the buildup state of readiness.

The sample consisted of 31 murderers out of a series of 65. The criteria for inclusion were:

1. Relative completeness of the studies.
2. Corroboration of the retrospective evidence.
3. Possible retrospective reconstruction of events.
4. Available medical, neurological and psychiatric evaluations.
5. Intact memory of the event or events. This selects out many murderers under the influence of alcohol and some drugs.

The 31 cases consisted of murderers in prisons in Texas, Minnesota, New Jersey and New York and mental hospitals in Texas, Minnesota, Saskatchewan, Massachusetts and New York. Twenty-three killed only 1 person and 8 killed 3, 5, 5, 6, 7, 12, 13, and 17 persons, respectively. Observations based on retrospective and reconstructed events are always difficult and fraught with potential error and the usual rearrangement of history as it is told and retold. This has been countered with careful and detailed interviewing of family members, relatives, neighbors, friends and associates. Medical, neurological and psychiatric evaluations are far from ideal in retrospective studies and not of the excellent quality desirable because of geographic inaccessibility and unavailability of such desirable evaluations in prisons, state and provincial mental hospitals and in rural areas. However, in present prospective evaluations of personal assaulters, not murderers, we are attempting to correct these deficiencies and to evaluate the risk factors for homicide.

PERSONALITY PATTERNS PREMURDER

These have been defined by collaborative investigations by several psychiatrists and corroboration by extensive interviewing of family members, friends, teachers, family physicians, neighbors and policemen and probation personnel in the areas where such persons reside.

Biological and maturational factors in personality evaluation are as significant as *social* and *environmental* factors. In our series 18 of the murderers, both single and multiple types, suffered marked parental deprivation because of deaths, absentee parents, and repeated placement in orphanages and foster homes, plus remorseless physical brutalization by parents. Nineteen with representatives in both single and multiple categories showed psychosexual confusion and gender defect, but not biological genital abnormality. Psychosexual confusion was characterized by chaotic sexual behavior, homosexuality as defined in the performance of the sexual act with children or not between consenting adults, absence of sexual impulse and action, or periodic repeated cross-dressing and passing. Genetic studies were not accomplished in this series, although no person resembled the XYY biological traits as described. Organic brain factors altering personality existed in four single and two multiple murderers. Temporal lobe epilepsy with clinically diagnosable repeated psychomotor seizures existed in two single murderers, idiopathic mental retardation was present in two single murderers, and organic brain syndrome caused by neoplasm was present in one multiple murderer. In another murderer of numerous persons organicity caused by early dementia related to central nervous system infection was present. Episodic behavioral dyscontrol as defined by Monroe (1) existed in eight single and three multiple murderers. Only four single murderers in this series had a history of alcohol usage and none murdered under the influence of alcohol, which, by statistical standards, makes this an unusual series. Corroboration of details of a murder are difficult to obtain and verification is impossible when amnesia for the event exists in several of those present at the time and the murderer has no memory for the events before or during the action. Two single murderers used drugs, but only for gaining the courage to accomplish the murder. One single murderer ingested a small amount of barbiturate and one multiple murderer sniffed two tubes of airplane glue after over a month's planning of the event. We classify episodic behavioral dyscontrol, alcohol and drugs and central nervous system abnormalities as short-circuiting events which rearrange the buildup state to the action state resulting from defect or alteration in the inhibitory capacities and failure of inherent restraint systems in the brain.

Maturational lag was induced in the life histories of five single murderers with delay in neurological maturation as evidenced by motor incoordination, marked diminution in sensory stimulation in critical developmental periods of childhood in highly abnormal early social environments of two persons, and early metabolic and infections processes were found in three persons—rubella in 1, prematurity in 1, and childhood diabetes in 1.

Social and environmental processes in childhood and adult experiences which resulted in what has been called high risk personality patterns abounded in this series. Defective male identification patterns with absent role model for patterning or repeated brutalization by the father in an inconsistent and unpredictably violent interaction between father and son existed in 18 of the 30, four of whom were murderers of numerous persons. Significant limitation in early socialization patterns with peers and playmates (2), loner type isolation (5), repeated impulse dyscontrol (16), animal cruelty (2), and unusual familiarity with weapons (13) were some examples of environmental contribution to high risk population with murderous impulses. Our results are similar to those of Glueck and Glueck (2), Robins (3), Brown (4), Daniels and co-workers (5).

A second phase—not always present—is the buildup state or state of readiness—often of hours' to weeks' duration and in rare instances of 1 or 2 years' duration. This state of readiness, by no means uniform, was universal in this series of preplanned and prearranged murders—both for murderers of single individuals as well as of multiple individuals. The *buildup state* consists of biological, cyclic, intrapsychic and social factors. In this series no hormonal studies were accomplished. The buildup of restlessness, increased motoric behavior and concomitant rise in anxiety level was described frequently (12). Three of the single and three multiple murderers had psychosomatic or psychophysiological symptom buildup before the event or events of the murder. Eight described a history of sexual impotence and five associated unusual sexual promiscuity after the event of murder.

Inconclusive evidence of cyclic phenomena exists in our studies, although correlations of plasma testosterone and history of aggression exist. Pokorny (6) failed to demonstrate positive correlations between lunar synodic cycling and homicide incidence. One murderess with a long history of premenstrual tension and instability did, in fact, murder her spouse 3 days premenstrually.

Intrapsychic buildup occurs in the absence of environmental interplay.

Episodic psychosis without external reality testing ability often driven by delusionally patterned thoughts was present in 15 of the murderers in our series, three of whom were multiple murderers. Content of the ideas was frequently expressed to other persons but derivative action was not often expressed or predictable. The concurrence of recognizable expectation levels exceeding performance leading to fear of and sense of failure is high enough to merit further study. Delusional ideas of the need to murder a named individual or individuals with characteristic detailed planning and processing of the act was present in eight murderers, five of whom were multiple—a physician with a list of persons, an exconvict with a list of guards, an adolescent with a family list, a parent with a family list, a young adult with a family list and a neighbor with a list of members of another family. Three murderers of one individual had named a spouse, a famous person, and an employee. In each instance reasons were stated and the buildup was accompanied by a planned progression of organized behavior, detailed and carefully executed goal-oriented purposive behavior despite delusional reasons and active delusional thinking sustained from 3 days to over 1 year in duration. In four instances detailed consultations with other persons, disguised as to goal but not as to methodology, were carried out in two instances, resulting in a change in plans. Stated fantasies as to the outcome following the event either verbally or in writing existed in two instances. Homicide notes were found in three instances by two persons.

An additional two persons not included above had delusional objects identified previously, but actually murdered persons who were misidentified at the time of the murder. One murderer recognized his mistake soon after the event, misidentifying a young male as the person who had introduced him to homosexuality and blaming him for his subsequent chaotic life situation. In only one instance in this series did a murderer have a sibling who had also murdered—not twins. Low self-esteem and depression were severe and noted in seven persons, three of whom were multiple murderers. Three of the single murderers who were depressed had recurrent depressions, but no periods of elation. Each had suffered severe personal losses (significant parent or parents) in early life, another of an idealized parent substitute of early adult life, two of the depressed murderers of multiple persons had lost girls they loved in the months before the murder and one had been taunted by his parents about having been jilted. The third had suffered significant multiple personal losses and separations in the 2 months preceding the murders.

The high incidence of significant and repeated personal humiliation (18) and sense of powerlessness (15) and personal inadequacy (11) cannot be overlooked. It is in this group that we postulate murder as a process

inexorably proceeding from the feeling of being cornered by a life
situation from which no foreseeable outlet exists. The usual pattern is a
series of "hurts," fantasied or real, plus repeated and memorable humili-
ations accompanied by severe feelings of shame at the seeming personal
inadequacy to extricate oneself from a powerless position. The recurrence
of a pattern of psychic hurts, verbal shaming and humiliation by significant parents before children's friends and other family members was re-
counted frequently and corroborated by family members who often stated
that the particular person was the scapegoat of the family or early identified as "different," defiant or the black sheep, with a stubborn resistance
to passive compliance with family expectations, be they a family of
hardened repetitive criminal behaviors in which most members had been
imprisoned or a family of overachievers in other fields of endeavor—inner
city or suburbia or rural. This pattern, in all instances, is a replay of a
familiar pattern, the chief difference being a more specific definition of
the role of the victim and his contribution to the plight of the tortured one.
Here the actions of the victim become important. An out of focus victim
may clearly identify himself by becoming the specific provocateur, or by
becoming the person whose eradication promises to ease the life situation,
or by actions which fuel the passions of the would-be murderer, and which
seem to indicate that without such action the hurt would be relieved.
Other patterns also exist. The study of victimology has contributed to our
understanding of the dyadic and triadic and group interaction of the
murderer and his victim or victims. Abrahamsen (7), Schafer (8–11), and
others have enlightened the role of the victim and the action of the
blaming of the victim.

Given the cornering series of life events and a personality pattern of
early brutalization by significant persons or a pattern of fostering by
parents of antisocial behavior from which parents gain vicarious gratification from the actions of the offspring, plus an arousal pattern of anger
at shame or humiliation by circumstance or potential victims plus stress
specific to the individual buildup, one can expect the emergence of
murderous feelings and actions which will overwhelm most inhibitory or
control systems. It is in this light that we perceive murder as a process
which leads to the event. The relative weightings of the various ingredients
is person-specific, and failure in one system, be it the biological, interpersonal, environmental or social control system, may lead to the action or
discharge phase.

This phase is followed by the action state in which the murder or
murders are accomplished, or the alternative state during which nonmurderous behavior releases the built-up readiness state and behaviors

other than murder displace or take the place of the action state leading to murder.

Murder by 31 persons was admitted incontrovertibly. Methods of murder included guns, pistols, rifles, shotguns, axes, choking or strangling, blunt instruments, forcible drowning, stalking and then shooting, stabbing, evisceration. In eight instances (five of one-person murderers and 3 of numerous person murderers) previous attempts at murder were reported—one murderer of numerous persons had made three previous specific attempts on lives of different individuals.

Only one of the murderers of multiple persons (six persons) again murdered, two at each event separated by several years.

The recidivism rate of persons in this series is therefore low, but some persons with lists are still under carefully structured environmental control.

ALTERNATIVE STATE—SUBSTITUTION FOR MURDEROUS ACTION

Physical nonmurderous action was often substituted for murderous impulse or threat. Instances of repeated personal assaults, rape in adolescence, multiple physical fights often associated with injuries as well as prefight threats, or threats made public by individuals, not members of gangs or groups, were common in the histories of murderers of single as well as numerous persons. The prior usage of alcohol and drugs to relieve the buildup phase at or near the emergence of the action state was common. In a few instances when judgment emerged, as it seemed to in a few individuals (self-induced environmental manipulation and control such as going on a trip away from the provocateurs or victim, escapes into longer periods alone in a cabin in the woods) one man recurrently visited a lake in the vicinity and would sit for hours and even days. Another substituted association with children, another became a scoutmaster, another sought strenuous nighttime employment because of the feelings of dyscontrol emerging at night, another walked a "plotting course" in a repetitious and stereotyped fashion. All such alternative states in this series were not successful eventually. Certainly many persons, however, do successfully employ the alternative state to prevent emergence of the action state.

SUMMARY

Selection of single or multiple persons for murder is not specifically related to personality, the buildup state, the events of the action state or the effectiveness of the discharge state. No predictive factors could be selected. Notable, however, was the careful and detailed planning for one or several murders by persons carrying delusional ideas but who were personally organized for hours to days to 1 or 2 years so that they could organize the plans for the action phase. The other factor which contributed was the episodic behavioral dyscontrol state and those persons with brain structural and functional alteration and the predictive clinical course of such persons. A more detailed neurological and electrophysiological study with correlation of experimental factors and psychological states in such persons ought to be productive in building alternative controls of behavior. Whether or not the crossing of the threshold of personal assault is predictive of murder is now being studied. Increase of the order of 20 percent in adolescents and young adults admitted to mental hospitals who have engaged in personal assault requires immediate and detailed evaluation of the possibility of progression to murder.

PREVENTION

Pediatricians, child care workers, playground and recreational specialists and school teachers should be taught to recognize early evidence of early socialization defects, loners and isolates and persons with episodic behavioral dyscontrol as well as the symptoms of brutalization. Careful and friendly early intervention in such persons and families together with the ready availability of trained persons to provide social, environmental, physical and therapeutic alternatives would prevent some murders. Further research into the biological and intrapsychic concomitants of mental illness—especially paranoia and delusional states—is indicated.

ACKNOWLEDGMENTS

I appreciate the valuable assistance of Drs. Stuart L. Brown, James Lomax and Norbert Mintz for their contributions to this study. Special appreciation to the Hogg Foundation for Mental Health for a grant and to Dr. Robert Sutherland, Director, for his help and continuing interest in this project is expressed and their help acknowledged.

REFERENCES

1. Monroe, R: Episodic Behavioral Disorders: A Psychodynamic and Neurophysiologic Analysis. Cambridge, Harvard University Press, 1970.
2. Glueck, S, Glueck, ET: Delinquents and Nondelinquents in Perspective. Cambridge, Harvard University Press, 1968.
3. Robins, LN: Deviant Children Grown Up: A Sociological and Psychiatric Study of Sociopathic Personality. Baltimore, Williams & Wilkins Co., 1966.
4. Brown, SL: The Automobile Death Syndrome. Med. Insight 2: (10): 38–49, 1970.
5. Daniels, DN, Gilula, MF, Ochberg, FM (eds): Violence and the Struggle for Existence. Boston, Little Brown & Co., 1970.
6. Pokorny, AD: Human violence: a comparison of homicide, aggravated assault, suicide, and attempted suicide. J Crim Law Criminol Police Sci 56: 488, 1965.

7. ABRAHAMSEN, D: The Psychology of Crime. New York, Columbia University Press, 1960.
8. SCHAFER, S: Compensation and Restitution to Victims of Crimes. Ed. 1. Montclair, New Jersey, Patterson Smith, 1970.
9. SCHAFER, S: Theories in Criminology. New York, Random House, 1969.
10. SCHAFER, S: Victim and His Criminal: A Study in Functional Responsibility. New York, Random House, 1968.
11. SCHAFER, S, KNUDTEN, D: Juvenile Delinquency: An Introduction. New York, Random House, 1970.

DISCUSSION

MR. HENRY F. GREEN (Washington, D.C.): Did these people give any thought to the possibility of imprisonment or the death penalty? Clearly, they all went ahead with committing murder, but were they restrained to any extent by the possible consequences? How does the extent of their attempts to avoid detection compare to their determination to achieve the act?

DR. SHERVERT H. FRAZIER (Belmont, Massachusetts): In this series, this factor was much dependent upon age, I think. The adolescents and young adults who murdered ran away, many of them to neighboring countries to try to escape detection. Whereas the awareness of consequences was present in a large number, I cannot say in exactly how many. I was impressed by the number who stated that given the same situation, with the same set of circumstances, they would still perform the same actions. They were not unaware of the consequences but recognized them and still were driven to the same behavior.

DR. ALFRED MESSER (Atlanta, Georgia): Do you have any thoughts on the homicide-suicide axis?

DR. FRAZIER: Yes, several persons not reported in this series, while planning homicides, took very direct steps toward getting themselves killed immediately in the events right after the act. Some of them actually wrote suicide notes. One person asked for the insurance returns to be given to mental health to investigate the causes of this kind of behavior.

DR. SALEEM SHAH (Rockville, Maryland): First of all, let me commend Dr. Frazier for his caution about generalizing from this data. Two questions: were these individuals convicted of murder, or were they charged and awaiting trial on another issue such as mental competence? Do you have information on the social class distribution of your sample?

DR. FRAZIER: First I will take the question of social class distribution. With this group, we made every attempt to get as many details as possible from representatives of all social classes, but the lower socioeconomic class is less represented in this series than the middle and upper middle classes. One reason is that lower class persons are not as willing to enter into the investigation process, to discuss themselves with strangers.

As for the charges, you, better than any of us here, are aware of the mishmash of the legal charges of murder. We all know that in many states, the charges are dropped as soon as an individual is admitted to a mental hospital, and therefore no charges exist. However, all of those in prison had been tried and had already recieved sentences. Five or six of them were at a maximum security part of a prison system. The place was supposedly mental hospital-oriented, but was certainly not an adequate treatment setting.

In some of the states where these studies were conducted, most murderers were kept in prison about 5 years or in a mental hospital from 18 months to 2 years. The ability to be released was significantly increased by being committed to a mental hospital.

DR. SHAH: In regard to the further studies you are doing, I would like to make a suggestion based on some experience in the legal-psychiatric setting. Our staff was often puzzled over why certain offenders who had committed other crimes had not engaged in violence, although the clinicians were ready to assume that they would have done so. It might be very interesting if your data, including the history, the psychiatric interview, the EEG, and other matters, were presented to judges, psychiatrists, or others, along with data on matched, nonviolent offenders. One might find that the base rates for a lot of indices of psychiatric or other pathology are fairly widely distributed, even among those who have not committed a violent act. Sometimes a murder happens when a bullet goes an inch in one direction rather than another.

Chapter 17

CONTROL OF VIOLENCE

LAWRENCE C. KOLB

Undoubtedly, the yearned for objective contained in the theme of this meeting of the Association—as well as a host of other meetings, symposia, conferences, discussion groups and publications—stems from a national concern of the means of *control of violence* (1). Violence is only one expression of the aggressive drive. Although man has achieved a myriad of complex representations of the aggressive drive, the pressing issue of the day is the ways men have evolved control of its destructive expression, particularly in violent acts against others or objects. My paper relates primarily to the ways that acquisition of, or impairment of, individual internalized mechanisms for the control of aggression impede or allow the eruption of violence.

Because of that unique function of the nervous system to record experience over time and progressively evolve new patterns of behavior to allow effective adaptations—which, for man, are primarily directed to life in social systems—the sources of knowledge as regards this development are all those chances of genetic inheritance, pre- and postnatal health which affect brain growth and its function. They determine to greater or lesser extent the brain's capacity to record the necessary social experiences which induce the control mechanisms inhibiting violent aggressiveness; that is, they establish the predispositions—firm, unstable, or deficient—within the growing individual, for learning effective social behavior.

The occurrence or absence of experience in human transactions, and their relative variations—which support or deny the growth of healthy controls of the aggressive drive—perhaps are of greater importance in establishing the predisposition to control in the growing personality than the action of the biological factors in setting the brain structure and function.

To understand the controls for violence, we must then address ourselves to those experiences in the lives of men which establish the formation of "conscience" or "superego," if you wish—a portion of personality functioning termed by Darwin as man's greatest achievement. The controlling portion of the personality, as Brosin (1) has reminded us, is thought to have its beginning some 4 to 5 centuries past in the early agri-

313

cultural societies of the world. Its functions facilitate the judgmental processes of the personality—the ego—in terms of release or inhibition of aggressive actions. It assists in defining that which is rewarding socially— not only in its immediacy, but also in terms of the future. It facilitates the establishment of and holding to a set of personal and social values—the ego ideal. When this portion of personality organization fails to evolve or is impaired in its functioning, the potential for destructive acting out against others exists.

Violence, as practiced by man in wars, property destruction, assassination, murder, assaults, rape and cruelty in mutilating others and the self, and suicide are expressions of aggressivity unique to his species. Such expressions of violence may be regarded as psychopathological only when they are expressive of abnormal development or impairment of function of the *individual* superego and ego. One may discern at least five patterns of maldevelopment. 1) In some, deficiency in brain growth leading to mental retardation may determine individual inability to absorb the learning of values from the family and cultural systems which lead to internalization of control of rage. 2) In others, severe emotional deprivation in early life, because of parental loss, neglect, or hatred, may impair the capacity of dependent attachment and thus the process of identification which determines the internalization of values. 3) In still others, parental discipline, or that provided in schools or other institutions, may be so brutal and hateful as to establish an identification with the aggressor, thus allowing acting out, later in life, of violence suffered by oneself toward others. 4) In the instance of some emotionally deprived children thirsting for additional support from the family or societal systems, frustration leads to reaction formations with denial of partially internalized social values. Children and adolescents reared to produce these formations may evolve a repetoire of shrewd and devious expressions of cruelty and destructiveness as a means of revenge and testing of others. 5) Still others, raised in seemingly healthy and socially conscious and law abiding families express violent or destructive behavior in narrowly defined forms because of superego deficit derived from some subtle communication of condoning behavior of parents or other authorities who unconsciously live out their destructive wishes through the acts of the young.

Socially sanctioned violent or destructive acts ordered and allowed by public authority in wartime may not be considered as psychopathological, nor may violent acts aroused in protection of self in the political interactions of various groups be so construed. As regards both latter categories of violent actions, certain individuals, predisposed to violence through impairment of superego formations, often indulge their individual psychopathology in overdetermined ways during wartime or in revolutionary periods. Eric Hoffer (3) epitomized well these psychopathological fringes when he stated with his characteristic penetration the following as the hangers-on of the mobs: "The poor, the misfits, the guilty, the selfish, the minorities, the sinners, the bored and the ambitious who visualize opportunities in its wake. . ."

Freud (4) first hypothesized that aggression was aroused when pleasure seeking or avoidance of pain was blocked—that is, aggression was the result of frustration. This hypothesis inspired Dollard (5) and his co-workers to elaborate a series of subsidiary hypotheses for which they found support in accounts of a variety of human actions. These hypotheses are pertinent to our current thinking about the management of violence. Therefore, allow me to repeat them:

1. Aggression is regulated by the ingroup.
2. Aggression is expressed against those who are competitors—actual or potential frustrators.
3. People who usually arouse only friendly feelings can produce marked aggression under certain circumstances.

As to the inhibition of aggression, Dollard and his co-workers postulated that:

1. The strength of inhibition of any act of aggression increases with the amount of punishment anticipated as a consequence of that act; a) injury to a loved object is punishment, b) anticipation of failure is equivalent to anticipation of punishment.
2. With the strength of *frustration* held constant, the greater the anticipation of *punishment* for a given act of aggression, the less apt the act is to occur.
3. With anticipation of *punishment* held constant, the greater the strength of *frustration,* the more apt the act is to occur.

Are these hypotheses valuable in application to everyday social problems, or even clinical problems? Man may express his aggression in activity or passivity; individually, in small groups, or in large collectives. He may express his aggression verbally through wit, sarcasm, scorn, obscenity, or silence. He may also do so through substituting another emotion toward the frustrating individual. He may substitute another person, himself, or some symbolic representation such as an inanimate object for the frustrating person.

He may discharge his aggressive impulses in games, arguments, defiant withdrawal, or creative sublimations. He may engage in violent rebellion or conscientiously conceived nonviolent protest and just as conscientiously conceived violent protest against presumed frustrators. He may use neurotic substitutions, masochism, depressive symptomatology, or schizophrenic withdrawal.

In man, aggression reveals itself actively in the motives to master, harm or destroy an object—or through passivity—to be mastered, harmed or destroyed. His aggressive drive may be modified as he fears the counter-actions of the object of aggression, leading to displacement and restriction of aims, sublimation, or by fusion with libidinal drive.

Yet the sources of aggression in deprivation and frustration are recognized as necessary for personality (ego) growth. Early in life, frustration produces only diffuse states of rage. That undifferentiated state of tension becomes directed and assumes forms of hostility toward others when the growing infant or child has developed a perceived attachment to another person. Direction of attack is a sign of personality organization, an adaptation of the early diffuse infantile protest.

Although much of the preceding has summarized the psychodynamics relating to evolution of conscience and control (superego and ego) functions within the personality, it is clear that the internalization of controls occurs in the sociodynamics of family life.

But beyond the sociodynamics of the family are those of the cultural institutions erected to support these controls. These are the supportive social processes contributing to child and family care, the system of justice in all its aspects, the legislative system, and the systems of belief distributed by the communications media including religious and political groups.

Are there sociodynamic factors today which magnify the sense of frustration in some and increase the potential for aggression? Rates for mental hospitalization, infant mortality, crime, drug addiction and all other indicators of anomie are higher for all groups who live in our urban slums. Here, too, in the social system of this country are the centers of life of those who suffer from the consequences of racism. Likewise, these urban areas are the center from which the most destructive violence has erupted within the past several years and has erupted in other societies for centuries.

On the basis of our accumulated knowledge, we may predict now that frustration levels will increase in all segments of human population where reasonable space, housing, health and educational services and effective justice fail in reasonably equitable distribution. So, too, we may predict that frustration levels will be enhanced among the disadvantaged in modern societies where the contrast in the rewards of life become conspicuously apparent to all levels of society through the use of such a powerful technological communication advance as television, a technology which enfranchises all including those living in the urban or rural ghettos. (Here, I emphasize an aspect of television contributing to the potential for violence different from that reported by Dr. Siegal who focused upon its potential for teaching violent acts to the young.)

We may predict as well that the precipitating events which release most commonly violent actions in predisposed personalities are:

1. The exposure to interpersonal situations leading to immediate threat to the security of the personality system usually in loss of a significant other person. That threat may be actual, fantasied or misperceived as in the psychotic mind. As mentioned before, violence in predatory and premeditated crime or that admitted through the permission of mobs or ordered in war are of another order where superego and social controls are nonexistent or are withdrawn in favor of the group aggression.

2. Acute forces impairing brain functions, intoxication largely, episodic dyscontrol as in epilepsy or caused by new growths, or other tissue destructive processes.

3. There is good evidence to demonstrate that where family and societal systems intrude and frustrate human behaviors related to oral and behavioral drives, the facilitating and associated violence and aggressivity increase. Witness the period of the 1920's when alcohol was, by law in the United States of America, denied. Our social system is not the first to test this hypothesis and discover its validity. Edicts have been promulgated at one time or another by various leaders as far back as the 4th century a.d., in attempts to restrict usage of such stimulants as coffee and tea (thought once to be aphrodisiac) as well as opium, heroin, peyote, mescaline (6), and so forth, as well as various food stuffs and forms of sex to no continuing avail. The only social effect has been the enhancement of the aggression and violence contained in the resulting illegitimate trade established to provide the interdicted oral or sexual behavior.

If those in government are, indeed, interested in fostering control of violence, the legislative programs and the actions of the executive and judicial branches will be so directed as to reduce the sources of increased frustration deriving from aggravations in the dynamic interchanges of the social system with individuals. The appropriate actions are clear, deriving from the information now available from history and science, and summarized briefly heretofore.

Beyond the internalization of control mechanisms, mention should be made of the necessity for internalization of ideals that may be achieved and thus allow, within the individual personality, a balance of guilt- and shame-free satisfactions.

Much more might be stated in regard to the sociodynamic importance of supporting general pleasurable activities as a means of control of violence. Unfortunately time will not allow me to expand this theme which pertains to support of the healthy socialized ego system. Here, too, the general actions to be taken by perceptive leaders, interested, informed and dedicated to social systems, seem reasonably obvious.

REFERENCES

1. KOLB, LC: Violence and aggression: An overview, in Dynamics of Violence, edited by Fawcett, J. Chicago, American Medical Association 1971, p. 7.
2. BERNARD, VW, CRANDELL, DL: Evidence for various hypotheses of social psychiatry, in Social Psychiatry, edited by Zubin, J, Freyhan, EA. New York, Grune & Stratton, 1968.
3. HOFFER, E: The True Believers. New York, Harper & Row, 1951.
4. FREUD, S: Psychoanal Study Child 3: 37, 1949.
5. DOLLARD, J, DOBB, LW, MILLER, NE, MOWRER, CH, SEARS, RR: Frustration and Aggression, New Haven, Conn., Yale University Press, 1939.
6. ORTEGA, L: Addiciones, Vicios y Estimulantes. Madrid, Alfaguara, 1966.

DISCUSSION

DR. JEROME FRANK (Baltimore, Maryland): It seems to me that Dr. Kolb's challenging last sentence should have been, at least partly, the topic of this conference. Yesterday, during the demonstration, I was thinking that we are inclined to focus on violence which is antisocial or rebellious or individual, forgetting that the real threat to survival today is violence that is organized and led by people who are highly socialized, come from intact families, have high I.Q.'s and no evidence of brain disease. Perhaps such a theme could be the basis for another conference.

Chapter 18

CRIME AND VIOLENCE IN THE UNITED STATES

RAMSEY CLARK

I am accepted as a generalist these days because I was once called Attorney General. A generalist is someone who knows more and more about less and less until he knows everything about nothing. I suppose I qualify. As a generalist you are not taken seriously or held responsible for what you say; and, because it cannot be disproved, you can make sweeping allegations.

Let me speak for a while about violence and our relation to it. The first thing society forgets is that crime, antisocial behavior, is the conduct of *people*. We create a mystique about crime. We fail to see ourselves as interdependent individuals comprising this society. For this reason, I have said, and I strongly believe, that crime reflects the character of all the people. In my judgement, a society has the capacity, in fact it has no higher duty, than to reduce antisocial conduct to a minimum. Yet this is perhaps the most vastly neglected field of activity in our time.

To me, antisocial conduct more clearly measures the quality of life, the moral temperature of a society, than any other index. It means we have people among us who care so little for others, people who are so unable to control themselves, that they destroy property or injure people. Although it would be impossible for us to agree on a moral philosophy or code, we cannot ignore this element. We need a definition on which we might be able to proceed. I suggest that we view morality as those qualities that many people have come to agree upon as desirable for making life more comfortable.

We like to think that we manage our affairs very well. But look around; see what little control there is. Some people like to look to the discipline of law. They believe that law can regiment and guide the conduct of our teeming and turbulent millions by mere dicta. I say that is utter nonsense. You cannot expect to have an appreciable impact on peoples' conduct by saying, "Do this because the law says so—or else." Obviously the problem is more complex.

It is not possible, by merely passing laws, to get people to behave. If they are behaving in ways that we do not like, let us examine the reasons. To merely look at the effect is not adequate in a mass, urban, technologically

319

advanced society. We must come to grips with the causes. I think the causes of antisocial conduct are fairly clear. It is probable that we do not want to see them because they seem so enormous, so difficult, and because their resolution will cause us to do things that we do not want to do.

Plato told us that poverty is the Mother of Crime. He meant poverty in the total range of human needs. What single factor in our society contributes more to antisocial conduct than our rationing of wealth? Deprivations in any area essential to the individual, his sense of who he is, what he wants to be, his dignity—any such—are the Mother of Crime.

Aristotle told us that the chief and universal cause of the revolutionary impulse is the desire for equality. I agree with him. What outrages an individual more than a sense of being the victim of inequality, of injustice? The deprivations which occur in the whole range of subjective and objective activities in society over a long period of time create rage. This anger can manifest itself in a loss of control and thus in a state of lawlessness.

We have to examine the quality of our society. We acknowledge that crime is both inflicted upon and inflicted by the poor. You can put it on a map. The previous speaker indicated this. It is the urban phenomenon in our urban society. If you want to improve your chances of not being a victim of robbery, move to a rural area. Chances of being a victim are $\frac{1}{35}$th less if you live outside of population centers of 25,000.

What happens if you are poor and living in Manhattan? Dr. Thomas S. Langer says that in his test group of 1034 children ages 3 to 18, 28 percent had what he called severe mental illness. They were unable to function in what he defined as one or more of five essential interpersonal relationships. Presently, 90 percent of the juvenile offenders in this country are school dropouts, and it is mostly the poor children who drop out.

Seventy-five percent of the juvenile offenders come from broken homes. After the Watts riots in August, 1965, Andy Bremer, who was then Assistant Secretary of Commerce and had the Bureau of Census under him, ran statistical tests for us. He discovered some interesting things about what was called the Curfew Zone of the city of Los Angeles. There were 485,000 people living within 45 square miles. Of the population under 18, only half lived with one or more of their natural parents.

When we look to the problems of alcoholism, drug addiction, mental retardation, and mental instability, we find that each problem has a high rate of recidivism. The common condition of these problems is that they repeat themselves. The majority of all traffic offenses in the United States are committed by people under the influence of alcohol. The 6 or 8 million alcoholics in this country constitute a complex social-medical problem.

Drug addiction is another. Some have suggested severe police measures. Do we think we can beat heroin out of the bloodstream of an addict or frighten it out of him with a gun?

The problems will not be solved by labeling and categorizing them. By simply dumping them on the criminal justice system, we will only further dehumanize ourselves. We must address ourselves to these problems because we are an interdependent people. What affects one aspect of society, affects us all.

The law can set some standards through a social compact: this is what we believe, this is what we are trying to do. Then, if there is general agreement among the people, it can take us a small way down the road. But the law cannot be effective unless it is respected; and it cannot be respected unless it is respectable. Law cannot compel respect. Respect for the law has to be won on the truth of circumstances.

How can we tell the child in the ghetto to respect the law? He lives with daily violations of law which threaten his health and safety. Where are most of the fires in Manhattan? The chance of being killed in a fire is 13 times greater for those who live in Harlem than for those on the upper East Side. He knows that. He knows about health and safety ordinances. He knows there are rats in his home. This child feels injustice. The truth seeps through, even in our complex times. Just as Aristotle said, people do not like inequality.

Historically, our reaction to discontent has been to use the two American methods of trying to enforce a rule of law: violence and segregation. In America we have glorified the power of violence and we have ignored its shame. We must examine our continuous glorification of violence from the first day we met the Indian. We must emphasize that violence is the ultimate human degradation. According to our theory of morality, what could be a greater cause of discomfort to people living together than violence? We must address the causes of violence and show that we do not believe in it. If the law is going to be effective, if it is going to be respected, if it is going to create among people a general will to obey it, it must possess a moral basis. It should not, itself, resort to violence.

Violence has no capacity as an interpersonal or international problem solver. It is no longer acceptable. We have expended too much of our cleverness and resources creating new and efficient means of killing.

As for segregation, we began segregating the Indians when we could no longer beat them into line on reservations. They are among the most deprived people in the United States. Their life expectancy is 20 years less than ours. Alaskan natives, the most segregated of all the native populations, have a life expectancy of 35.3 years. Malnutrition is the basic cause.

Their daily caloric intake is less than one-half of what is medically recommended. These 60,000 human beings are part of this society; we are interdependent. When they suffer, we suffer. What affects them, affects us all.

The specialists in this society have failed to realize that they have to work within the framework of all our needs. Examine the field of mental health. What are your priorities? What is the law doing to help? How much time is spent determining whether an individual is legally sane? What an absurd piece of business for intelligent people. We lawyers have the same argument about *de jure* and *de facto* segregation. What difference can it make to a child in a segregated school? *De facto, de jure,* private, public, what difference do the words make? Grown men on the witness stand cleverly argue with each other about legal sanity. For what end? We bend the powers of keen intellect to petty causes.

When a person commits an offense that injures someone, society has a basis for coming to grips with him. First it is necessary to determine only whether he did commit a crime. Any other concept is based on punishment. If he did it, then you have to try to address the causes of his problem. Is he an alcoholic? Is he an addict? Is he mentally retarded? Twenty-five percent of our prison population is mentally retarded, certainly a commentary on our national lack of attention to the causes of crime. We must work with the fundamental causes, the specific problems of the individual.

We will address greed, we will address racism, we will address fear. You need to tell us about that. But you need priorities. Clearly, a high priority is working with people who have committed an antisocial act. We can make a difference for them. But where do we? Show me one prison system where we make more than a gesture. Prisons do not work. No institution in our society is a greater failure. I think prisons manufacture crime.

I do not believe in operant conditioning. I do not think it can work. If we allow ourselves to think we can structure a situation and through operant conditioning get people to behave the way we want them to, we have badly misjudged our capacity to control and to cope. Instead, we must send resources to people who have been involved in antisocial conduct previously. There we could make an enormous difference. Eighty percent of all serious crime is committed by the recidivist. Why don't we work in this context?

Beyond that, you have to be the people who address themselves to societal mental health. If automobiles are going to drive us crazy, you have to tell us. Then, perhaps, we can come to grips with technology. Last year we produced more cars than babies. Is there anything within the automotive industry telling it to make fewer cars? It is the same with television. Will watching television all the time make us a vacant-headed people? You have to tell us. Somehow you must organize your skills and resources. You must find people who can address themselves to the problems which affect our entire society.

You must tell us how to be gentle. You must tell us the many ways in which technology is making us violent. You must explore everything which is dehumanizing in our society. You have to help lead us to a time when we can again see ourselves as a community.

We have gone beyond Auden's "Age of Anxiety." We are in an age of incoherence and we are moving toward unintelligibility. We need to grab hold. We have to see that the law cannot solve these problems for us. It can only help to create priorities and move us forward.

DISCUSSION

DR. SALEEM SHAH (Rockville, Maryland): I think this audience would agree with your ideas. My question pertains to the fact that in many areas we already have enough information. For example, we have known for many years that drunken drivers kill nearly twice as many people as are murdered. We also know that people subjected to involuntary civil commitment because they are mentally unstable kill only a fraction of the people killed by drunk drivers. Do I understand you to say that we need greater social commitment on the part of professionals to implement policy consistent with the known facts?

MR. RAMSEY CLARK (Washington, D.C.): The problem is that we make artificial distinctions which result in the segregation of the mentally ill, the retarded, the elderly, prisoners, blacks; but our labels do not help society. There is no pragmatic difference between what happens to the person who is civilly committed and the person who is criminally committed. Both are confined in institutions.

I talk constantly about the horror of prison confinement. Compare the confinement of those we describe as mentally ill. I think we have no right to confine people who have not inflicted some injury. We must approach the problem in a different way.

The factors implicit in forceful confinement depreciate your chances of working effectively. You can offer services to those who need them. You can hope to work with them and their families. But first you must get them to accept your good faith, for only the self-motivated will be able to work effectively with the available services. Then we can begin to make a difference.

ASSOCIATION FOR RESEARCH IN NERVOUS AND MENTAL DISEASE

Sustaining Members—1972

ANDERSON, SAMUEL W., 722 W. 168 St., New York, NY 10032

BARD, PHILIP, 725 N. Wolfe St., Baltimore, MD 21205

BATKIN, STANLEY, School of Medicine, Univ. of Hawaii, Honolulu, HA 96822

BICKFORD, REGINALD C., Dept. of Neurosciences, Univ. of California, San Diego, CAL 92037

BULLARD, DEXTER M., Chestnut Lodge, Rockville, MD 20853

DENCKLA, MARTHA B., 710 W. 168 St., New York, NY 10032

DONNELLY, JOHN, 200 Retreat Ave., Hartford, CT 06106 |

DYKEN, PAUL R., Dept. of Neurology, Section of Child Neurology, Medical College of Georgia, Augusta, GA 30902

DILDEN, DONALD H., The Wistar Inst., 36th and Spruce Sts., Philadelphia, PA 19104

ELLIOTT, FRANK A., 807 Spruce St., Philadelphia, PA 19107

HAMMILL, JAMES F., 710 W. 168 St., New York, NY 10032

HOFFMAN, JULIUS, 7805 Green Twig Rd., Bethesda, MD 20034

KLEE, CLAUDE ELISE B., 4517 Traymore St., Bethesda, MD 20014

KURTZKE, JOHN F., 7509 Salem Rd., Falls Church, VA 22043

LEVIN, JULES D., 1530 W. Spruce Court, River Hills, WI 53217

LEVY, DAVID M., 47 E. 77 St., New York, NY 10021

LIEBERMAN, JAMES S., Univ. of California School of Medicine, Dept. of Neurology, Davis, CA 95616

LORAND, SANDOR, 40 Central Park S., New York, NY 10019

MUMFORD, ROBERT S., 137 E. 66 St., New York, NY 10021

RATINOV, GERALD, 808 Memorial Prof. Bldg., Houston, TX 77025

ROSENBERG, ROGER N., 2237 Soledad Rancho Rd., San Diego, CA 92109

SAMUELS, STANLEY, 550 First Ave., New York, NY 10016

SCHEAR, MYRNA J., 710 W. 168 St., New York, NY 10032

SCHILDKRAUT, JOSEPH J., Mass. Mental Health Ctr., 74 Fenwood Rd., Boston, MA 02115

SEELYE, EDWARD E., 21 Bloomingdale Rd., White Plains, NY 10605

SUMMERS, DAVID C., 559 Prospect St., Maplewood, NJ 07040

THOMPSON, RAYMOND K., 803 Cathedral St., Baltimore, MD 21201

VORIS, HAROLD C., Mercy Medical Center, 25 St. Prarie Ave., Chicago, IL 60616

WARREN, PORTER H., 21 Bloomingdale Rd., White Plains, NY 10605

Senior Members—1972

ACKERLY, SPAFFORD, 206 E. Chestnut St., Louisville, KY 40202

ADLER, ALEXANDRA, 30 Park Ave., New York, NY 10016

BAILEY, PEARCE, 982 McCleary St., Delray Beach, FL 33444

BALSER, BENJAMIN H., 137 E. 66 St., New York, NY 10021

BRACELAND, FRANCIS J., 200 Retreat Ave., Hartford, CT 06106

BINGER, CARL, 21 Lowell St., Cambridge, MA 02138

BOWMAN, KARL M., Alaska Psychiatric Inst., 2500 Providence Ave., Anchorage, AK 99504

BROWDER, R. JEFFERSON, 200 Hicks St., Brooklyn, NY 11201

CHAMBERLAIN, OLIN B., Old Town Rd., Route 8, Charleston, SC 29407

CURRAN, FRANK J., 11 E. 87 St., New York, NY 10028
DAVIDOFF, LEO M., 73 Marshall Ridge Rd., New Canaan, CT 06840
ECHLIN, FRANCIS A., P.O. Box 342, New Paltz, NY 12561
EPSTEIN, JOSEPH, 340 E. 64th St., Yonkers, NY 10705
EVANS, JOSEPH P., Univ. of Chicago Hospital, Chicago, IL 60637
FOX, JAMES C., JR., 85 Jefferson St., Hartford, CT 06106
FREMONT-SMITH, FRANK, 16 E. 52nd St., Suite 804, New York, NY 10022
GAMMON, GEORGE D., Vet. Administration Hospital, Ann Arbor, MI 48105
GROFF, ROBERT A., Medical Tower, Suite 2306–08, 255 S. 17th St., Philadelphia, PA 19103
HAMILL, RALPH C., 8 S. Michigan Ave., Chicago, IL 60603
HARE, CLARENCE C., 880 Painted Bunting Lane, Vero Beach, FL 32960
HELDT, THOMAS J., 17 Poplar Park, Pleasant Ridge, MI 48069
HODGSON, JOHN S., 13 Jefferson Rd., Chestnut Hill, MA 02167
HOEFER, PAUL F. A., 710 W. 168th St., New York, NY 10032
HUDDLESON, JAMES R., Park Royal Convalescent Home, 2430 N.W. Marshall St., Portland, OR 97210
HUNT, EDWARD L., 330 Ocean Ave., Lawrence, NY 11559
JOHNSON, GEORGE S., 1960 Vallejo St., San Francisco, CA 94123
KUBIE, LAWRENCE S., Wheeler Lane, Route 1, P.O. Box 91-I, Sparks, MD 21152
LEAVITT, P. H., 1527 Pine St., Philadelphia, PA 19102
LITTLEJOHN, WILMOT, 2629 Aberdeen Rd., Birmingham, AL 35223
McKENNA, JOHN B., 6 Mourlyn Rd., Hanover, NH 03755
McKINNEY, JOHN M., Bridgehampton, Long Island, NY 11932
MASON, VERNE R., P.O. Box 2306, Miami Beach, FL 33140
MAYBARDUK, PETER K., 320 N. Main St., Orlando, FL
MELLA, HUGO, 333 Glebe Rd., Arlington, VA 22204
MENNINGER, KARL A., The Menninger Foundation, Box 829, Topeka, KS 66601
MERRITT, H. HOUSTON, 710 W. 168th St., New York, NY 10032
MERWARTH, HAROLD R., 30 Eighth Ave., Brooklyn, NY 11217
MEYERS, RUSSELL, Highland Clinic, P.O. Box 681, Williamson, WV 25661
MOORE, MATTHEW T., 1813 Delancey Pl., Philadelphia, PA 19103
OLDBERG, ERIC, 901 Hawthorne Pl., Lake Forest, IL 60045
PENFELD, WILDER, Montreal Neurological Inst., 3801 University St., Montreal, Canada
RAPHEAL, THEOPHILE, Univ. of Michigan Health Service, Ann Arbor, MI 48104
RAY, BRONSON S., 525 E. 58th St., New York, NY 10021
REBACK, SAMUEL, 100 Central Ave., Staten Island, NY 10301
REESE, HANS H., 3421 Circle Clos, Madison, WI 53705
ROYER, J. ELLIOTT, 1569 Jackson St., Oakland, CA 94612
SCARFF, JOHN E., 761 W. 231st St., Riverdale, NY 10471
SCOTT, MICHAEL, 3401 N. Broad St., Philadelphia, PA 19140
SIBERMANN, MAXIMILIAN, 893 Park Ave., New York, NY 10021
SOLOMON, ALFRED P., 30 Michigan Ave., Chicago, IL 60602
SOLOMON, HARRY G., 74 Fenwood Rd., Boston, MA 02115
SPIEGEL, ERNEST A., Temple Univ. Medical School, Broad and Ontario Sts., Philadelphia, PA 19140
TERHUNE, WILLIAM B., Silver Hill, Box 1177, New Canaan, CT 06840
WAGGONER, RAYMOND W., University Hospital, Neuropsychiatric Unit, Ann Arbor, MI 48104
WEIL, ARTHUR, 104-40 Green Blvd., Suite 17G, Forest Hills, NY 11375
WHOLEY, CORNELIUS, 121 University St., Pittsburgh, PA 15213
YORSHIS, MORRIS, 158 Main St., Andover, MA 01810

Active Members—1972

ABRAMS, RICHARD, 142 Columbia Heights, Brooklyn, NY 11201

ADAMS, RAYMOND D., Kennedy Laboratory, Massachusetts General Hospital, Boston, MA 02114

ADELMAN, LESTER S., Dept. of Pathology, Univ. of Virginia School of Medicine, Charlottesville, VA 22903

AGRANOFF, BERNARD W., 2960 Overridge Dr., Ann Arbor, MI 48104

AIRD, ROBERT B., Univ. of California School of Medicine, Dept. of Neurology, San Francisco, CA 94122

ALAMPRESE, DONATO J., St. Agnes Medical Center, Suite 306, Wilkens & Pine Heights Ave., Baltimore, MD 21229

ALEXANDER, EBEN, JR., Bowman Gray School of Medicine, Winston-Salem, NC 27103

ALEXANDER, LEO, 433 Marlborough St., Boston, MA 02115

ALLEN, JAMES N., Div. of Neurology, Rm. N-924, 410 W. 10 St., Columbus, OH 43210

ALLEN, MARSHALL B., JR., Medical College of Georgia, 1459 Gwinnett St., Augusta, GA 30903

ALLEN, RICHARD J., Univ. of Michigan Medical Center, Dept. of Pediatrics, Ann Arbor, MI 48104

ALLENTUCK, SAMUEL, 521 Park Ave., New York, NY 10021

ALPERS, BERNARD J., 111 N. 49 St., Philadelphia, PA 19139

ALTER, MILTON, Veterans Hospital, Dept. of Neurology, 54 E. 48 Avenue So., Minneapolis, MN 55417

ALVORD, ELLSWORTH C., JR., 5547 Windermere Rd., Seattle, WA 98105

AMOLS, WILLIAM, The Mary Imogene Bassett Hospital, Cooperstown, NY 13326

ANDERSON, MILTON H., 3700 Bellemeade Ave., Suite 109, Evansville, IN 47715

ANDERSON, PAUL J., Dir. of Neuropathology, Mt. Sinai School of Medicine, 100 St., and Fifth Ave., New York, NY 10029

ANDERSON, SAMUEL W., New York Psychiatric Inst., 722 W. 168 St., New York, NY 10032

ANDERSON, WILLIAM W., 457 Remillard Dr., Hillsborough, CA 94022

ANDY, ORLANDO J., Univ. of Mississippi Medical Center, Jackson, MS 39216

ANGRIST, BURTON, Dept. of Psychiatry, N.Y. University Medical Center, 550 First Ave., New York, NY 10016

ANSARI, KHURSHED A., V. Ad. Hospital, 54 St. & 48 Ave. So., Minneapolis, MN 55417

ARIEFF, ALEX J., 5733 N. Sheridan Rd., Chicago, IL 60626

ARING, CHARLES D., Cincinnati General Hospital, Dept. of Neurology, Cincinnati, OH 45206

ARMSTRONG, CATHERINE, 19-56 Lincoln Place, Ossining, NY 10562

ARNOLD, JESSE O., #406, 27 Elm St., Worcester, MA 01608

ARNOT, ROBERT E., 350 Beacon St., Boston, MA 02115

ARONSON, STANLEY M., 164 Summit Ave., The Miriam Hospital, Providence, RI 02906

ASCHER, ABRAHAM H., 2755 Bedford Ave., Brooklyn, NY 11210

AUSTIN, JAMES H., 128 S. Fairfax, Denver, CO 80220

AUTH, THOMAS L., 3759 Northampton N.W., Washington, DC 20015

BADAL, DANIEL W., 11328 Euclid Ave., Cleveland, OH 44106

BAILEY, ORVILLE T., Univ. of Illinois College of Medicine, Neuropsychiatric Inst. 912 S. Wood St., Chicago, IL 60612

BAKER, A. B., Univ. of Minnesota School of Medicine, Minneapolis, MN 55414

BAKER, JOHN B., 1111 Delafield St., Waukesha, WI 53186

BAKER, ROBERT N., 700 Loveland Dr., Omaha, NE 68114

BAKER, WALTER W., Eastern Pennsylvania Psychiatric Inst., Philadelphia, PA 19129

BALDESSARINA, ROSS J., Psychiatric Res. Laboratory, Massachusetts General Hospital, Boston, MA 02114

BARD, PHILIP, 725 N. Wolfe St., Baltimore, MD 21205

BARLOW, CHARLES F., 300 Longwood Ave., Boston, MA 02115

BARLOW, JOHN S., Massachusetts General Hospital, Boston, MA 02114

BARNETT, H. J. M., 1571 Gloucester Rd., London 72, Ontario, Canada

BARRETT, ROBERT E., 71 E. 77 St., New York, NY 10021

BARRON, KEVIN D., Dept. of Neurology, Albany Medical College, Albany, NY 12208

BARTECEK, ADOLF, 108 E. 81 St., New York, NY 10028

BARTLE, HARVEY, JR., 864 County Line Rd., Bryn Mawr, PA 19010

BASKA, RICHARD E., 751 E. 63 St., Kansas City, MO 64110

BATKIN, STANLEY, School of Medicine, Univ. of Hawaii, Honolulu, HI 96822

BATTISTA, ARTHUR A., N.Y. University Medical School, 550 First Ave., New York, NY 10016

BAUER, WILLIAM R., 5 Severance Circle, Cleveland Heights, OH 44118

BAZAR, PHILIP S., First National Bank Bldg., Suite 502, Montgomery, AL 36104

BELL, H. CRAIG, 1335 Highland Ave., Abington, PA 19001

BELL, ROBERT L., 51 S. 12 St., Coatesville, PA 19320

BENDER, LAURETTA, Psychiatric Inst., 722 W. 168 St., New York, NY 10032

BENNETT, IVAN F., 8452 Green Braes North Dr., Indianapolis, IN 46234

BENSON, D. FRANK, 770 Boylston St., Boston, MA 02199

BERG, LEONARD, Queeny Tower Bldg., Suite 5108, 4989 Barnes Hospital Plaza, St. Louis, MO 63110

BERG, SEYMOUR, 129 E. 80 St., New York, NY 10021

BERMAN, AARON J., 135 E. Parkway, Brooklyn, NY 11238

BERMAN, PETER H., Children's Hospital of Pennsylvania, 1740 Bainbridge St., Philadelphia, PA 19146

BERRY, RICHARD G., 1025 Walnut St., Philadelphia, PA 19107

BERTRAND, CLAUDE, 1392 Sherbrooke St. East, Montreal 24, Quebec, Canada

BICKFORD, REGINALD C., Dept. of Neurosciences, Univ. of California, San Diego, La Jolla, CA 92037

BIEHL, JOSEPH PARK, Cincinnati General Hospital, 3231 Burnett Ave., Cincinnati, OH 45229

BIELE, FLORA H., 1103 Spruce St., Philadelphia, PA 19107

BLACK, SAMUEL P. W., Univ. of Missouri Hospital, Dept. of Surgery, Columbia, MO 65201

BLAU, ABRAM, 47 E. 88 St., New York, NY 10028

BLISS, EUGENE L., Univ. of Utah Medical Center, Salt Lake City, UT 84112

BLOCK, JEROME M., 1 E. 87 St., New York, NY 10028

BOHN, Z. STEPHEN, 3800 Woodward Ave., Detroit, MI 48201

BOLDREY, EDWIN B., Univ. of California Medical School, San Francisco, CA 94122

BOOTH, CARL B., 28 Mohawk Rd., Yonkers, NY 10710

BORKOWSKI, WINSLOW J., 1324 Red Rambler Rd., Jenkintown, PA 19046

BORRUS, JOSEPH C., 184 Livingston Ave., New Brunswick, NJ 08902

BOSCHENSTEIN, FRANK, 710 W. 168 St., New York, NY 10032

BOSHES, BENJAMIN, 251 E. Chicago Ave., Suite 930, Chicago, IL 60611

BOSHES, LOUIS D., 30 N. Michigan Ave., Chicago, IL 60602

BOUZARTH, WILLIAM F., Episcopal Hospital, Front and Lehigh Sts., Philadelphia, PA 19135

BRANNON, WILLIAM, JR., 8920 Copenhaver Dr., Potomac, MD 20854

BRAUN, CARL W., 1090 Amsterdam Ave., New York, NY 10032

BRAY, PATRICK F., Univ. of Utah Medical Center, Dept. of Pediatrics, Salt Lake City, UT 84112

BRENDLER, SAMUEL J., 10 Hospital Dr., Holyoke, MA 01040

BRENNAN, JOHN H., Boston Clinical Assoc., 280 Washington St., Brighton, MA 02135

BRIDGER, WAGNER H., Albert Einstein College of Med., Eastchester Rd., New York, NY 10061

BRIDGES, THOMAS, JR., 710 W. 168 St., New York, NY 10032

BRODY, MATTHEW, 41 Eastern Parkway, Brooklyn, NY 11238

BROOKS, VERNON B., Univ. of Western Ontario, Dept. of Physiology, London 72, Ontario, Canada

BROSIN, HENRY W., 240 Sierra Vista Dr., Tuscon, AZ 85719

BROWN, A. JAMES, 710 W. 168 St., New York, NY 10032

BROWN, JASON W., 124 Marquand Ave., Bronxville, NY 10708

BROWN, JAMES MADISON, U.S. Naval Hospital, Charleston, SC 29408

BROWN, JOE R., 102-110 Second Ave., S.W., Rochester, MN 55901

BROWN, MEYER, 636 Church St., Evanston, IL 60201

BROWN, WARREN T., 3200 Silver S.W., Albuquerque, NM 87106

BROWN, WILLIAM, 37-48 90 St., Jackson Heights, NY 11372

BROWNE-MAYERS, A. N., 17 W. 54 St., New York, NY 10019

BRUUN, BERTEL, 52 E. 73 St., New York, NY 10021

BRUST, JOHN C. M., 710 W. 168 St., New York, NY 10032

BUCKLEY, PAUL J., 159 Palisades Ave., Bogota, NJ 07603

BULLARD, DEXTER M., Chestnut Lodge, Rockville, MD 20853

BUSCHKE, HERMAN, Dept. of Neurology, Albert Einstein College of Medicine, 1300 Morris Park Ave., Bronx, NY 10461

BUSSE, EWALD W., Duke Univ. School of Medicine, Dept. of Psychiatry, Durham, NC 27706

BYERS, RANDOLPH K., 300 Longwood Ave., Boston, MA 02115

CALVERLEY, JOHN R., Univ. of Texas School of Medicine, Galveston, TX 77660

CANTOR, FREDRIC K., V.A. Hospital, Neurology Service, 50 Irving St., N.W., Washington, DC 20422

CARES, REUBEN M., Kings Park State Hospital, Kings Park, NY 11754

CAREY, JOSHUA H., 1218 Bourbon St., New Orleans, LA 70116

CARLSON, EARL R., P.O. Box 2834, Pompano Beach, FL 33062

CARTER, SIDNEY, 710 W. 168 St., New York, NY 10032

CARTON, CHARLES A., 465 N. Roxbury Dr., Beverly Hills, CA 90210

CASH, PAUL T., 1405 Woodland, Des Moines, IA 50314

CASSIDY, ROBERT J., 1541 Union St., Schenectady, NY 12309

CATTANACH, GEORGE S., 115 E. 61 St., New York, NY 10021

CATTELL, JAMES P., 160 E. 84 St., New York, NY 10028

CAVENESS, WILLIAM F., National Inst. of Health, NINDB, Bldg. 363, Bethesda, MD 20014

CHAMBERLIN, HARRIE R., Univ. of N.C. School of Medicine, Dept. of Pediatrics, Chapel Hill, NC 27514

CHARLTON, MAURICE H., Univ. of Rochester, 260 Crittenden Blvd., Rochester, NY 14642

CHASE, RICHARD A., Johns Hopkins Univ. School of Medicine, Dept. of Psychiatry, Baltimore, MD 21205

CHASE, THOMAS N., NIMH, 9000 Rockville Pike, Bethesda, MD 20014

CHRZANOWSKI, GERARD, 250 E. 87 St., New York, NY 10028

CHURCHILL, JOHN A., National Institute of Research Health, 7550 Wisconsin, Perinatal Branch, Bethesda, MD 20014

CHUSID, JOSEPH C., St. Vincent's Hospital, New York, NY 10011

CLARK, WILLIAM K., 5323 Harry Hines Blvd., Dallas, TX 75235

COBB, CULLY A., JR., 539 Medical Arts Bldg., Nashville, TN 37212

CODDON, DAVID R., 1031 Fifth Ave., New York, NY 10028

COHEN, IRVIN M., 1405 Herman Professional Bldg., Houston, TX 77025

COHEN, MAYNARD M., Presbyterian-St. Luke Hospital, Dept. of Neurology, 1753 W. Congress Pkwy., Chicago, IL 60612

COHEN, NORMAN H., Dept. of Neurology, New York Medical College, 1249 Fifth Ave., New York, NY 10029

COHEN, ROBERT A., 4514 Dorset Ave., Chevy Chase, MD 20015

COHEN, SIDNEY M., 710 W. 168 St., New York, NY 10032

COHEN, ROBERT, 7221 Pyle Rd., Locust Ridge, Bethesda, MD 20034

COLE, EDWIN M., 275 Charles St., Boston, MA 02115

COLE, MALVIN, 246 S. Washington, Casper, WY 82601

COLE, MONROE, Bowman-Gray School of Medicine, Winston-Salem, NC 27103

COLLINS, WILLIAM F., JR., Yale Univ. School of Medicine, 333 Cedar St., New Haven, CT 06510

COOK, ALBERT W., 200 Hicks St., Brooklyn, NY 11201

CORRELL, JAMES W., 710 W. 168 St., New York, NY 10032

COSTA, ERMINIO, NIMH, Div. of Special Health Res., St. Elizabeth Hospital, WAW Bldg., Washington, DC 20032

COTE, LUCIEN, 630 W. 168 St., New York, NY 10032

COTTON, JOHN M., 421 W. 113 St., St. Luke's Hospital, New York, NY 10025

COTZIAS, GEORGE C., Brookhaven National Lab., Upton, L. I., NY 11973

COURSIN, DAVID B., Research Inst., St. Joseph's Hospital, Lancaster, PA 17604

COX, ARIX W., Dept. of Psychoneurology, Tulane Medical School, 1430 Tulane Ave., New Orleans, LA 70112

CRITIDES, SAMUEL D., 8-12 Clifton Pl., Jersey City, NJ 07304

CULLETON, JAMES F., 421 Huguenot St., New Rochelle, NY 10801

CURRY, HIRAM B., 536 N. Hobcaw Dr., Mt. Pleasant, SC 29464

CUTLER, ROBERT W. P., 5529 Cornell Ave., Chicago, IL 60637

DALE, ROBERT T., 5544 Tenth Ave. So., Minneapolis, MN 55417

DANFORTH, ROBERT C., 700 N. Water St., Milwaukee, WI 53202

DAVEY, LYCURGUS M., 2 Church St. So., New Haven, CT 06519

DAVIS, COURTLAND H., JR., Bowman-Gray School of Medicine, Winston-Salem, NC 27103

DAVIS, JEAN P., 3003 Good Hope Rd., W., Milwaukee, WI 53209

DAVIS, JOHN M., Tennessee Neuropsychiatric Central State Psychiatric Hospital, Nashville, TN 37217

DAWSON, DAVID M., 41 Monument St., Concord, MA 01742

DEFRIES, ZIRA, 40 E. 83 St., New York, NY 10028

DEICHELMANN, STEPHEN J., 305 Dreshertown Rd., Ft. Washington, PA 19034

DEJONG, RUSSELL N., Univ. Hospital, Ann Arbor, MI 48104

DE LA TORRE, ERNESTO, 1900 S. Hawthorne Rd., Suite 256, Winston-Salem, NC 27103

DE LA TORRE, JACK C., Univ. of Chicago Hospital, Div. of Neurological Surgery, Chicago, IL 60637

DEMUTH, EDWIN L., 14 Soundview Ave., White Plains, NY 10606

DEMYER, WILLIAM E., Indiana Univ. Medical Center, Indianapolis, IN 46207

DENAPOLI, ROBERT A., 710 W. 168 St., New York, NY 10032

DENBO, ELIC A., 300 Broadway, Suite 907, Stevens Bldg., Camden, NJ 08103

DENNY-BROWN, DEREK E., 3 Mercer Circle, Cambridge, MA 02138

DENCKLA, MARTHA B., 710 W. 168 St., New York, NY 10032

DERBY, BENNETT M., V.A. Hospital, First Ave. at E. 24 St., New York, NY 10010

D'ERRICO, ALBERT, 3707 Gaston St., Dallas, TX 75246

DICKEL, HERMAN A., Portland Medical Center, Suite 1308, 511 S.W. Tenth Ave., Portland, OR 97205

DILLON, HAROLD, 275 S. 19 St., Philadelphia, PA 19103

DODGE, PHILIP R., Dept. of Pediatrics, Washington Univ., 500 S. Kingshighway, St. Louis, MO 63110

DONNELLY, JOHN 200 Retreat Ave., Hartford, CT 06106

DONNENFELD, HYMAN, St. Vincent's Hospital, 153 W. 11 St., New York, NY 10011

DOW, ROBERT S., 2525 N.W. Lovejoy, Portland, OR 97210

DOYLE, ARTHUR M., N. York General Hospital, 4001 Leslie St., Suite 805D, Willowdale, Ontario, Canada

DRAYER, CALVIN S., 811 Lafayette Rd., Bryn Mawr, PA 19010

DREIFUSS, FRITZ E., Univ. of Virginia Hospital, Charlottesville, VA 22903

DREW, ARTHUR L., JR., Indiana Univ. Medical Center, 111 W. Michigan, Indianapolis, IN 46202

DRIBBEN, IRVING S., Albany Medical Center Hospital, Albany, NY 12208

DUFFY, PHILIP D., 75 Prospect St., Demarest, NJ 07627

DUNSMORE, REMBRANDT H., 85 Jefferson St., Hartford, CT 06106

DUNSTONE, H. CARTER, 101 Three Rivers Apt., Fort Wayne, IN 46802

DUTY, JOSEPH E., 3204 W. River Rd., Toledo, OH 43614

DUVOISIN, ROGER C., 1212 Fifth Ave., New York, NY 10029

DYKEN, MARK L., Indiana Univ. Medical Center, 1100 W. Michigan, Indianapolis, IN 46202

DYKEN, PAUL R., Dept. of Neurology, Section of Child Neurology, Medical College of Georgia, Augusta, GA 30902

EARLE, KENNETH M., Armed Forces Inst. of Pathology, Washington, DC 20306

EBERHART, JOHN C., NIMH, Clinical Center, Room 3N-242, Bethesda, MD 20014

EBIN, JUDAH, 101 S.E. 3rd St., Permanent Savings Bldg., Evansville, IN 47708

ECKER, ARTHUR D., 407 University Ave., Syracuse, NY 13210

EFFRON, ABRAHAM S., 220 E. 33 St., Paterson, NJ 07504

EGANA, ENRIQUE, Instituteo de Medicine Experimental Hospital Clinico, S. Vincente, Santiago, Chile

EICHMAN, PETER L., 5033 La Crosse St., Madison, WI 53701

EISENBERG, LEON, 1 Sparks Pl., Cambridge, MA 02138

EISENDORFER, ARNOLD, 11 E. 68 St., New York, NY 10021

ELIZAN, TERESITA S., Mt. Sinai Hospital School of Medicine, Dept. of Neuro. Fifth Ave. and 100th Sts., New York, NY 10029

ELKES, JOEL, Johns Hopkins Univ. School of Medicine, Dept. of Psychiatry, Baltimore, MD 21205

ELLINGSON, ROBERT J., Nebraska Psychiatric Inst., 602 S. 45 St., Omaha, NE 68105

ELLIOTT, FRANK A., 807 Spruce St., Philadelphia, PA 19107

ELLISON, GEORGE W., Dept. of Neurology, UCLA Center for Health Sciences, Los Angeles, CA 90024

ELMORE, JOHN D., Suite 510 Professional Bldg., 800 Montclair Rd., Birmingham, AL 35213

ENGISCH, ROBERT R., P.O. Box 106, Williston, VT 05495

EPSTEIN, SAMUEL H., 220 Marlborough St., Boston, MA 02116

ERKULVRAWATR, SAMARD, Dept. of Neurology, 180F, V.A. Hospital, Augusta, GA 30904

ESSER, ROBERT A., 240 North St., Harrison, NY 10528

EVANS, HARRISON S., Loma Linda University, Loma Linda, CA 92354
EVERTS, WILLIAM H., 2910 N. Flagler Dr., West Palm Beach, FL 33407

FAHN, STANLEY, Dept. of Neurology 710 W. 168 St., New York, NY 10032
FAILLACE, LOUIS A., Univ. of Texas Medical School at Houston, 102 Jesse Jones Library Bldg., Houston, TX 77025
FARMER, THOMAS W., Univ. of N.C. School of Medicine, Chapel Hill, NC 27514
FARMER, RODNEY A., 200 Township Line Rd., Elins Park, PA 19177
FEIGIN, IRWIN H., 54-24 Brownvale Lane, Douglaston, NY 11362
FEINBERG, IRWIN, Chief of Psychiatry, Ft. Miley V.A. Hospital, 42 Ave. and Clement St., San Francisco, CA 94121
FELDMAN, DANIEL S., Dept. of Neurology, Medical College of Georgia, Augusta, GA 20902
FELDMAN, ROBERT C., 74 Rita Rd., Braintree, MA 02184
FELIX, ROBERT H., St. Louis Univ. School of Medicine, 1402 S. Grand Blvd., St. Louis, MO 63104
FERINGA, EARL R., 1030 Cedar Bend Dr., Ann Arbor, MI 48105
FERMAGLICH, JOSEPH, Georgetown Univ. Medical Center, 3800 Reservoir Rd., N.W., Washington, DC 20007
FERRIS, GREGORY S., 1542 Tulane Ave., New Orleans, LA 70112
FIELDS, WILLIAM S., 6301 Almeda Rd., Houston, TX 77021
FIEVE, RONALD R., 722 W. 168 St., New York, NY 10032
FINK, MAXIMILIAN, Dept. of Psychiatry, S.U.N.Y. at Stony Brook, Stony Brook, NY 11790
FINKELHOR, HOWARD B., Mellon Pavilion, 4815 Liberty Ave., Pittsburgh, PA 15224
FINLEY, KNOX H., 450 Sutter St., San Francisco, CA 94108
FINNEY, JOSEPH C., Dept. of Educational Psychology, Univ. of Kentucky, Lexington, KY 40506
FISH, BARBARA, 16428 Sloan Dr., Los Angeles, CA 90049
FISH, DAVID J., 355 Thayer St., Providence, RI 02906
FISHMAN, DONALD, Hahnemann Hospital, 230 N. Broad St., Philadelphia, PA 19102
FISHMAN, ROBERT A., Univ. of California, San Francisco Medical Center, Dept. of Neurology, San Francisco, CA 94122
FLANIGAN, STEVENSON, Univ. of Arkansas School of Medicine, Little Rock, AR 71655
FLICKER, DAVID J., 606 S. Orange St. at S. Kingman Rd., So. Orange, NJ 07079
FLOWERS, HILAND L., 2780 Arlington Ave., New York, NY 10463
FOLEY, ARCHIE R., 142 E. 38 St., New York, NY 10016
FOLEY, JOSEPH M., Univ. Hospital, Cleveland, OH 44106
FOGELSON, M. HAROLD, 295 Erkenbrecker Ave., Cincinnati, OH 45229
FORD, HAMILTON, 200 University Blvd., Galveston, TX 77550
FORREST, DAVID V., 155 W. 68 St., New York, NY 10032
FORSTER, FRANCIS M., Univ. Hospital, Univ. of Wisconsin, Madison, WI 53706
FRAZIER, SHERVERT H., McLean Hospital, 115 Mill St., Belmont, MA 02178
FREED, HERBERT, 255 S. 17 St., Philadelphia, PA 19103
FREEDMAN, DAVID A., 1200 Moursund Ave., Houston, TX 77025
FREEDMAN, HOWARD, 175 Eastern Pkwy, Brooklyn, NY 11238
FREIMAN, ISRAEL S., 37 W. 70 St., New York, NY 11023
FRIEDHOFF, ARNOLD J., 550 First Ave., New York, NY 10016
FRIEDMAN, ARNOLD P., 71 E. 77 St., New York, NY 10021
FRIMMER, ISIDORE, 1227 Grand Concourse, Bronx, NY 10452
FROSCH, WILLIAM A., N.Y. University Medical Center, 550 First Ave., New York, NY 10016
FUNKHOUSER, JAMES B., 2 Albemarle Ave., Richmond, VA 23226

GABAY, SABIT, V.A. Hospital, Biochemical Research Lab., Brockton, MA 02401
GAELEN, LESLIE H., 550 Washington Ave., San Diego, CA 92103
GALBRAITH, JAMES C., Medical College of Alabama, Birmingham, AL 35205
GAMBOA, EUGENIA T., 710 W. 168 St., New York, NY 10032
GAMEZ, GILBERTO L., 45-13 St., New Manila, Quezon City, Philippines
GANG, KENNETH M., 30 Greenridge Ave., White Plains, NY 10605
GARCIA, JULIO H., Anatomic Pathology Laboratory, Div. of Neuropathology, Univ. of
    Maryland Hospital, 22 S. Greene St., Baltimore, MD 21201
GAROFALO, MICHAEL, JR., St. Vincent's Hospital, 153 W. 11 St., New York, NY 10011
GARVIN, JOHN S., 912 S. Wood St., Chicago, IL 60612
GASSEL, M. MICHAEL, 425 Warren Dr., San Francisco, CA 94131
GATES, EDWARD M., The Harbin Clinic, Rome, GA 30161
GATFIELD, P. D., Children's Psychiatric Research Inst., London, Ontario, Canada
GELLER, LESTER M., Div. of Neuropathology, College of Physicians and Surgeons, 630 W
    168 St., New York, NY 10032
GERSHON, SAMUEL, 82 Dartmouth St., Forest Hills, NY 11375
GESCHWIND, NORMAN, 137 Clinton Rd., Brookline, MA 02146
GILDEA, EDWIN F., 4940 Audubon Ave., St. Louis, MO 63110
GILDEN, DONALD H., The Wistar Inst., 36 and Spruce Sts., Philadelphia, PA 19104
GILLEN, H. WILLIAM, 1601 Doctor's Circle, Wilmington, NC 28401
GILMAN, SID, College of Physicians and Surgeons, Dept. of Neurology, 630 W. 168 St.,
    New York, NY 10032
GILROY, JOHN, Harper Hospital, 3825 Brush St., Detroit, MI 48201
GLASER, GILBERT H., Yale Univ. School of Medicine, 333 Cedar St., New Haven, CT
    06510
GLUSMAN, MURRAY, 722 W. 168 St., New York, NY 10032
GOLD, ARNOLD P., 710 W. 168 St., New York, NY 10032
GOLD, MAX, 47 Plaza St., Brooklyn, NY 11217
GOLDBERG, HAROLD H., 280 Prospect Ave., Hackensack, NJ 07601
GOLDENSOHN, ELI S., 710 W. 168 St., New York, NY 10032
GOLDIN, GERALD S., 111 E. 210 St., Bronx, NY 10467
GOLDIN, GURSTON D., 166 E. 63 St., New York, NY 10021
GOLDMAN, DOUGLAS, 179 E. McMillan St., Cincinnati, OH 45219
GOLDSTEIN, MURRAY, NINDS, NIH, Bethesda, MD 20014
GOLDSTEIN, NORMAN P., Mayo Clinic, Rochester, MN 55901
GOMEZ, ANTONIO J., 425 Dorset St., Apt. 18, So., Burlington, VT 05401
GOMEZ, MANUEL R., Mayo Clinic, Rochester, MN 55901
GOTTSCHALK, LOUIS A., College of Medicine, Univ. of California Irvine, Irvine, CA 92664
GRAUBERT, DAVID N., 3 Shelter Rock Rd., Manhasset, L.I., NY 11030
GRAY, GEORGE H., JR., 133 Warwick Dr., Pittsburgh, PA 15241
GREEN, DAVID, 930 Madison Ave., Albany, NY 12208
GREEN, HARRY, Smith, Kline, and French Lab., Philadelphia, PA 19101
GREEN, LAWRENCE, 315 Maple Ave., Swarthmore, PA 19081
GREEN, JOSEPH B., Medical College of Georgia, Augusta, GA 30902
GREEN, MARTIN A., 1 Barstow Rd., Great Neck, NY 11021
GREENBERG, ALVIN D., 2 Church St., New Haven, CT 11576
GREENBERG, I. MELBOURNE, 62 The Hemlocks, Roslyn Estate, Roslyn, NY 11576
GREENE, JUSTIN L., 164 E. 72 St., New York, NY 10021
GREENHILL, MAURICE H., 70 Hampton Rd., Scarsdale, NY 10583
GREER, MELVIN, Univ. of Florida School of Medicine, Gainesville, FL 32601

GRINKER, ROY R., SR., 910 N. Lake Shore Dr., Chicago, IL 60611

GROSSMAN, ROBERT, Albert Einstein College of Medicine, Dept. of Neurosurgery, 1300 Morris Park Ave., Bronx, NY 10461

GRUENBERG, ERNEST, 722 W. 168 St., New York, NY 10032

GUMNIT, ROBERT J., Div. of Neurology, 640 Jackson St., St. Paul, MN 55101

GURDJIAN, E. S., 3800 Woodward Ave., #808, Detroit, MI 48201

GURIAN, HARVEY, Mary Imogene Bassett Hospital, Cooperstown, NY 13326

GUTTMAN, LUDWIG, Route 7, Box 514, Morgantown, WV 26505

GUTTMAN, SAMUEL A., Hunters Green, Pennington, NJ 08534

GUZE, SAMUEL, Washington Univ. School of Medicine, Dept. of Psychiatry, 4940 Audubon Ave., St. Louis, MO 63110

HAASE, GUNTER R., 799 Robinhood Dr., Rosemont, PA 19010

HAMBURG, DAVID A., Stanford Univ. School of Medicine, Dept. of Psychiatry, Stanford, CA 94305

HAMILTON, FRANCIS J., 21 Bloomingdale Rd., White Plains, NY 10605

HAMLIN, HANNIBAL, 270 Benefit St., Providence, RI 02903

HAMMILL, JAMES F., 710 W. 168 St., New York, NY 10032

HAND, MORTON H., 1620 Ditmas Ave., Brooklyn, NY 11226

HANNA, GEORGE R., Univ. of Virginia School of Medicine, Div. of Neurology, Charlottesville, VA 22904

HANSON, PEGGY A., 2777 Rosendale Rd., Niskayuna, NY 12309

HARDING, GEORGE T., 445 E. Granville Rd., Worthington, OH 44106

HARPER, EDWARD O., 2040 Abington Rd., Cleveland, OH 44106

HARRIS, HENRY E., 123 S. Munn Ave., East Orange, NJ 07018

HARTER, DONALD H., 710 W. 168 St., New York, NY 10032

HASENBUSH, LESTER L., 315 Buckminster Rd., Brookline, MA 02146

HASS, WILLIAM KARL, N.Y. University School of Medicine, 550 First Ave., New York, NY 10016

HAWKINS, J. ROBERT, 411 Oak St., Suite 201, Cincinnati, OH 45219

HAYMAKER, WEBB, NASA Ames Research Center, Moffett Field, CA 94035

HAYWARD, JAMES NEIL, Dept. of Neurology, UCLA School of Medicine, 405 Highland Ave., Los Angeles, CA 90024

HEATH, ROBERT G., Tulane Univ. School of Medicine, 1430 Tulane Ave., New Orleans, LA 70112

HEDLEY-WHYTE, E. TESSA, Childrens Hospital Medical Center, 300 Longwood Ave., Boston, MA 02115

HEIMAN, MARCEL, 1148 Fifth Ave., New York, NY 10028

HEILMAN, KENNETH M., Div. of Neurology, Univ. of Florida College of Medicine, Gainesville, FL 32601

HELFER, LEWIS M., 208 Medical Professional Bldg. 1303 N. McCullough, San Antonio, TX 75212

HELLER, IRVING H., 3801 University St., Montreal 112, Quebec, Canada

HERRMANN, CHRISTIAN, JR., Univ. of California Medical Center, Los Angeles, CA 90024

HILLS, JOHN R., New England Medical Center, 171 Harrison Ave., Boston, MA 02111

HIMWICH, HAROLD E., Galesburg State Res. Hospital, Galesburg, IL 61401

HINSEY, JOSEPH C., Chateau Lorraine, Apt. 5-M, Scarsdale, NY 10583

HINTERBUCHNER, LADISLAV, Brooklyn Cumberland Medical Center, 39 Auburn Pl., Brooklyn, NY 11205

HOAGLAND, HUDSON, 222 Maple Ave., Shrewsbury, MA 01545

HOEHN, MARGARET, 3851 S. Xanthia St., Denver, CO 80237
HOENIG, EUGENE M., N.Y. Medical College, Center for Chronic Diseases, Bird S. Coler Hospital, Roosevelt Is., NY 10017
HOFFMAN, JULIUS, 7805 Green Twig Rd., Bethesda, MD 20034
HOFFMAN, STEPHEN F., 926 Mt. Kisco Dr., San Antonio, TX 78213
HOGAN, EDWARD L., Dept. of Neurology, Medical Univ. of S. Carolina, 80 Barre St., Charleston, SC 29401
HOLMES, THOMAS H., Univ. of Washington, Dept. of Psychiatry, University Hospital, Seattle, WA 98105
HOMMES, OTTO R., Radbout University Hospital, Nymegan, Netherlands
HORENSTEIN, SIMON, 1221 S. Grand Blvd., St. Louis, MO 63104
HORST, ELMER L., 1134 Penn Ave., Wyomissing, PA 19610
HORWITZ, SAMUEL J., 5 Severance Circle, Cleveland Heights, OH 44116
HOUFEK, EDWARD E., 417 Security Bank Bldg., Sheboygan, WI 53081
HOUSEPIAN, EDGAR M., 710 W. 168 St., New York, NY 10032
HUBBARD, OSCAR H., 53-47 97 St., Corona, NY 11368
HUBER, WARREN V., Dir. of Neurology Serv. 112L, V.A. Central Office, Washington, DC 20420
HUDSON, ARTHUR, 8 Doncaster Ave., London, Ontario, Canada
HUDSON, ROBERT J., Physt. Bldg., 121 University Pl., Pittsburgh, PA 15213
HUERTAS, JORGE, 11555 Arroyo Oaks, Los Altos Hills, CA 94022
HULBURT, MARGARET, (R.N.) RFD 2, Petersburg, NY 12138
HUNTER, RALPH W., Hitchcock Clinic, Hanover, NH 03755

IVEY, EVELYN P., Arthur Brisbane Child Treatment Center, P.O. Box 625, Farmingdale, NJ 07727

JACOBS, ERWIN M., 7 Fox St., Poughkeepsie, NY 12601
JACOBS, LAWRENCE D., The Dent Neurologic Inst., Millard Fillmore Hospital, 3 Gates Circle, Buffalo, NY 14209
JACOBSON, SHERWOOD ARTHUR, 328 E. 18 St., New York, NY 10003
JAFFE, JOSEPH, 722 W. 168 St., New York, NY 10032
JARCHO, LEONARD W., Univ. of Utah Medical Center, Dept. of Neurology, 3 E. 512, Salt Lake City, UT 84112
JASPER, HERBERT H., 804 Upper Lansdowne Ave., Westmount 217 P. Quebec, Canada
JENKINS, RAMON B., Dept. of Neurology, 110 Irving St., Washington Hospital, Washington, DC 20010
JEUB, ROBERT P., 1747 Medical Arts Bldg., Minneapolis, MN 55402
JOHNS, THOMAS R., II, Univ. of Virginia Hospital, Charlottesville, VA 22903
JONAS, SARAN, 566 First Ave., New York, NY 10016
JOYNT, ROBERT J., Univ. Hospital, Dept. of Neurology, Iowa City, IA 52240

KAELBER, WILLIAM W., Basic Science Bldg., Univ. of Iowa, Iowa City, IA 52242
KAELBING, RUDOLF, 1386 Friar Lane, Columbus, OH 43221
KALINOWSKY, LOTHAR B., 115 E. 82 St., New York, NY 10028
KANDEL, ERIC R., Public Health Res. Institute, 455 First Ave., New York, NY 10016
KAPLAN, HAROLD I., 50 E. 78 St., New York, NY 10020
KAPLAN, HARRY A., 57 Montague St., Brooklyn, NY 11201
KAPLAN, LAWRENCE I., 812 Park Ave., New York, NY 10021
KARLINER, WILLIAM, 20 Franklin Rd., Scarsdale, NY 10583

KAUFMAN, MOSES R., 19 E. 98 St., New York, NY 10029
KAWI, ALI A., Downstate Medical Center, 450 Clarkson Ave., Brooklyn, NY 11203
KEILL, STUART L., NYS Dept. of Mental Hygiene, Two World Trade Ctr.–56th floor, New York, NY 10047
KELLER, N. J. A., 1008 Elm Ave., Takoma Park, MD 20012
KENNARD, MARGARET A., 130 Tarrytown Rd., Manchester, NH 03103
KENNEDY, CHARLES, 5115 Allan Terrace, Bethesda, MD 20016
KETY, SEYMOUR S., Dept. of Psychiatry, Mass. General Hospital, Boston, MA 02114
KING, ARTHUR B., 728 S. Main St., Athens, PA 18810
KLEE, CLAUDE ELISE P., 4517 Traymore St., Bethesda, MD 20014
KLINE, NATHAN S., Rockland State Hospital, Orangeburg, NY 10962
KOENIG, HAROLD, V.A. Research Hospital, 333 E. Huron St., Chicago, IL 60611
KOENIGSBERGER, M. R., 27 Rodney Pl., Demarest, NJ 07627
KOFMAN, OSCAR, 99 Avenue Rd., Ste. 608, Toronto, Ontario, Canada
KOKMAN, EMRE, Dept. of Neurology, University Hospital, Ann Arbor, MI 48104
KOLB, LAWRENCE C., Psychiatric Inst., 722 W. 168 St., New York, NY 10032
KOEPPEN, ARNULF H., 23 Salem Rd., Delmar, NY 12054
KOLODNY, EDWIN H., E.K.S. Center for Mental Retardation, 200 Trapelo Rd., Waltham, MA 02154
KOPIN, IRWIN J., NIMH, Laboratory of Clinical Science, Bethesda, MD 20014
KOREIN, JULIUS, 25 E. 83 St., New York, NY 10028
KOTT, EDNA, Dept. of Neurology, Beilinson Hospital, Petah Tikva, Israel
KRAL, VOJTECH, Dept. of Psychiatry, University Hospital, 339 Windermere Rd., London, Ontario, Canada
KREIGER, HOWARD P., 960 Park Ave., New York, NY 10028
KUBIK, CHARLES S., Lincoln Rd., Lincoln, MA 01773
KURTZKE, JOHN F., 7509 Salem Rd., Falls Church, VA 22043

LAIDLAW, ROBERT W., 563 Park Ave., New York, NY 10021
LAKE, GEORGE L., 520 Franklin Ave., Garden City, NY 11530
LAKKE, JOHANNES, P.W.F., Lokveenweg 8, Haren (Gr.), Netherlands
LAMBROS, VASILIOS, 623 W. Duarte Rd., Arcadia, CA 91006
LANDAU, WILLIAM M., Washington Univ. Dept. of Neurology, 6605 Euclid Ave., School of Medicine, St. Louis, MO 63110
LANDRY, CHRISTOPHER L., 170 Merrimack St., Lowell, MA 01852
LANE, MARK H., 1010 Los Lomas Rd., N.E., Albuquerque, NM 87106
LANGFITT, THOMAS W., Pennsylvania Hospital, 34th and Spruce Sts., Philadelphia, PA 19107
LANGWORTHY, ORTHELLO, 112 Melrose Avenue E., Baltimore, MD 21212
LAPHAM, LOWELL W., Dept. of Pathology, Univ. of Rochester Medical Center, 260 Crittenden Blvd., Rochester, NY 14642
LAPOVSKY, ARTHUR J., 887 Ocean Ave., Brooklyn, NY 11226
LAWYER, TIFFANY, JR., Montefiore Hospital, New York, NY 10467
LAYZER, ROBERT, Univ. of California School of Medicine, Dept. of Neurology, San Francisco, CA 94122
LEBENSOHN, ZIGMOND M., 2015 R St., N.W., Suite 101, Washington, DC 20009
LEHRER, GERARD M., Mt. Sinai Hospital, Dept. of Neurology, 11 E. 100 St., New York NY 10029
LEOPOLD, ROBERT L., Dept. of Community Medicine, Univ. of Pennsylvania, 36th and Hamilton Walk, Philadelphia, PA 19104

Lesse, Stanley, 15 W. 81 St., New York, NY 10024

Levens, Arthur J., 3819 Roseneath St., Olney, MD 20832

Levin, Grant, 2300 Sutter St., San Francisco, CA 95115

Levin, Jules D., 1530 W. Spruce Court, River Hills, WI 53217

Levin, Paul M., 1227 Medical Arts Bldg., Dallas, TX 75201

Levy, Daniel, 810 King St., Hamilton, Ontario 22, Canada

Levy, David M., 47 E. 77 St., New York, NY 10021

Levy, Irwin, Queeny Tower Bldg., Suite 5108, 4989 Barnes Hospital Plaza, St. Louis, MO 63110

Levy, Lewis L., 111 Park St., New Haven, CT 06511

Levy, Sol, 407 Paulsen Medical and Dental Bldg., Spokane, WA 99201

Lewis, Linda D., 710 W. 168 St., New York, NY 10032

Lewis, Nolan D. C., Route #5, Frederick, MD 21701

Liberson, Wladimir T., Box #28, V.A. Hospital, Hines, IL 60141

Lieberman, Abraham N., 566 First Ave., New York, NY 10016

Lieberman, James S., Dept. of Neurology, Univ. of California School of Medicine, Davis, CA 95616

Lifshitz, Kenneth, 22 Waverly Pl., Monsey, NY 10952

Lindemann, Erich, Stanford Medical Center, Stanford, CA 94305

Lipin, Theodore, 11 E. 87 St., New York, NY 10028

Lipkin, Lewis E., 9913 Belhaven Rd., Bethesda, MD 20034

Liss, Leopold, Dept. of Pathology, 320 W. 10 Ave., Columbus, OH 43210

Livingston, E. Arthur, 125 E. 87 St., New York, NY 10028

Lhamon, William T., 525 E. 68 St., New York, NY 10021

Livingston, Kenneth E., The Wellesley Hospital, 160 Wellesley St., E., Toronto, 5 Ontario, Canada

Locascio, Nicholas R., 139 Westminster Dr., Yonkers, NY 10710

Locksley, Herbert B., Univ. Hospital, Div. of Neurosurgery, Iowa City, IA 52240

Loeser, Eugene W., 10 Parrott Mill Rd., Chatham, NJ 07928

Loman, Julius, 10 Hammond Pond Pkwy., Chestnut Hill, MA 02167

Lombroso, Cesare T., 300 Longwood Ave., Boston, MA 02115

London, Jack, 114-20 Queens Blvd., Forest Hills, NY 11375

Long, W. L., 2038 Locust St., Philadelphia, PA 19103

Lorand, Sandor, 40 Central Park S., New York, NY 10019

Lorenz, Albert A., Box 224, Eau Claire, WI 54701

Lorenzo, Antonio V., Children's Hospital Medical Center, Pediatrics Res. Bldg., Boston, MA 02115

Loscalzo, Anthony, 137 E. 36 St., New York, NY 10016

Low, Niels L., 710 W. 168 St., New York, NY 10032

Lowenbach, Hans, Duke Hospital, Durham, NC 27706

Lowis, Samuel, 475 Commonwealth Ave., Boston, MA 02115

Lubic, Lowell G., 1878 Shaw Ave., Pittsburgh, PA 15217

Luton, Frank H., Vanderbilt Univ. Hospital, Nashville, TN 37212

McCaman, Richard E., Div. of Neurosciences, City of Hope Medical Center, Duatre CA 91010

McDowell, Fletcher H., New York Hospital-Cornell Medical Center, 1300 York Avenue, New York, NY 10016

McGovern, John P., 6655 Travis St., Houston, TX 77025

McGrath, John F., 3 E. 68 St., New York, NY 10021

McHenry, John T., Wayne State Univ. College of Medicine, 3825 Brush St., Detroit, MI 48201

McHugh, Paul R., 21 Bloomingdale Rd., White Plains, NY 10605

McKinney, William M., Dept. of Neurology, Bowman-Gray School of Medicine, Winston-Salem, NC 27103

McKnight, William K., 21 Bloomingdale Rd., White Plains, NY 10605

McLaurin, Robert L., Cincinnati General Hospital, Cincinnati, OH 45229

McMasters, Robert E., Univ. of Texas Medical School at San Antonio, 7702 Floyd Curl Dr., San Antonio, TX 78229

McNaughton, Francis L., 3801 University St., Montreal, Canada

McNerney, John C., 83 Morgan St., Stamford, CT 06903

MacPherson, Donald J., 1101 Beacon St., Brookline, MA 02146

Madonick, Moses J., 1882 Grand Concourse, New York, NY 10057

Madow, Leo, Medical College of Pennsylvania, 3300 Henry Ave., Philadelphia, PA 19129

Magee, Kenneth R., Univ. Hospital, Dept. of Neurology, 1313 E. Ann St., Ann Arbor, MI 48104

Magladery, John W., The Johns Hopkins Hospital, 601 N. Broadway, Baltimore, MD 21205

Malitz, Sidney, 722 W. 168 St., New York, NY 10032

Maltby, George L., 31 Bramhall St., Portland, ME 04102

Mancall, Elliott L., Dept. of Medicine, Hahnemann Medical College, 230 Broad St., Philadelphia, PA 19102

Mandel, Martin M., Benson Manor, Suite 110, Township Line, Washington Lane, Jenkintown, PA 19024

Marcus, Elliott M., 171 Harrison Ave., Boston, MA 02111

Margolis, George, Dartmouth Medical School, Dept. of Pathology, Hanover, NH 03755

Margulies, Murray E., 1002 Avenue "J", Brooklyn, NY 11230

Maringer, Simon, 1225 Park Ave., New York, NY 10028

Markham, Charles H., Dept. of Neurology, UCLA School of Medicine, Los Angeles, CA 90024

Marotta, Joseph T., 8 Peebles Ave., Don Mills, Ontario, Canada

Marshall, Curtis, 103 Medical Arts Bldg., Baltimore, MD 21201

Martin, Herbert L., DeGoesbriand Memorial Hospital, Burlington, VT 05401

Masland, Richard L., 710 W. 168 St., New York, NY 10032

Mastri, Angeline R., 1770 Bryant Ave. S., Minneapolis, MN 55043

Matthews, Richard J., Pharmakon Lab., 1140 Quincy Ave., Scranton, PA 18510

Matthysse, Steven, Res. 4, Massachusetts General Hospital, Boston, MA 02114

Mattson, Richard, Yale Univ. School of Medicine, Sect. of Neurology, New Haven, CT 06510

Meisel, Arthur M., 90 Eighth Ave., Brooklyn, NY 11215

Meislin, Jack, 5 Howard Dr., Spring Valley, NY 10977

Mello, Nancy K., 560 North St., S.W., Apt. N912, Washington, DC 20024

Meltzer, Theodore, 123 E. 37 St., New York, NY 10016

Mendelson, Jack H., Boston City Hospital, 818 Harrison Ave., Boston, MA 02118

Menken, Matthew, 7 Wirt St., New Brunswick, NJ 08901

Merlis, Jerome K., University Hospital, Baltimore, MD 21201

Merlis, Sidney, Carleton Ave., Central Islip, NY 11722

Michael, Stanley, 21 Bloomingdale Rd., White Plains, NY 10605

Michels, Robert, 722 W. 168 St., New York, NY 10032

Michelsen, Jost J., 710 W. 168 St., New York, NY 10032

MICKEL, HUBERT S., 300 Longwood Ave., Boston, MA 02115
MILLER, CLAUDE H., 7 Park Ave., New York, NY 10017
MILLER, JAMES R., 175 Riverside Dr., New York, NY 10024
MILLER, LEROY, 717 Encino Pl. N.E., Albuquerque, NM 87106
MILLER, RAYMOND, 1725 W. Harrison St., Chicago, IL 60612
MILLER, ROBERT B., Fairfield Hills Hospital, Newton, CT 06470
MILLET, JOHN P., 45 East End Ave., New York, NY 10028
MILLICHAP, J. GORDON, 720 N. Michigan, Suite 1620, Chicago, IL 60611
MILLIKAN, CLARK H., Mayo Clinic, Rochester, MN 55901
MILNER, BRENDA, Montreal Neurological Inst., 3801 University St., Montreal, 112, Quebec, Canada
MITCHELL, CLIFFORD L., Riker Labs. Inc., 3M Center Bldg., 218-2, St. Paul, MN 55101
MONCKTON, GEORGE, Univ. Hospital, Edmonton, Alberta, Canada
MONES, ROBERT J., 1212 Fifth Ave., New York, NY 10029
MOORE, DONALD F., 1315 W. Tenth St., Indianapolis, IN 46202
MOOSSY, JOHN, Dept. of Pathology (Neuro), Univ. of Pittsburgh, Pittsburgh, PA 15213
MORRIS, CHARLES E., Univ. of N.C. School of Medicine, Chapel Hill, NC 27514
MORTON, BENJAMIN F., Baptist Medical Center-Professional Bldg., 801 Princeton Ave., Suite 601, Birmingham, AL 35211
MOSOVICH, ABRAHAM, Arenales 2198, Buenos Aires, Argentina
MOUNT, LESTER A., 710 W. 168 St., New York, NY 10032
MULFORD, EDWIN H., II, 5 Elmcrest Terrace, Norwalk, CT 06850
MUMFORD, ROBERT S., 137 E. 66 St., New York, NY 10021
MUNSAT, THEODORE L., Div. of Neurology, UCLA School of Medicine, Los Angeles, CA 90024

NAGLER, BENEDICT, Lynchburgh Training School and Hospital, P.O. Box 1098, Lynchburg, VA 24505
NARDINI, JOHN E., 5921 Bradley Blvd., Bethesda, MD 20014
NASHOLD, BLAINE, Duke Medical Center, Durham, NC 27706
NATHANSON, MORTON, 1035 Park Ave., New York, NY 10028
NEGRIN, JUAN, JR., 108 E. 81 St., New York, NY 10028
NELLHAUS, GERARD, Univ. of Colorado Medical Center, 4200 E. 9th Ave., Denver, CO 80220
NETSKY, MARTIN G., Univ. of VA, School of Medicine, Dept. of Pathology, Charlottesville, VA 22903
NEUMANN, JAMES W., 2929 Baltimore, Suite 215, Kansas City, MO 64108
NIELSEN, AAGE, 3800 Woodward St., Detroit, MI 48229
NISWANDER, G. DONALD, 105 Pleasant St., Concord, NH 03301
NORSA, LUIGIA, 155 E. 76 St., New York, NY 10021
NURNBERGER, JOHN I., Indiana Univ. Medical Center, 1100 W. Michigan, Indianapolis, IN 46202

O'BRIEN, JOSEPH L., 710 W. 168 St., New York, NY 10032
O'DOHERTY, DESMOND S., Georgetown Univ., Dept. of Neurology, Washington, DC 20007
OKAZAKI, HARUO, Mayo Clinic, Rochester, MN 55902
O'LEARY, JAMES L., Washington Univ. School of Medicine, Dept. of Neurology, 6605 Euclid Ave., St. Louis, MO 63110
OLSEN, AXEL K., 1700 Benjamin Franklin Pkwy., The Windsor, Suite 2307, Philadelphia, PA 19103

O'Neil, Jane F., 21 Bloomingdale Rd., White Plains, NY 10605
O'Reilly, Sean, George Washington Univ. Medical Center, 2150 Pennsylvania Ave., N.W., Washington, DC 20037
Ornsteen, A. M., 2007 Delancey Pl., Philadelphia, PA 19103
Osborne, Raymond L., 140 E. 54 St., New York, NY 10022
Osler, Geoffrey F., 1175 York Ave., New York, NY 10021

Pacella, Bernard L., 115 E. 61 St., New York, NY 10021
Paddison, Richard M., 1542 Tulane Ave., New Orleans, LA 70112
Page, W. Randolph, 4900 St. Charles Ave., New Orleans, LA 70101
Palmer, Edwin J., 1130 Second St. S.W., Roanoke, VA 24016
Parker, Joseph B., Box 3167, Duke Univ. Medical Center, Durham, NC 27706
Parr, Justin L., Hahnemann Hospital, 230 N. Broad St., Philadelphia, PA 19152
Pasik, Pedro, The Mt. Sinai Hospital, New York, NY 10029
Pasik, Tauba, The Mt. Sinai Hospital, New York, NY 10029
Patel, Aneel N., Towers of Colonie, Bldg. 3, Apt. 332, 424 Sand Creek Rd., Albany, NY 12205
Payne, Charles A., 185 Mimosa St., Santa Maria, Rio Piedras, PR 00927
Pearson, Manuel M., 111 N. 49 St., Philadelphia, PA 19139
Penn, Audrey S., Dept. of Neurology, 710 W. 168 St., New York, NY 10032
Penry, James Kiffin, 502 Mannakee St., Rockville, MD 20850
Perlo, Vincent P., 275 Charles St., Boston, MA 02114
Perret, George, University Hospital, Iowa City, IA 52240
Peters, Henry A., 1300 University Ave., Madison, WI 53706
Peterson, Arthur L., 111 N. 49 St., Philadelphia, PA 19139
Pfeiffer, Carl C., Renner Bldg., N.J.N.P.I., Box 1000, Princeton, NJ 08540
Pfeiffer, John B., Jr., Duke Univ. School of Medicine, Durham, NC 27706
Pietri, Raoul, 601 Grand Ave., Asbury Park, NJ 07712
Pinney, Edward L., Jr., 148 E. 78 St., New York, NY 10021
Pisetsky, Joseph E., 26 Braemar Ave., New Rochelle, NY 10804
Pittman, Hal W., 302 W. Thomas Rd., Phoenix, AZ 85103
Pitts, Ferris N., Jr., Finn, Irvin and Pitts, Ltd., 1035 Bellevue Ave., Suite 202, St. Louis, MO 63117
Platman, Stanley, 80 Goodrich St., Buffalo, NY 14203
Plum, Fred, N.Y. Hospital-Cornell Medical Center, Dept. of Neurology, New York, NY 10021
Pollack, Seymour L., 511 Edgewood Dr., New Castle, IN 47362
Pollack, George H., 180 N. Michigan Ave., Chicago, IL 60601
Pope, Alfred, Longwood Towers, Brookline, MA 02146
Porter, Huntington, 171 Harrison Ave., Boston, MA 02111
Poser, Charles M., De Goesbriand Univ. Medical Center Hospital of Vt., Burlington, VT 05401
Prince, David A., Dept. of Neurology, Stanford Univ. Medical Center, Stanford, CA 94305
Prockop, Leon, Philadelphia General Hospital, Philadelphia, PA 19104

Quinn, Philip, 280 Washington St., Brighton, MA 02135

Raine, Cedric S., Dept. of Neuropathology, Albert Einstein College of Medicine, 1300 Morris Park Ave., Bronx, NY 10461

RAINER, JOHN D., 722 W. 168 St., New York, NY 10032
RANDT, CLARK T., 550 First Ave., New York, NY 10016
RANSOHOFF, JOSEPH, 550 First Ave., New York, NY 10016
RAPIN, ISABELLE, Albert Einstein College of Medicine, Bronx, NY 10461
RASMUSSEN, THEODORE, 3801 University St., Montreal, Canada
RATINOV, GERALD, 808 Memorial Professional Bldg., Houston, TX 77025
RAU, RAYMOND L., 3515 Fifth Ave., 600 Medical Center Bldg., Pittsburgh, PA 15213
REIS, DONALD J., Cornell University-Medical College, 1300 York Ave., New York, NY 10021
REIVICH, MARTIN, Dept. of Neurology, Univ. of Pennsylvania, Philadelphia, PA 19104
RHEE, SANG C., Box 64, 710 W. 168 St., New York, NY 10032
RICHARDSON, EDWARD P., JR., Massachusetts General Hospital, Boston, MA 02114
RICHARDSON, J. CLIFFORD, 170 St. George St., Toronto, Canada
RICHARDSON, ROY B., 50 Alexander St., Apt. 304, Toronto 5, Canada
RICHTER, CURT, The Johns Hopkins Medical School, Henry Phipps Clinic, Baltimore, MD 21205
RICHTER, RALPH W., 700 W. 168 St., New York, NY 10032
RINSLEY, DONALD B., Adolescent Unit, Dir. of Children's Section, Topeka State Hospital, 2700 W. Sixth St., Topeka, KS 66606
RIOCH, DAVID McK., Walter Reed Army Inst. of Research, Div. of Neuro-Psychiatry, Washington, DC 20212
ROBB, PRESTON, 3801 University St., Montreal 2, Canada
ROBERTS, LAMAR, 138 S.W. 15th St., Ocala, FL 32670
ROBERTS, M. P., JR., Div. of Neurosurgery, Univ. of Connecticut School of Medicine, 2 Holcomb St., Hartford, CT 06112
ROBIE, THEODORE R., 1 Upper Mountain Ave., Montclair, NJ 07042
ROBINS, ALVIN L., 205 Engle St., Englewood, NJ 07631
ROBINS, ELI, Washington Univ. School of Medicine, Dept. of Psychiatry, 4940 Audubon Ave., St. Louis, MO 63110
ROBINSON, FRANKLIN, 100 York St., New Haven, CT 05511
RODIN, ERNEST A., Lafayette Clinic, 951 E. Lafayette, Detroit, MI 48207
ROEMER, EDWARD P., 1194 Oxford Rd., San Marino, CA 91108
ROFFWARG, HOWARD P., 390 West End Ave., New York, NY 10024
ROIZIN, LEON, 722 W. 168 St., New York, NY 10032
ROMANUL, FLAVIU C. A., Boston Univ. School of Medicine, 80 E. Concord St., Boston, MA 02118
ROMANO, JOHN, Strong Memorial Hospital, 260 Crittenden Blvd., Rochester, NY 14620
ROME, HOWARD P., 622 Fifth St., Rochester, MN 55901
ROSALES, REMEDIOS K., 54 Ellis Rd., W. Newton, MA 02105
ROSE, AUGUSTUS S., Univ. of California Medical Center, Los Angeles, CA 90024
ROSEMAN, EPHRAIM, Louisville General Hospital, 323 E. Chestnut St., Louisville, KY 40202
ROSENBERG, ROGER N., 2237 Soledad Rancho Rd., San Diego, CA 92109
ROSENBERG, SEYMOUR J., 18 Hasketh St., Chevy Chase, MD 20075
ROSENBLUM, JAY A., 226 E. 68 St., New York, NY 10021
ROSOMOFF, HUBERT L., Dept. of Neurological Surgery, Univ. of Miami, P.O. Box 875, Biscayne Annex, Miami, FL 33152
ROSS, ALEXANDER T., Indiana Univ. Medical Center, Indianapolis, IN 46207
ROTHBALLER, ALAN B., 1249 Fifth Ave., New York NY 10029
ROTTERSMAN, WILLIAM, 490 Peachtree St., N.E., Suite 368-C, Atlanta, GA 30308
ROVIT, RICHARD L., St. Vincent's Hospital and Medical Center, Dept. of Neurology, 153 W. 11th St., New York, NY 10011

ROWLAND, LEWIS P., 710 W. 168 St., New York, NY 10032
RUBIN, SIDNEY, 133 Esplanade Dr., Rochester, NY 14610
RUESCH, JURGEN, Univ. of California School of Medicine, San Francisco, CA 94122
RUMBERG, JOAN, 55 Hampton Oval, New Rochelle, NY 10805
RUSHTON, JOSEPH C., 200 First St., Rochester, MN 55901
RYAN, JAMES, 722 W. 168 St., New York, NY 10032

SABRA, ALBERT B., Weizman Inst. of Science, Behovor, Israel
SABRA, FUAD, American University, Beirut, Lebanon
SACKLER, MORTIMER, 15 E. 62 St., New York, NY 10021
SACKLER, RAYMOND, 15 E. 62 St., New York, NY 10021
SAENZ-ARROYO, LUIS, Montes Urales No. 717, Lomas de Chapultepec, Mexico, DF
SAHS, ADOLPH L., University Hospital, Iowa City, IA 52240
SALAAN, MARIA ZABRIENSKA, Massachusetts General Hospital, Neurology Dept., Boston, MA 02114
SAMSON, FREDERICK E., JR., Dir., Kansas Ctr. for Mental Retardation, Univ. of Kansas Medical Center, Kansas City, KS 66103
SAMUELS, STANLEY, 550 First Ave., New York, NY 10016
SATTERFIELD, JAMES H., Dir. of Research Gateway Hospital, 1891 Effie St., Los Angeles, CA 90026
SATTIN, ALBERT, Dept. of Biochemistry, Maudsley Hospital, Denmark Hill, London S.E. 5, England
SCANLON, WILSON, G., 709 Lomax St., Jacksonville, FL 32204
SCHACHTER, JEROME M., 3 Park Ave., Binghamton, NY 13903
SCHACHTER, JOSEPH, 201 DeSota St., Pittsburgh, PA 15213
SCHAERER, JACQUES P., 777 S. New Dallas Rd., St. Louis, MO 63131
SCHARF, JOHN H., 555 Park Ave., New York, NY 10021
SCHATZ, NORMAN J., 255 S. 17 St., Philadelphia, PA 19103
SCHEAR, MYRNA J., 710 W. 168 St., New York, NY 10032
SCHEINBERG, LABE C., Albert Einstein College of Medicine, Eastchester Rd., New York, NY 10061
SCHEINBERG, PERITZ, The Institute, Jackson Memorial Hospital, Miami, FL 33136
SCHILDKRAUT, JOSEPH L., Massachusetts Mental Health Center, 74 Fenwood Rd., Boston, MA 02115
SCHLESINGER, EDWARD B., 710 W. 168 St., New York, NY 10032
SCHLEZINGER, NATHAN S., 255 S. 17 St., Philadelphia, PA 19103
SCHMIDT, RICHARD P., Univ. of Florida College of Medicine, Gainesville, FL 32601
SCHNECK, STUART A., Univ. of Colorado Medical Center, Div. of Neurology, 4200 E. 9th Ave., Denver, CO 80220
SCHNEIDER, RICHARD C., University Hospital, Dept. of Neurosurgery, Ann Arbor, MI 48104
SCHNITKER, MAX T., 425 Jefferson Ave., Toledo, OH 43603
SCHUELEIN, MARIANNE, 3208 44 St., N.W., Washington, DC 20016
SCHUMACHER, GEORGE A., Dept. of Neurology, DeGoesbriand Unit, Univ. of Vt. College of Medicine, Burlington, VT 05401
SCHWARTZ, HENRY G., Barnes Hospital Plaza, St. Louis, MO 63110
SCHWARTZ, JAMES F., Emory Univ. School of Medicine, Atlanta, GA 30303
SCIARRA, DANIEL, 710 W. 168 St., New York, NY 10032
SCOVILLE, WILLIAM B., 85 Jefferson St., Hartford, CT 06106
SEELYE, EDWARD E., 21 Bloomingdale Ave., White Plains, NY 10605
SELVERSTONE, BERTRAM, 205 Waterman St., Providence, RI 02906

SENCER, WALTER, 1185 Park Ave., New York, NY 10028

SENERCHIA, FRED F., JR., 38 Aberdeen Rd., Elizabeth, NJ 07208

SENGSTAKEN, ROBERT W., 166 E. Main St., Huntington, NY 11743

SHANDS, HARLEY C., Roosevelt Hospital, 428 W. 59 St., New York, NY 10019

SCHANZER, STEFAN, 710 Park Ave., New York, NY 10021

SHAPIRO, MORTIMER F., 960 Park Ave., New York, NY 10028

SHAPIRO, SIDNEY K., 1218 Medical Arts Bldg., Minnaepolis, MN 55402

SHARP, LEWIS A., 165 E. 35 St., New York, NY 10016

SHENKIN, HENRY A., Episcopal Hospital, Front St. and Lehigh Avenue, Philadelphia, PA 19125

SHIELD, JAMES A., 212 W. Franklin St., Richmond, VA 23220

SHOPSIN, BARON, Dept. of Psychiatry, Neuropsychopharmacology, Research Unit, N.Y. Univ. Medical Center, New York, NY 10016

SHUTER, ELI R., 1221 S. Grand Bldv., St. Louis, MO 63104

SIBLEY, WILLIAM A., 7949 E. Mable Dr., Tucson, AZ 85715

SIEKERT, ROBERT G., Mayo Clinic, 200 First St., Rochester, MN 55901

SILBERBERG, DONALD H., Univ. of Pennsylvania Hospital, Dept. of Neurology, Philadelphia, PA 19104

SILLER, EVERARD J., The University of Texas Medical School, Dept. of Physiology and Medicine, Sect. of Neurosciences, 6703 Floyd Curl Dr., San Antonio, TX 78229

SILVERMAN, ALBERT J., Dept. of Psychiatry, Univ. of Michigan Medical School, Ann Arbor, MI 48104

SILVERMAN, DANIEL, 408 Waring Rd., Elkins Park, PA 19117

SILVERSTEIN, ALEXANDER, 1829 Pine St., Philadelphia, PA 19103

SILVERSTEIN, ALLEN, 215 Blauvelt Ave., Ho-Ho-Kus, NJ 07423

SIMMS, LEON M., 1187 Ocean Ave., Brooklyn, NY 11230

SIMON, BENJAMIN, 10 Hawthorne Pl., Charles River Park, Boston, MA 02114

SIMON, John L., P.O. Box 6102, Loiza St. Station, Santurce, P.R. 00914

SIMPSON, JOHN F., Dept. of Neurology, Univ. of Michigan Medical School, Ann Arbor MI 48104

SINGER, ROBERT P., 811 Horsepen Rd., Richmond, VA 23229

SIRIS, JOSEPH H., 10 Split Rock Dr., Great Neck, NY 11024

SKULTETY, F. MILES, Univ. of Nebraska College of Medicine, Dept. of Surgery, 42 St. and Dewey Ave., Omaha, NE 68105

SLOANE, R. BRUCE, Univ. of S. California, Los Angeles, CA 90033

SLOSBERG, PAUL S., 1040 Park Ave., New York, NY 10029

SMITH, BERNARD H., 462 Grider St., Buffalo, NY 14215

SMITH, BUSHNELL, The Chetwynd, Apt. 608, Rosemont, PA 19010

SMITH, GERARD P., 21 Bloomingdale Rd., White Plains, NY 10605

SMYTHIES, JOHN RAYMOND, Mandsley Hospital, Denmark Hill, London, England

SNYDER, SOLOMON, Dept. of Pharmacology, Johns Hopkins Univ., Baltimore, MD 21205

SOBIN, ALLAN J., 60 Plaza St., Brooklyn, NY 11238

SOKOLOFF, LOUIS, NIMH, Bethesda, MD 20014

SOLOMON, SEYMOUR, Montefiore Hospital, New York, NY 10467

SORIANO, VICTOR, Calle Buenos Aires 363, Montevideo, Uruguay

SPOTNITZ, HYMAN, 41 Central Park W., New York, NY 10023

SPROFKIN, BERTRAM H., 237 Medical Arts Bldg., Nashville, TN 37212

STAFFORD, WALTER F., JR., 24 Tudor Pl., Buffalo, NY 14222

STALEY, ROBERT W., 538 Medical Arts Bldg., Pittsburgh, PA 15213

STARBUCK, HELEN L., 384 Post St., San Francisco, CA 94108

STEIN, AARON, 1140 Fifth Ave., New York, NY 10028

STELLAR, STANLEY, St. Barnabas Hospital, 3rd and 183rd Sts., New York, NY 100Ľ*⁄*

STERN, LAWRENCE Z., Arizona Medical Center, 1501 N. Campbell Ave., Tucson, AZ 85724

STERN, MARVIN, 184 Rugby Rd., Brooklyn, NY 11226

STEWART, MARK ARMSTRONG, Child Psychiatry Serv., 500 Newton Rd., Iowa City, IA 52240

STOWELL, AVERILL, 11511 S. Peoria, Tulsa, OK 74120

STRACHAN, JOYCE S. H., 2050 Seward Ave., APT. 1F, BRONX, NY 10473

STROBOS, ROBERT B. J., New York Medical College, Dept. of Neurology, Fifth Ave. at 105 St., New York, NY 10029

STROEBEL, CHARLES F., Dir. Psychophysiology, Inst. of Living, 400 Washington St. Hartford, CT 06102

STUNKARD, ALBERT J., Dept. of Psychiatry, Stanford Univ. School of Medicine, Stanford, CA 94305

SUGERMAN, A. ARTHUR, 125 Roxboro Rd., Trenton, NJ 08638

SULLIVAN, JOHN F., New England Center Hospital, Boston, MA 02111

SUMMERS, DAVID C., 559 Prospect St., Maplewood, NJ 07040

SUMMERS, THOMAS B., 1403 Woodland Ave., Doctor's Park, Des Moines, IA 50309

SUNG, JOO HO, Univ.of Minnesota School of Medicine, Div. of Neurology, Minneapolis, MN 55414

SUTER, CARY G., Medical College of Va., 1200 E. Broad St., Richmond, VA 23219

SUVER, PHILLIP J., 510 Cobb Medical Center, Seattle, WA 98101

SWANSON, AUGUST G., Dir. of Academic Affairs, Assn. of American Medical Colleges, ℀1 DuPont Circle N.W., Suite 20, Washington, DC 20036

SWEET, WILLIAM H., 35 Chestnut Pl., Brookline, MA 02135

TALBERT, O. RHETT, Medical College Hospital, 55 Doughty St., Charleston, SC 29403

TAREN, JAMES A., Sect. of Neurosurgery, Univ. of Michigan Medical Center, Ann Arbor, MI 48104

TARLOV, ISADORE M., 1034 Fifth Ave., New York, NY 10028

TASKER, WILLIAM G., Philadelphia Children's Hospital, 1740 Bainbridge, Philadelphia, PA 19146

TAYLOR, JUDITH M., 27 Hampton Rd., Scarsdale, NY 10583

TAYLOR, MICHAEL, 9 Convent Pl., Hartsdale, NY 10530

TERRY, ROBERT D., Albert Einstein College of Medicine, Eastchester Rd. and Morris Park Ave., Bronx, NY 10461

THOMAS, MADISON H., 330 Ninth Ave., Salt Lake City, UT 84103

THOMPSON, GEORGE N., 2010 Wilshire Blvd., Los Angeles, CA 90057

THOMPSON, HARTWELL G., Charleston Div. West Virginia University Medical Center, Charleston, WV 25326

THOMPSON, LLOYD J., Kingmill Rd., Chapel Hill, NC 27514

THOMPSON, RAYMOND K., 803 Cathedral St., Baltimore, MD 21201

THORNER, MELVIN W., Neurology Service, (180) V.A. Hospital, Downey, IL 60064

TIMBERLAKE, WILLIAM H., Lemuel Shattuck Hъspital, 170 Morton St., Jamaica Plains, MA 02130

TISSENBAUM, MORRIS J., 67 E. Cheshire Pl., Staten Island, NY 10301

TOOLE, JAMES F., Bowman-Gray School of Medicine, Dept. of Neurology, Winston-Salem, NC 27103

TORNAY, ANTHONY S., 2038 Locust St., Philadelphia, PA 19103

TOURLENTES, THOMAS T., Dir. CCMHC, 2701 17 St., Rock Island, IL 61201
TOURTELLOTTE, WALLACE W., 1229 Chautaugua Blvd., Pacific Palisades, CA 90272
TRAWICK, JOHN D., 1204 Heyburn Bldg., Louisville, KY 40202
TRUFANT, SAMUEL A., Cincinnati General Hospital, Cincinnati, OH 45229
TUCKER, JOLYON S., 85 Jefferson St., Hartford, CT 06103
TUCKER, WEIR M., 212 W. Franklin St., Richmond, VA 23220
TURNER, ARTHUR J., 425 E. Wisconsin Ave., Milwaukee, WI 53202
TURNER, OSCAR A., 1009 Boardman-Canfield Rd., Boardman, OH 44512
TWITCHELL, THOMAS E., 171 Harrison Ave., Boston, MA 02111
TYLER, H. RICHARD, 169 Fisher Ave., Brookline, MA 02146

ULLMAN, MONTAGUE, Maimonides Hospital, Dept. of Psychiatry, 4802 Tenth Ave., Brooklyn, NY 11219

VALSAMIS, MARIUS P., 681 Clarkson Ave., Brooklyn, NY 11203
VAN ALLEN, MAURICE W., University Hospital, Dept. of Neurology, Iowa City, IA 52240
VAN BOGAERT, LUDO, Institut Bunge, 59 Rue Filip Williot, Berchem, Anvers, Belgium
VAN DEN NOORT, STANLEY, 1800 Port Taggart Pl., Newport Beach, CA 92660
VANDER EECKEN, HENRY, Coupre 27 Ghent, Belgium
VICALE, CARMINE T., 710 W. 168 St., New York, NY 10032

WACHS, HIRSH, Allegheny General Hospital, 320 E. North Ave., Pittsburgh, PA 15212
WADSWORTH, RICHARD C., 187 Juniper St., Bangor, ME 04401
WALKER, HERBERT E., 165 E. 35 St., Suite 6F, New York, NY 10016
WALLNER, JULIUS M., 1405 E. Ann St., Ann Arbor, MI 48104
WALTZ, ARTHUR G., Univ. of Minnesota Hospital, Minneapolis, MN 55455
WARD, ARTHUR A., JR., Univ. of Washington School of Medicine, Seattle, Wash 98105
WARD, JAMES W., Vanderbilt Medical School, Dept. of Anatomy, Nashville, TN 37203
WARNER, FRANCIS J., P.O. Box 523, Philadelphia, PA 19105
WARREN, PORTER, 21 Bloomingdale Rd., White Plains, NY 10605
WATSON, ROBERT, 1026 Donaghey Bldg.,Little Rock, AR 72201
WATTERS, GORDON V., Dept. of Neurology, The Montreal Children's Hospital, 2300 Tupper St., Montreal 108, Quebec, Canada
WEBSTER, HENRY DEF., Lab. of Neuropathology, Neuroscience Bldg., 26, NIH, Bethesda, MD 20014
WEICKHARDT, GEORGE D., 5225 Burke Dr., Alexandria, VA 22309
WEINER, HERBERT, Montefiore Hospital, Div. of Psychiatry, New York, NY 10461
WEINER, LEWIS M., 927 Northfield Rd., Woodmere, NY 11498
WEISS, ARTHUR H., 910 Park Ave., New York, NY 10021
WEISS, DESO A., 1680 York Ave., New York, NY 10028
WEISSMAN, WILLIAM K., 5 W. 86 St., 18C, New York, NY 10024
WEITZMAN, ELLIOT D., Montefiore Hospital, Dept. of Neurology, Bronx, NY 10467
WELLS, CHARLES E., Vanderbilt Univ. School of Medicine, Nashville, TN 37203
WERNER, GERHARD, Dept. of Pharmacology, Univ. of Pittsburgh, School of Medicine, Pittsburgh, PA 15213
WEST, LOUIS JOLYON, 760 Westwood Plaza, Los Angeles, CA 99024
WHARTON, RALPH N., 40 E. 62 St., New York, NY 10021
WHELAN, JOSEPH L., 820 Arlington Dr., Petoskey, MI 49770
WHITCOMB, BENJAMIN B., 85 Jefferson St., Hartford, CT 60106
WHITE, HARRY HOUSTON, Dept. of Neurology, University of Missouri Medical Center Columbia, MO 65201

WHITEHORN, JOHN C., 210 Northfield, Baltimore, MD 21210

WHITSELL, LEON J., 909 Hyde St., San Francisco, CA 94109

WHITTIER, JOHN R., Creedmoor Institute, Box 12, Station 60, Jamaica, NY 11427

WIEDMAN, OTTO G., 31 Woodland St., Hartford, CT 06105

WIKLER, ABRAHAM, Univ. of Kentucky College of Medicine, Dept. of Psychiatry, Lexington, KY 40506

WILLIAMS, ERNEST Y., 5208 Colorado Ave., Washington, DC 20011

WILLIAMS, ROBERT L., Dept. of Psychiatry, Baylor College of Medicine, Texas Medical Center, Houston, TX 77025

WILLIAMS, SHIRLEY Y., Norwalk Hospital, Norwalk, CT 06852

WILLNER, HERMAN H., 675 Old Country Rd., Westbury, NY 11590

WILSON, WILLIAM P., Duke Univ. Medical Center, Box 3355, Durham, NC 27710

WILSON, WILLIAM W., 561 Fairthorne St., Philadelphia, PA 19128

WINOKUR, GEORGE, Iowa Psychopathic Hospital, Iowa City, IA 52240

WITTSON, CECIL L., 9651 N. 29 St., Omaha, NE 68112

WOLF, ABNER, 630 W. 168 St., New York, NY 10032

WOLF, SHELDON MARK, Southern California Permanente Medical Group, 4900 Sunset Blvd., Los Angeles, CA 90027

WOOD, ERNEST H., 710 W. 168 St., New York, NY 10032

WOODALL, J. MARTIN, 1020 Center St., Boston, MA 02130

WOOLSEY, JOYCE E., Dept. of Neurology, St. Louis Univ. School of Medicine, 1325 S. Grand Ave., St. Louis, MO 63103

WOOLSEY, ROBERT M., St. Lousi Univ. School of Medicine, Dept. of Neurology, St. Louis, MO 63103

WRIGHT, R. LEWIS, 4908 Monument Ave., Richmond, VA 23230

YAHR, MELVIN, 710 W., 168 St., New York, NY 10032

YAKOVLEV, PAUL I., 21 Addington Rd., Brookline, MA 02133

YASKIN, H. EDWARD, The Raben Bldg., Suite 22, 807Haddon Ave., Haddonfield, NJ 08033

YATSU, FRANK, San Francisco General Hospital, Rm. 4521, 22nd and Potrero Sts., San Francisco, CA 94110

ZEIFERT, MARK, 1065 South St., Fresno, CA 93721

ZFASS, ISADORE S., 2502 Monument Ave., Richmond, VA 23220

ZIEGLER, FREDERICK M., Community Hospital of the Monterey Peninsula, Box HH Carmel, CA 93921

ZIER, ADOLFO, 663 Queen Anne Rd., Teaneck, NJ 07666

ZIMMERMAN, EARL A., 710 W. 168 St., New York, NY 10032

ZIMMERMAN, HARRY H., Dept. of Pathology, Montefiore Hospital & Medical Center, 111 E. 210 St., Bronx, NY 10467

ZITRIN, ARTHUR, N.Y. University School of Medicine, 550 First Ave., New York, NY 10016

Associate Members—1972

BACH, L. M. N., Univ. of Nevada Sch. of Medical Sciences, Div. of Biomedical Sciences, Reno, NV 89507

BARR, MURRAY L., University of Western Ontario, Department of Anatomy, 346 South Street, London, Ontario, Canada

BEACH, FRANK A., University of California, Department of Psychology, Berkeley, CA 94704

BERRY, CHARLES M., Seton Hall College of Medicine, Department of Anatomy, Jersey City, NJ 07304

BODIAN, DAVID, 709 N. Wolfe St., Baltimore, MD 21205

BOTELHO, STELLA Y., University of Pennsylvania, Department of Physiology, Philadelphia, PA 19104

BREMER, FREDERIC, 115 Bd. de Waterloo, Brussels, Belgium

BRONK, DETLEV W., National Academy of Sciences, 2101 Constitution Avenue, Washington, DC 20025

BROOKS, CHANDLER, 450 Clarkson Avenue, Brooklyn, NY 11203

BURR, HAROLD S., Sterling Hall of Medicine, New Haven, CT 06510

CAMPBELL, BERRY, Functional Correlates-B, University of California, Irvine, CA 92664

CARPENTER, MALCOLM B., 185 Delhi Road, Scarsdale, NY 10583

CHAMBERS, WILLIAM W., University of Pennsylvania School of Medicine, Department of Anatomy, Philadelphia, PA 19104

CHATFIELD, PAUL O., Harvard Medical School, Department of Physiology, 25 Shattuck St., Boston, MA 02115

COMROE, JULIUS H., JR., Cardiovascular Research Institute, University of California, San Francisco, CA 94122

COWEN, DAVID, 630 W. 168th St., New York, NY 10032

CROSBY, ELIZABETH C., 5502 Kresge Medical Research, University of Michigan, Ann Arbor, MI 48104

DAVIS, HALLOWELL, Central Institute for the Deaf, 818 S. Kingshighway, St. Louis, MO 63110

DURELL, JACK, The Psychiatric Institute, 2141 K Street N.W., Washington, DC 20037

ELLIOTT, K. A. C., McGill University, Department of Biochemistry, 3801 University St., Montreal, Canada

FLEXNER, LOUIS B., University of Pennsylvania School of Medicine, Department of Anatomy, Philadelphia, PA 19104

FOLCH-PI, JORDI, Research Laboratory, McLean Hospital, Belmont, MA 02178

FREYGANG, WALTER H., JR., National Institutes of Health, Bethesda, MD 20014

FUORTES, M. G. F., Route 1, Layhill, Silver Spring, MD 20906

GATES, REGINALD H., 46 Lincoln House, Basil, Knightsbridge, S.W. 3, London, England

GRENELL, ROBERT G., University of Maryland School of Medicine, Baltimore, MD 21201

GRUNDFEST, HARRY, 630 W. 168th St., New York, NY 10032

HEBB, D. O., McGill University, Department of Psychology, Montreal 2, Canada

HENRY, CHARLES E., Cleveland Clinic, Department of Neurology, 2020 E. 93rd St., Cleveland, OH 44106

HINES, MARION, 1514 Berwick Road, Ruxton, MD 21204

HOVDE, CHRISTIAN A. (REV.), Bishop Anderson Foundation, 714 S. Marshfield Avenue, Chicago, IL 60612

KABAT, ELVIN A., 710 W. 168th St., New York, NY 10032

KIES, MARION W., National Institute of Mental Health, Laboratory of Cerebral Metabolism, Bethesda, MD 20014

KLÜVER, HENRICH, 305 Culver Hall, University of Chicago, Chicago, IL 60637

LABROSSE, ELWOOD H., Department of Surgery, University of Maryland Medical School, Baltimore, MD 21201

LARRABEE, MARTIN G., The Johns Hopkins University, Department of Biophysics, Baltimore, MD 21218

LASSER, ARTHUR M., 80 E. Concord St., Boston, MA 02118

LILLY, JOHN C., Communication Research Institute, 3430 Main Highway, Coconut Grove, FL 33133

LIVINGSTON, ROBERT B., University of California, Department of Neurosurgery, San Diego, CA 92037

LLOYD, DAVID P. C., Rockefeller Institute for Medical Research, 66th St. and York Ave., New York, NY 10021

LOWRY, OLIVER H., Washington University School of Medicine, Euclid Ave. and Kingshighway, St. Louis, MO 63110

McCOUCH, GRAYSON P., R.D. 4, Westchester, PA 19380

MAGOUN, HORACE W., University of California School of Medicine, Los Angeles, CA 90024

MALMO, ROBERT B., 1025 Pine Avenue, Montreal 2, Canada

MANERY, JEANNE F., University of Toronto, Department of Biochemistry, Toronto, Canada

MARQUIS, DONALD G., Massachusetts Institute of Technology, Cambridge, MA 02139

METTLER, FRED A., Pippin Hill, Blairstown, NJ 07825

NACHMANSOHN, DAVID, 630 W. 168th St., New York, NY 10032

NASTUK, WILLIAM L., College of Physicians and Surgeons, Department of Physiology, 630 W. 168th St., New York, NY 10032

NEUMANN, META A. (Miss), St. Elizabeth's Hospital, Blackborn Laboratory, Washington DC 20020

PASAMANICK, BENJAMIN, 44 Holland Avenue, Albany, NY 12208

PERLIN, SEYMOUR, Montefiore Hospital, Division of Psychiatry, 210th St. and Bainbridge Ave., Bronx, NY 10467

ROOFE, PAUL G., University of Kansas School of Medicine, Department of Anatomy, Lawrence, KS 66044

ROOTE, WALTER S., Department of Physiology, 630 W. 168th St., New York, NY 10032

RUCH, THEODORE C., University of Washington School of Medicine, Seattle, WA 98105

SABIN, ALBERT B., President of the Weizman Institute of Science, Rehovor, Israel

SIEBENS, ARTHUR A., 350 Henry Street Brooklyn, NY 11202

SINGER, MARCUS, Western Reserve University School of Medicine, Department of Anatomy, Cleveland, OH 44106

SMITH, WILBUR K., 260 Crittenden Boulevard, Rochester, NY 14620

SNIDER, RAY S., Center for Brain Research, University of Rochester, River Station, Rochester, NY 14627

SNYDER, LAURENCE H., University of Oklahoma, Graduate College, Norman, OK 73069

SPERRY, WARREN M., 722 W. 168th St., New York, NY 10032

SPRAGUE, JAMES M., University of Pennsylvania School of Medicine, Department of Anatomy, Philadelphia, PA 19104

TEUBER, HANS-LUKAS, Porter Place, Dobbs Ferry, NY 10522

TRUEX, RAYMOND S., Temple University School of Medicine and Hospital, Broad and Ontario Streets, Philadelphia, PA 19140

WAGMAN, IRVING H., University of California, National Center for Primate Biology, Third and Parnassus Sts., Davis, CA 95616

WANG, S. C., 630 W. 168th St., New York, NY 10032

WEISS, PAUL A., Rockefeller Institute for Medical Research, 66th St. and York Ave., New York, NY 10021

WINDLE, WILLIAM F., Institute of Rehabilitation Medicine, 400 E. 34th St., New York, NY 10016

WOODBURY, DIXON M., 6834 Crestview Circle, Bountiful, UT 84010

WOOLSEY, CLINTON M., University of Wisconsin Medical School, Madison, WI 53706

ZUBIN, JOSEPH, 722 W. 168th St., New York, NY 10032

INDEX